REMOTE AND RURAL DEMENTIA CARE

Policy, Research and Practice

Edited by Anthea Innes, Debra Morgan
and Jane Farmer

First published in Great Britain in 2020 by

Policy Press
University of Bristol
1-9 Old Park Hill
Bristol
BS2 8BB
UK
t: +44 (0)117 954 5940
pp-info@bristol.ac.uk
www.policypress.co.uk

North America office:
Policy Press
c/o The University of Chicago Press
1427 East 60th Street
Chicago, IL 60637, USA
t: +1 773 702 7700
f: +1 773-702-9756
sales@press.uchicago.edu
www.press.uchicago.edu

© Policy Press 2020

British Library Cataloguing in Publication Data
A catalogue record for this book is available from the British Library

Library of Congress Cataloging-in-Publication Data
A catalog record for this book has been requested

ISBN 978-1-4473-4495-7 hardcover
ISBN 978-1-4473-4497-1 ePub
ISBN 978-1-4473-4496-4 ePdf

Cover design by Qube Design Associates, Bristol
Front cover image: GettyImages-984036492
Printed and bound in Great Britain by CPI Group (UK) Ltd,
Croydon, CR0 4YY
Policy Press uses environmentally responsible print partners

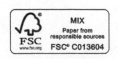

Contents

List of figures and tables

Figures

Tables

Notes on contributors

Stefanie Auer is a clinical and health psychologist. She worked at New York University on the development of test measures. In Austria, she and her team developed the Dementia Service Centre Model at MAS Alzheimerhilfe in 2001. Since 2015, she has been Professor of Dementia Studies at Danube University Krems, Austria.

Michael Bauer is an honorary senior research fellow at the Australian Institute for Primary Care and Ageing, La Trobe University, Melbourne, Australia. His research interests include residential aged care, dementia, sexuality, staff–family relationships and older people's use of computer-aided manufacturing technology.

Irene Blackberry is Director and John Richards Chair of Rural Ageing and Aged Care Research at the John Richards Centre for Rural Ageing Research, La Trobe University, Melbourne, Australia. Her research interests span dementia, ageing, aged care, rural health, chronic disease, access to care and technology.

Jessica M. Chiovitte is a research associate in the Memory Keepers Medical Discovery Team – Health Equity, University of Minnesota Medical School Duluth, USA. Her research interests are health equity, Indigenous health and ageing, implementation science and evaluation, trauma-informed and strengths-based approaches, and community-based participatory research.

Hilary Davis is a senior research fellow at the Centre for Social Impact, Swinburne University of Technology, Melbourne, Australia. Her research interests cover dementia, human–computer interaction, digital storytelling, social media and rural community health service delivery.

Jane Farmer is Research Professor of Health and Social Innovation and Director of the Social Innovation Research Institute at Swinburne University of Technology, Melbourne, Australia. The Institute focuses on the nexus of new technology, design thinking, data analytics and social and health challenges. Professor Farmer has a background in information science, community co-design, social enterprise and co-production research, mainly in rural health and community services.

Sharon Grant is a senior lecturer in the Department of Psychological Sciences at Swinburne University of Technology, Melbourne, Australia. Her research interests span industrial and organisational psychology, personality psychology and health-related aspects of social psychology. Her published work focuses on occupational stress, coping and strain; personality and work; and subjective and psychological wellbeing.

Ben Hicks is a research fellow at the Centre for Dementia Studies at Brighton and Sussex Medical School, UK. His research interests include supporting the social inclusion of people with dementia through the use of creative psychosocial initiatives including arts and gaming technology.

Margit Höfler received a doctoral degree in experimental psychology from the University of Graz, Austria, in 2010, and worked as a postdoctoral researcher at Graz University of Technology and the University of Graz, Austria. Since 2017, she has been a senior researcher at Danube University Krems, Austria.

Andy Hyde is the founder and Director of Go Upstream, based in Edinburgh, Scotland. He leads the development of Go Upstream, creating opportunities for travel service providers to work together with people with dementia, developing a new understanding of travel challenges and a process for designing more inclusive and enabling services. Go Upstream wishes to acknowledge the support of the Life Changes Trust.

Anthea Innes is Professor of Dementia and Coles-Medlock Director, Salford Institute for Dementia, University of Salford, UK. She is a social scientist who has specialised in the area of dementia for the past 20 years. At the core of her work is a concern to engage with the lived experiences of those affected by dementia, namely those diagnosed with the condition, their family members and professional care supporters. Her research interests span the care continuum from pre-diagnosis to end of life. Her particular research topics include rurality, technology and creative approaches to supporting those living with dementia.

Kristen M. Jacklin is Professor of Medical Anthropology in the Department of Family Medicine and Biobehavioral Health and Associate Director, Memory Keepers Medical Discovery Team – Health Equity, University of Minnesota Medical School Duluth, USA. Her research interests are health equity, Indigenous health and ageing, cognitive health and dementia, diabetes, Indigenous health education and community-based participatory research.

Andrew Kirk is Professor of Neurology at the University of Saskatchewan, Canada. His research and clinical interests have included language, construction, hemispatial neglect and accessible care for those with dementia. In 2004, he co-founded the Rural and Remote Memory Clinic at the University of Saskatchewan.

Oyvind Kirkevold is Assistant Research Director at the Norwegian National Advisory Unit on Ageing and Health, a researcher at the Research Centre for Age-Related Functional Decline and Diseases at Innlandet Hospital Trust, Norway, and Professor of Clinical Nursing in the Department of Health Sciences at the Norwegian University of Science and Technology.

Julie Kosteniuk is a research associate in the Canadian Centre for Health and Safety in Agriculture within the College of Medicine at the University of Saskatchewan, Canada. Her research and publications focus is on primary health care and rural health services, particularly for individuals with dementia and their families.

Kari Midtbo Kristiansen is Executive Manager at the Norwegian Advisory Unit on Ageing and Health. She is a member of the Nordic Dementia Network, and was involved in the planning and implementation of the Norwegian Dementia Plan 2020.

Fiona Marshall is a senior research fellow at the University of Nottingham, UK. As a health ethnographer, she has an interest in ageing in place. She has undertaken applied organisational research with older people, families, providers and policy makers. Her work includes cross-disciplinary and mixed-methods studies in rural and remote regions. She contributes to UK rural economic, health and dementia policy.

Nancy McAdam is a person living with dementia in remote and rural Scotland. She has been active in advocating for people living with dementia for the past 15 years. She was an early member of the Scottish Dementia Working Group and is currently a member of Scottish Dementia Alumni.

Debra Morgan is Professor and Chair in Rural Health Delivery at the Canadian Centre for Health and Safety in Agriculture, University of Saskatchewan, Canada; lead researcher for the Rural Dementia Action Research (RaDAR) team; and Director of the Rural and Remote Memory Clinic. Her research focuses on rural and remote health service delivery for dementia, including specialist and primary health care services.

Gary Naglie is a professor in the Department of Medicine and the Institute of Health Policy, Management and Evaluation at the University of Toronto, Canada. He is Vice President of Medical Services and Chief of Staff, and Chief of the Department of Medicine at Baycrest Health Sciences, and is a scientist at Baycrest's Rotman Research Institute. His research interests focus on driving in older adults and persons with dementia.

Megan E. O'Connell is an associate professor in the Department of Psychology, University of Saskatchewan, Canada, and a clinical psychologist in the Rural and Remote Memory Clinic. Her current programmes of research include neuropsychological measurement relevant to dementia and evaluation of telehealth for caregiver support, exercise interventions and cognitive rehabilitation.

Eamon O'Shea is a professor in the School of Business and Economics at the National University of Ireland (NUI) Galway. He was founder-director of the Irish Centre for Social Gerontology and is currently Director of the Centre for Economic and Social Research on Dementia at NUI Galway. His research interests are focused on the economics of ageing, rural gerontology and dementia. His work has been influential in setting the agenda for reform of services and policies for older people in Ireland. Professor O'Shea is the holder of a Health Research Board Leader award in dementia. The award provides the research framework to support the implementation of the National Dementia Strategy in Ireland.

Mark Rapoport is Professor of Psychiatry at the University of Toronto, Canada, and a geriatric neuropsychiatrist at Sunnybrook Health Sciences Centre, Toronto. His research interests lie in driving in older adulthood and dementia.

Paulina Ratajczak gained a Master's degree in statistics at the University of Vienna, Austria. Since 2015, she has worked as a research assistant in the Centre for Dementia Studies, Danube University Krems, Austria.

Helen Rochford-Brennan is a person with dementia living in remote and rural Ireland. She is Chairperson of the European Working Group of People with Dementia and is the group's nominee to the Board of Alzheimer Europe. She is also former Chair of the Irish Dementia Working Group. She is on the Monitoring Committee of Ireland's National Dementia Strategy and is a Global Dementia Ambassador.

Edith Span received a Master's degree in social work from the University of Applied Sciences in Salzburg, Austria. At MAS Alzheimerhilfe, she participated in the development of the Dementia Service Centre Model since 2001.

Norma Stewart is Professor Emerita in the College of Nursing, University of Saskatchewan, Canada. She works with the RaDAR team led by Debra Morgan and is a Co-Principal Investigator on a national survey of nursing practice in rural and remote areas of Canada.

Kieran Walsh is Professor of Ageing and Public Policy and Director of the Irish Centre for Social Gerontology, NUI Galway. His research interests and expertise focus on social exclusion in later life; the relative nature of disadvantage in cross-national contexts; place and life-course transitions; and informal and formal infrastructures of care.

Clare Wilding is a research fellow at John Richards Centre for Rural Ageing Research, La Trobe University, Melbourne, Australia. Her research interests span dementia, technology, healthy ageing in rural and remote areas, digital literacy, health literacy, ageing well, occupational science, dementia-friendly communities and age-friendly communities.

Margaret Winbolt is a senior research fellow at the Australian Institute for Primary Care and Ageing, La Trobe University, Melbourne, Australia. Her research interests focus on care of people living with dementia.

Acknowledgements

The editors would like to acknowledge the support of their respective institutions in providing the time to work on this book. Anthea Innes has also received support from the Coles-Medlock Foundation while working on this book. In addition, thanks to Lesley Waring and Carolyn Wallace for their assistance in preparing the manuscript for the publishers.

The authors of Chapter 2 would like to thank Kate Swaffer, Chief Executive Officer of Dementia Alliance International, and Katrin Seeher, Technical Officer, Department of Mental Health and Substance Abuse, World Health Organization, for providing information for this chapter, much of which we have incorporated. The authors of Chapter 3 acknowledge funding from the Foundation for Rural and Regional Renewal, Australian Government Department of Health and the Sandhurst Trust.

In Chapter 5, funding for the Rural and Remote Memory Clinic research demonstration project was provided by the Canadian Institutes of Health Research through a New Emerging Team grant and an Applied Chair in Health Services and Policy Research Chair award to Debra Morgan. The rural primary health care research was funded by the Saskatchewan Health Research Foundation through a partnership with the Canadian Institutes of Health Research, in support of the Canadian Consortium on Neurodegeneration in Aging (CCNA).

The work in Chapter 6 was supported by the following grants: (1) Fonds Gesundes Österreich and County of Upper Austria: Gesund Länger Pflegen, Project No. 599/III/83 (2002–05); (2) County of Upper Austria: Six Dementia Service Centres (2002–currently); (3) Austrian National Bank: Activity Program for Persons Living in a Nursing Home, Project No. 10569 (2004–05); (4) Fonds Gesundes Österreich and County of Upper Austria: Project No. 1481/III/2 (2008–10); (5) County of Upper Austria and Austrian National Insurance Company: Evaluation of the Model of the Dementia Service Centers (2013–17); (6) Fonds Gesundes Österreich Einsatz Demenz (Police Project): Project No. 2442 (2014–17). The authors of Chapter 6 would like to express gratitude to the entire team for their wonderful work, all social workers and psychologists: Maria Reitner, Yvonne Roithinger-Donabauer, Rosa Handlbauer, Karin Laschalt, Nicole Moser, Stefanie Plötzeneder, Doris Prieschl, Sandra Spack, Roland Sperling, Carmen Viereckl, Sabine Weber and Julia

Wimmer-Elias. Currently, about 50 trainers support the team with the provision of stage-specific training sessions and guiding families in daily life challenges. Their contribution and enthusiasm makes all the difference and inspires the life of persons living with dementia and their families.

The authors of Chapter 8 would like to acknowledge all the men, their care partners and the volunteers who participated in the research, as well as Age UK Dorchester and Bournemouth University, which part-funded the doctoral study.

The author of Chapter 9 would like to acknowledge the Connection Space Community Interest Company, Matlock, Derbyshire, UK, which shared photographs of activities, as well as the multiple organisations and families who provided support and shared their aspirations with the author as part of the Scaling the Peaks Research Study, and the Alzheimer's Society for funding the author's work from 2015 to 2019 as part of the Senior Research Fellowship Scheme (AS-SF-2014-005). The study is registered with the NIHR IRAS 188103. The views of the author may not necessarily reflect those of the Alzheimer's Society.

The authors of Chapter 10 would like to acknowledge that the research of Mark Rapoport and Gary Naglie was funded by the CCNA. The CCNA is supported by a grant from the Canadian Institutes of Health Research with funding from several partners. Gary Naglie is supported by the George, Margaret and Gary Hunt Family Chair in Geriatric Medicine, University of Toronto. Mark Rapoport receives research support from the Sunnybrook Psychiatry Partnership in Toronto. The development of Go Upstream has been supported by a grant from the Life Changes Trust. The authors of Chapter 10 also wish to thank Sara Sanford and Elaine Stasiulis for their work in collecting and presenting qualitative data on driving cessation and dementia.

The authors of Chapter 11 would like to acknowledge the intellectual contributions of Wayne Warry and Melissa Blind, University of Minnesota Medical School Duluth, and of Karen Pitawanakwat, RN Community Researcher, and Elder Jerry Otowadjiwan, from the Wikwemikong Unceded Reserve. Having worked closely with the authors for many years on research into Indigenous dementia, their ideas and words are impossible to disentangle from this chapter. Most notably, the authors would like to acknowledge the Indigenous people and communities who have welcomed researchers into their territories and who have shared their lives, experiences and knowledge. Miigwech.

The author of Chapter 12 would like to acknowledge the support of Clodagh Whelan from the Alzheimer Society of Ireland.

The author of Chapter 13 would like to acknowledge the support of her friends at the iPad class, the many local groups she attends with the support of her friends, and the other people with dementia she has met along the way who have become her firm friends.

Introduction

1

Remote and rural dementia care: why is this important for policy, research, practice and the lived experience of dementia?

Anthea Innes, Debra Morgan and Jane Farmer

This book is the first edited collection to focus on dementia in remote and rural areas. Drawing on examples of research studies and innovative practice from remote and rural locations globally, it highlights the implications of living with dementia in remote and rural areas for dementia policy, practice and future research. The chapters represent countries with considerable experience and expertise in developing support and services for their rural and remote populations, such as Canada, Australia, the UK, Ireland and Austria. However, many other countries have rural geographies and ageing populations, and are likely to face similar challenges of meeting the needs of people living with dementia in remote and rural areas. To promote knowledge translation, the book's contributors share ideas from their countries to help practitioners working in challenging geographical landscapes anywhere as they strive to provide the highest standards of support for those living with dementia. The book draws on research conducted in different countries with longstanding histories of conducting remote and rural dementia research, and as such it is a resource for academics who teach or research rurality and dementia. The edited structure allows international examples of innovative research/practice in the remote and rural dementia field to be showcased with the implications of such national examples to be considered in relation to research, policy and practice globally. In this way, we hope that you, the reader, will find this edited collection to be a resource, whether you are a student, practitioner, policy influencer or academic, to assist you in enhancing the experience of living with dementia in remote and rural areas in the future.

Dementia has been defined by the World Health Organization as:

> ... an umbrella term for several diseases that are mostly progressive, affecting memory, other cognitive abilities and behaviour, and that interfere significantly with a person's ability to maintain the activities of daily living. (WHO, 2017c: 5)

Although the symptoms of dementia may be similar, how these are experienced and the impact on individuals' lives can vary significantly. The experience of dementia is one that is fraught with challenges for the person diagnosed with dementia, and for families, friends and communities. It may require coming to terms with new identity and functionality and may require significant adaptation and resilience at individual, family and community levels (Innes et al, 2011). An international consensus report from 2005 estimated that there were 24.3 million people worldwide living with dementia, with an additional 4.6 million new diagnoses per year (Ferri et al, 2005). More recent data from 2015 estimated that there were 46.8 million people with dementia internationally, with 9.9 million new cases per year (ADI, 2015). Thus, the number of people affected by dementia across the globe is rising and will continue to rise into the 21st century due to people living longer and the use of more sophisticated diagnostic processes (ADI, 2015). Policy drivers to improve diagnosis have accelerated the rising numbers of people identified with dementia. Thirty-two countries were reported to have a national dementia strategy in 2018 (ADI, 2018), with Canada releasing its strategy in 2019, making the current total 33, with other countries also with strategies in development. Remote and rural geographies create a distinct challenge when developing policies and strategies for many countries (Pot and Petrea, 2013). Given that rural places internationally tend to have older populations compared with urban places (United Nations, 2015), coupled with trends in some countries for retirement migration to rural locations either for high amenity or affordability – depending on the nature of the rural place (Pennington, 2013) – there is an increased value in learning from research and practice in rural dementia care in different locations to enable practitioners, academics and policy makers to address the challenges of rural service provision in the communities and countries where they live and work.

Policy, research, practice and lived experiences are part of the process of bringing about change, and hopefully improvements in dementia care. These four factors do not sit in isolation from one another; rather,

Figure 1.1: Factors for change in remote and rural dementia care

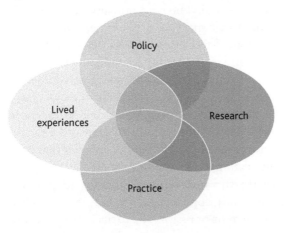

they impact on and are affected by progress and developments in each area, as demonstrated in Figure 1.1.

This book is organised into four sections: policy drivers, research evidence, practice challenges and lived experiences. Each section of the book highlights the influence of rurality on the service provision solutions that are appropriate, and how to address the quality of life and/ or care needs of those living with dementia in challenging geographical landscapes. The importance of hearing the views and experiences of those living with dementia, their care supporters and professional care providers has been our starting point when we have been working in this area, and we have a section in the book that focuses on living with dementia with two chapters written by people living with dementia in rural settings. Nancy McAdam and Helen Rochford-Brennan demonstrate clearly how rural dwelling influences their experiences of life with dementia. Policy, research and practice innovations are all well and good, but if there is no benefit to those living with dementia, then such efforts by policy makers, influencers and researchers, and the practice innovations that are often informed and inform policy and research, are arguably not as effective as required.

We have elected to focus on 'remote' and 'rural' dementia care rather than comparisons between urban and rural areas. However, what constitutes rural or urban varies according to country classification systems. For example, in Scotland alone (Scottish Government, 2018), there are four different classifications of rural and urban. One is based on settlement size: urban (over 3,000 people) and rural (less than 3,000 people). Another makes a distinction between density of population and travel times to urban centres. In Canada (Statistics Canada, 2017), the term 'population centres' is based on levels of population density: less than 1,000 people is defined as rural. The commonality in definitions across countries are population density and the time and distance from less densely populated areas to population centres. The lack of geographical accessibility to, and distance from, the urban service hubs are central to the challenges of supporting people living with dementia and their families. Learning from and adapting successful initiatives from different locations is one way we can all work together to promote living well with dementia in rural areas. This book provides a forum for sharing and learning from initiatives in different countries that have begun to address dementia care in rural and remote areas.

Chapter authors draw on the research and policy and practice evidence from urban areas where appropriate, but our concern with this book is to address the current omission of a focus on remote and rural dementia care. Systematic reviews devoted to dementia care in rural areas (Innes et al, 2011; Morgan et al, 2011) demonstrate that formal or informal dementia care provision in rural areas is challenging, with a mismatch in support needs and support available. In a recent UK rural dementia-friendly communities guide (Bould et al, 2018), the foreword reminds us that 'the impact for people living with dementia in rural areas is often greater due to geographical, financial and transportation constraints which can make accessing support and guidance difficult' (Hughes, 2018). However, despite this recognition, remote and rural dementia care has been slow to emerge as an area requiring focus and attention. Remote and rural dementia care is increasing in importance as evidenced by recent large research programmes in two of the editors' countries (Canada and Australia), with some of the earliest research about dementia in rural areas undertaken in the other editor's location (Scotland). The prevalence of dementia is increasing most rapidly in developing countries with a predominantly rural population base (ADI, 2015). This book is therefore ahead of the curve in terms of this being an important area for current research and future studies.

We hope this book challenges practitioners, policy makers and other academics to fully consider the needs of those who do not live in urban centres with their associated service hubs and available workforce. By drawing attention to the challenges of geographic landscapes, rural cultures and norms, the staff development and support needs of families, and the impact rurality has on the lived experience of dementia, it can be seen that remote and rural dementia care offers challenges and the opportunity for creative solutions. This book is the first collection to bring together research evidence from academics based in countries that have pioneered rural dementia research and practice initiatives. As such, the book disseminates research evidence to practice, policy and academic audiences, but in a thematic and structured way designed to challenge thinking, reconsider practice and to enable those working in rural areas to learn from existing research, policy and practice evidence.

The first part of the book sets out some of the varying policy contexts surrounding remote and rural dementia care. Chapter 2 focuses on challenges and policy in low- and middle-income countries (LMICs), informed by interviews with representatives from the World Health Organization (WHO) and Dementia Alliance International (DAI). WHO's *Global action plan on the public response to dementia 2017–2025* and toolkits for training community workers and supporting carers form a robust foundation on which individual countries can build their national dementia planning (WHO, 2017a, 2017b). It can be a struggle to prioritise dementia policy as LMICs often prioritise other basic health issues, such as child health, over dementia. To push for national dementia planning, the role of civil society and, importantly, the voices of people living with dementia, are significant. The case of DAI is one example where technology has been significant in allowing connection between civil society actors across the world, highlighting that rural connectivity policy is significant to health as rural societies wrestle with globalisation, urbanisation and consequent health service accessibility challenges.

Chapter 3 portrays an array of funding mechanisms and initiatives in Australia. While dementia was declared a national health priority in 2012 and allocated substantial government funding, this chapter highlights that Australia's complex health funding and jurisdictional arrangements have the potential to confuse not only service users, but also service providers. Some services are directly funded from the federal government, others from state governments. Services can also be provided by local government and non-governmental agencies such as the Royal Flying Doctor Service. The chapter depicts efforts to empower people with dementia, their carer partners and supporters, and health practitioners to navigate the complex service landscape using technology. My Aged Care is a governmental portal to services. To contextualise this for rural areas, government has provided funding to research studies such as Verily Connect, a technology intended to connect people to services and to each other.

Norway's organised and systematic approach to dementia policy and services is depicted in Chapter 4. Norway was an early leader in committing to develop a national dementia plan in 2007, delivered in 2015 and refreshed in 2020. The authors depict holistic services organised as a result of national planning, including day programmes, guidelines and the Dementia ABC educational programme. The chapter highlights particular challenges of delivering the same level and quality of services regardless of location. It also highlights rural innovations designed to help, including dementia work groups, where small groups of practitioners organise care and support together, so that people with dementia only have to deal with a limited number of service providers and can build continuing relationships.

The second section of the book presents examples of research evidence drawn from Canada, Austria and Ireland.

Chapter 5 discusses rural dementia care in Canada, focusing on the research conducted by the Rural Dementia Action Research (RaDAR) team in the western province of Saskatchewan. This community-based participatory research programme has developed interventions to address priorities identified by stakeholders. The interdisciplinary, one-stop Rural and Remote Memory Clinic provides access to specialist assessment and diagnosis for rural people with complex atypical dementias, and uses telehealth videoconferencing for follow-up appointments, to reduce travel burden. A longitudinal clinic database supports numerous interdisciplinary research projects. To build capacity for dementia diagnosis and management in rural communities, the team partnered with primary healthcare teams to design and implement rural primary healthcare memory clinics.

Chapter 6 also discusses a model of rural dementia care: the Dementia Services Centres (DSCs) that have been implemented in six centres in rural Upper Austria. The main goals are to provide early detection of dementia, delaying institutionalisation, and reducing the burden of support providers. The DSCs are easily accessible and visible in communities, providing local services such as screening, referral to a specialist for diagnosis, and post-diagnostic support and education for the person with dementia and family caregivers. Programmes for individuals living with dementia focus on maintaining functioning and providing opportunities for social interaction. A database was established early in the DSC programme to provide evidence supporting the model.

Chapter 7 discusses the challenges of rural dementia care in Ireland where there is differentiation in the policies supporting care in urban and rural areas that has led to a process of social exclusion and policy fragmentation that impacts directly on the experiences of people living with dementia in rural areas. How to address this and to promote living well with dementia in rural Ireland is therefore challenging when there is a dearth of health and social care support systems in place.

The third part of the book is a collection of chapters that draw out practice implications based on research evidence.

Chapter 8 discusses two issues: providing support suitable for older men with dementia in rural areas, and the role technology can play in providing such support. Drawing on the example of 'tech groups' in rural England, the authors demonstrate that considering the gendered nature of experiences of dementia is important and that a group using technology as a means to initiate and sustain an enjoyable group environment was so popular with participants that the groups secured funding to continue as community programmes following the conclusion of the research.

Farm-based care is the topic of Chapter 9, and a delightful example of a creative approach to using the natural resources in rural communities to the advantage of people living with dementia. It demonstrates how local resources have been harnessed to provide maximum benefits to people living in these communities. Activities offered relate to the seasons, the weather and the local landscape, and as such are relevant to providers and participants of farm-based care everywhere.

Chapter 10 discusses an issue that is often difficult for people living with dementia, particularly in rural areas, to accept: the loss of a driving licence and of the ability to drive. Drawing on public transport examples from Scotland, the authors consider the research evidence, the practical challenges presented by the inability to continue to drive, and how public transport has the potential to provide an alternative mobility solution and yet is often limited in rural areas. The ability to continue to contribute to community life and access a range of services, not just health services, but amenities we may take for granted, such as a local shop, can therefore be severely curtailed.

Chapter 11 articulates a cultural safety framework lens through which to view experiences of dementia and subsequent responses with appropriate support and services. The chapter focuses on issues arising from research with Indigenous communities in Canada, but will resonate with people from communities or backgrounds that may be constructed as 'different' in some way from the mainstream population, be they from an Indigenous community, or, for example, a minority ethnic or cultural group.

The final section of the book focuses on lived experiences of dementia and a future agenda for rural dementia care. Chapters 12 and 13 provide a stark reminder that our key concern should be to listen and respond to the needs of those experiencing dementia. Helen Rochford-Brennan describes how living in a rural community brings both community support and challenges of geography in accessing formal services. Her suggestions for other people diagnosed with dementia in rural areas, as well as researchers and practitioners, provide a compelling message to remember that remote and rural dementia care needs to put those living with dementia as its core concern.

Nancy McAdam moved to a rural community in the Highland region of Scotland around the time of her diagnosis. Her experiences demonstrate that life does indeed continue with a diagnosis of dementia, and that living in a rural area has enabled her to live well with her dementia. The drawbacks of limited transport and sometimes poor weather conditions, leading to being cut off for short periods of time, are in her experience offset by the benefits of living in a peaceful and quiet environment with support systems to access groups and friends and practical assistance firmly in her control and actioned via a robust local support network and a strong family who, although they live some distance away, provide her with the practical support and personal connections she requires to function well with dementia.

This book draws on examples of research, practice and policy commentary to highlight the dimensions of living with dementia in remote and rural areas around the world. As such, it provides a unique and contemporary resource for teaching, research, policy and practice around rurality and dementia. This topic is significant as, in many countries, the percentages of older people in the population and of people with dementia are rising (Chertkow, 2018). Alongside this, forces of globalisation over the past 40 years have led to decline of economic opportunities in rural areas internationally, with concomitant out-migration of youth, leading to ageing rural populations outside metropolitan areas and rural metropolitan commuting zones (Phillipson, 2010). This means that ageing and dementia are rising phenomena in rural areas (Dal Bello-Haas et al, 2014; Sharma and Bothra, 2018). Further, following the 2008 global financial crisis, in many countries, there has been an increase in public sector retrenchment, forcing 'efficiency measures' of downsizing of rural services, centralisation of services to urban hubs and increasing online service provision (Halseth et al, 2019). Professionalisation and specialisation in health also means that career-oriented practitioners are drawn to cities to work in high-volume health and care settings (Laurence et al, 2010). For rural places, this 'perfect storm' of interconnected forces has resulted in unsustainable traditional service models for all kinds of services and increasing calls for innovative ways to provide rural services (Halseth et al, 2019). As dementia has been on the rise during this period, the pressure on 'traditional' rural dementia services is even more severe (Szymczynska et al, 2011; Herron et al, 2016). However, given the evidence that has surfaced in editing this book, it could be said that there is no such thing as a traditional 'typical' rural dementia service model and that consequently, this is fertile ground for the novel ways to provide services that are emerging around the world, some of which are documented in this book. Given this emergence of different models to meet rural needs coupled with WHO's *Global action plan on the public response to dementia 2017–2025* (WHO, 2017a), which provides a foundational policy blueprint and toolkits, now seems an opportune time to 'take the temperature' of international remote and rural dementia care. New ways to provide services, new policy responses, the rise of civil society and the need to adapt or change existing systems perhaps mean this is a crossroads and that coordinated appropriate rural care will be more available, to more people, in the future.

Taken together, this edited collection demonstrates the common challenges that remote and rural landscapes pose for people living with dementia and those providing support services. It highlights the range of country-specific solutions that have emerged in response to these challenges and includes accounts from people living with dementia that demonstrate that living in remote or rural places can contribute to wellbeing in dementia.

References

ADI (Alzheimer's Disease International) (2015) *World Alzheimer report 2015: The global impact of dementia. An analysis of prevalence, incidence, cost and trends*, London: ADI. Available from: www.alz.co.uk/research/ WorldAlzheimerReport2015.pdf

ADI (2018) *From plan to impact: Progress towards targets of the global action plan on dementia*, London: Alzheimer's Disease International. Available from: www.alz.co.uk/adi/pdf/from-plan-to-impact-2018.pdf?2

Bould, E., Ball, A., Donoghue, T., Jenkins, C., Sherriff, I. and the Prime Minister's Rural Dementia Task and Finish Group Members (2018) *Dementia-friendly rural communities guide: A practical guide for rural communities to support people affected by dementia*, London: Alzheimer's Society. Available from: www.alzheimers.org.uk/get-involved/ dementia-friendly-communities/rural-communities

Chertkow, H. (2018) 'An action plan to face the challenge of dementia: international statement on dementia from IAP for Health', *Journal of Prevention of Alzheimer's Disease*, 5(3): 207–12.

Dal Bello-Haas, V., Cammer, A., Morgan, D., Stewart, N. and Kosteniuk, J. (2014) 'Rural and remote dementia care challenges and needs: perspectives of formal and informal care providers residing in Saskatchewan', *Rural and Remote Health*, 14: 2747.

Ferri, C.P., Prince, M., Brayne, C., Brodaty, H., Fratiglioni, L., Ganguli, M., Hall, K., Hasegawa, K., Hendrie, H., Huang, Y., Jorm, A., Mathers, C., Menezes, P.R., Rimmer, E., Scazufca, M., and Alzheimer's Disease International (2005) 'Global prevalence of dementia: a Delphi consensus study', *The Lancet*, 366(9503): 2112–17.

Halseth, G., Markey, S. and Ryser, L. (2019) *Service provision and rural sustainability*, Abingdon: Routledge.

Herron, R.V., Rosenberg, M.W. and Skinner, M.W. (2016) 'The dynamics of voluntarism in rural dementia care', *Health & Place*, 41: 34–41.

Hughes, J. (2018) 'Foreword', in E. Bould, A. Ball, T. Donoghue, C. Jenkins, I. Sherriff and the Prime Minister's Rural Dementia Task and Finish Group Members (eds) *Dementia-friendly rural communities guide: A practical guide for rural communities to support people affected by dementia*, London: Alzheimer's Society. Available from: www. alzheimers.org.uk/get-involved/dementia-friendly-communities/ rural-communities

Innes, A., Morgan, D. and Kosteniuk, J. (2011) 'Dementia care in rural and remote settings: a systematic review of informal/family caregiving', *Maturitas*, 68(1): 34–46.

Laurence, C.O., Williamson, V., Sumner, K.E. and Fleming, J. (2010) '"Latte rural": the tangible and intangible factors important in the choice of a rural practice by recent GP graduates', *Rural and Remote Health*, 10(2): 1316.

Morgan, D., Innes, A. and Kosteniuk, J. (2011) 'Dementia care in rural and remote settings: a systematic review of formal or paid care', *Maturitas*, 68(1): 17–33.

Pennington, J. (2013) *Moving on: Migration trends in later life*, London: IPPR. Available from: www.ippr.org/files/images/media/ files/publication/2013/06/moving-on-older-people_June2013_ 10898.pdf?noredirect=1

Phillipson, C. (2010) 'Globalisation, global ageing and intergenerational change', in M. Izuhara (ed) *Ageing and intergenerational relations*, Bristol: Policy Press, pp 13–28.

Pot, A.M. and Petrea, I. (2013) *Improving dementia care worldwide: Ideas and advice on developing and implementing a national dementia plan*, London: Bupa/ADI. Available from: www.alz.co.uk/sites/default/ files/pdfs/global-dementia-plan-report-ENGLISH.pdf

Scottish Government (2018) 'Scottish Government Urban Rural Classification'. Available from: www2.gov.scot/Topics/Statistics/ About/Methodology/UrbanRuralClassification

Sharma, S. and Bothra, M. (2018) 'Changing demographics and dementia: a reflection on the challenges ahead for India', *Nursing and Healthcare*, 2: 1–8.

Statistics Canada (2017) 'Population Centre and Rural Area Classification 2016'. Available from: www.statcan.gc.ca/eng/subjects/standard/pcrac/2016/introduction

Szymczynska, P., Innes, A., Mason, A. and Stark, C. (2011) 'A review of diagnostic process and postdiagnostic support for people with dementia in rural areas', *Journal of Primary Care and Community Health*, 2(4): 262–76.

United Nations (2015) *World population ageing 2015*, New York, NY: United Nations. Available from: www.un.org/en/development/desa/population/publications/pdf/ageing/WPA2015_Report.pdf

WHO (World Health Organization) (2017a) *Global action plan on the public health response to dementia 2017–2025*, Geneva: WHO.

WHO (2017b) *Dementia: Toolkit for community workers in low- and middle-income countries. Guide for community-based management and care of people with dementia*, Manila: World Health Organization Regional Office for the Western Pacific.

WHO (2017c) *Dementia: number of people affected to triple in next 30 years*. Available from: www.who.int/news-room/detail/07-12-2017-dementia-number-of-people-affected-to-triple-in-next-30-years

PART I

Policy drivers

2

The future of dementia care in rural areas of the world

Jane Farmer and Sharon Grant

Introduction

The purpose of this chapter is to consider the issues experienced by people with dementia, their carers and families – and the issues of providing services for people with dementia – in rural areas around the world. The chapter endeavours to focus in particular on issues for low- and middle-income countries (LMICs), also sometimes referred to here as developing countries. The chapter seeks to highlight issues in rural experiences of dementia that policy makers in resource-depleted settings need to consider at national and regional levels. The chapter specifically acknowledges supra-national efforts to improve experiences of dementia and care, and to influence development of dementia-specific policy, and considers the specific role of these efforts for rural places. This includes supra-national policy organisations – primarily the leadership of the World Health Organization (WHO) – and civil society and research organisations that advocate for people with dementia to have their voice heard and that drive knowledge and solutions about, for and with, people with dementia in LMIC settings.

While across the world 'rural' is differentiated from 'urban' by its distance from large centres of services and amenities coupled with sparse population distribution, rural places are highly diverse internationally and can be so even within one country setting. Thus, as discussed, 'the nature, context and needs of rural communities and rural practice will differ around the world. Local solutions will require … local initiatives' (WONCA, 2014: 1).

While rural places differ around the world, they tend to share some key features that are essential to understand and acknowledge when making and applying rural policy. In social terms, rural places tend to have cultural norms and values that, due to small populations repeatedly interacting, become strongly enforced and reinforced, making it hard to be different. Difference can be stigmatised and people strive to 'fit in', which drives attempts to be resilient and get through rather than to show weakness. Gender roles and power dynamics can be strongly enforced, with formal and informal leaders having significant power. Internationally, people in rural areas tend to experience higher levels of poverty, and lower levels of education and access to welfare compared with those in urban areas. Transportation and technology-related imbalances result in rural dwellers experiencing spatial social exclusion (Strasser et al, 2016; Salemink et al, 2017). With considerable disruption to traditional major industries such as agriculture, mining, fishing and forestry, 'the rural decline' is widely discussed (Strasser, 2003). Alongside this are the increasing effects of climate change.

Given this international rural backdrop, we proceed to explore a range of issues specific to experiences of dementia in rural areas, focusing on experiences in LMICs. This particular lens is significant as it highlights the challenge of dementia internationally in rural places, while, to date, much work on developing knowledge and solutions has been situated in high-income countries. The size of the challenge is highlighted in the *World Alzheimer Report 2015* statistics that predict a rise of 56 per cent in the number of older people with dementia living in high-income countries by 2050. This percentage is dwarfed by predicted rises of 185 per cent in middle-income countries and 239 per cent in low-income countries (Prince et al, 2015). The *World Alzheimer Report 2011* (Prince et al, 2011a) estimated that, in high-income countries, less than 50 per cent of dementia cases receive a diagnosis. This figure is less than 90 per cent in LMICs. Given that many individuals live with dementia for several years, the costs of disability associated with dementia for stretched health systems in LMICs are high. For example, for Latin America and China, the direct costs of disability from dementia exceed those from depression, diabetes or ischaemic heart disease (Sousa et al, 2010). The implication is, and will continue to be for some time, that the majority of people with dementia living in developing countries are unlikely to be receiving care beyond that available from family or the community. A key issue is the extent to which countries recognise dementia as a significant non-communicable disease and are organised to address it. There is a woeful international response to mental and neurological disorders: although one in ten people has a mental health problem, only one per cent of the international health workforce provides mental healthcare (Keynejad et al, 2017). Problems of access to trained workers are most acute for those living in poverty in rural areas of LMICs.

Policy, research and civil action is thus imperative to tackle the many challenges experienced by those with dementia and the families and communities that support them. We now consider some specific challenges for people living in rural areas of LMICs in relation to developing relevant dementia policy.

Rural poverty and its effects on living with dementia

Many countries lack universal healthcare and social welfare, thus social protection in old age is dependent on a complex interaction involving health, living arrangements, family support and income sources. Caring for a person with dementia increases financial stress for families (Gurayah, 2015), particularly in collective cultures, where families have close kinship ties and are obliged to support each other. Prince and colleagues (2008: 338) reported that, in countries with low pension coverage, 25 per cent or more of older people are reliant on family finance transfers, with a 'substantial minority' reporting food insecurity. In such countries, many older people work for as long as possible, as there is little employment insurance (Prince et al, 2008). The authors describe a rise of dependency anxiety among older people in developing countries who do not want to be a burden on relatives and try to maintain independence from family (Prince et al, 2008). A study by the 10/66 Research Group found that a considerable number of older people in developing country settings live alone, without access to family supports (Sousa et al, 2010). This is likely to be a particular problem in rural areas as young people must migrate out to access employment and education. Many people in rural areas of LMICs already have precarious finances due to lack of employment opportunities. Thus, people with dementia may be living in extreme poverty in households that lack basic amenities such as electricity, running toilets, cooking equipment and adequate living space (Benade, 2012).

Unreceptive environments and lack of culturally appropriate tools

Underdiagnosis of dementia is reported globally, but WHO (2018) reports that, in many countries, lack of societal awareness or acceptance of dementia as a condition exacerbates the problem, also precluding regional prevalence estimates (Mkhonto and Hanssen, 2018). The use of different methods and screening tools around the globe further complicates estimation and benchmarking (de Jager et al, 2017).

Although Alzheimer's disease accounts for 60 to 70 per cent of dementia cases, there are different dementia subtypes (WHO, 2017a). Accurate diagnosis requires comprehensive clinical assessment, as diagnostic profiles are not 100 per cent distinct and a range of methods are required (Maestre, 2012), including a review of the individual's medical history; cognitive, neurological and physical assessments; and interviews with carers to obtain lived experience information about cognitive functioning (ADI and DA, 2014). Accurate diagnosis is likely well out of reach in situations where access to specialists and diagnostic equipment is poor, likely to particularly affect under-served rural places. People with dementia are also less likely to receive a diagnosis for comorbid health conditions which, left untreated, can accelerate cognitive decline (WHO, 2017b). Underdiagnosis represents a barrier to understanding the urgency of dementia policy and putting dementia care in place, as prevalence estimates have implications for assessing resource needs (de Jager et al, 2017).

Early diagnosis is especially problematic in rural areas of LMICs due to lack of access to universal healthcare and basic public services in many settings; few qualified specialist workers or access to aged care; and tensions between western biomedical thinking about conditions and traditional cultures, beliefs and practices. These combine to make an unreceptive environment for information and advice about dementia.

Beyond this, the tools and practices of dementia diagnosis and care may be culturally insensitive. For example, standard diagnostic tools may be unavailable or untested for local cultural appropriateness and languages (Prince et al, 2009). Providing a Chinese example, Chen and colleagues (2014) noted that while diagnostic tools are available in Chinese translation, these are not widely accessible in rural areas of China and the Community Screening Instrument for Dementia, though validated for some LMIC settings (Prince et al 2011b), is untested in Chinese clinics for those with low literacy. We note that Kristen Jacklin, of the Indigenous Cognition and Aging Awareness Exchange, is undertaking valuable work on culturally appropriate tools for assessment and diagnosis in Canadian Indigenous communities (see Chapter 11 of this book).

Stigma – a particularly rural problem?

The way that dementia is regarded within a society – as a health condition or 'just a normal part of ageing' – affects the way that society responds in policy, resources and services and thus affects the experience of those with dementia. Lack of recognition of dementia as a condition can be associated with stigmatisation (ADI and DA, 2014). Beliefs embedded in some cultures can intensify stigma, with the condition blamed on the person's life behaviours or even with sinister forces (Guerchet et al, 2017; Mkhonto and Hanssen, 2018). These entrenched traditional beliefs can endure over longer time spans in rural places as mentioned earlier in this chapter, due to the culture norms of small communities and local power structures. For example, a rural South African study found that in some places community members, including healthcare practitioners, linked dementia to witchcraft or retribution for mistakes in previous life (Mkhonto and Hanssen, 2018). Stigma linked to such beliefs perpetuates fear and shunning of individuals with dementia, leading to discrimination, social isolation, violence and even homicide. Mkhonto and Hanssen noted that there are substantial numbers of isolated, low-status older women living in rural areas, and this group tends to attract blame and stigma. Such women can be labelled as 'witches', with researchers describing the phenomenon of older women with dementia living isolated in separate: 'villages consisting of simple huts where they [women with dementia] have no support and living conditions are extremely poor' (Mkhonto and Hanssen, 2018: 173). From 2010 to 2015, 76 cases of witch killings appeared before South African courts and in Tanzania, witch killings are estimated at 500 older women per year. This is described as 'Africa's hidden war on women' (Mkhonto and Hanssen, 2018: 170; see also Ferreira and Kalula, 2009; Hari, 2009). Ingstad (1990) noted that such traditional beliefs can be hard to alter as they are a deep-seated part of group identity and belonging.

Varying levels of stigma is a widespread phenomenon associated with the kinds of entrenched traditional cultural practices that are more associated with life in rural places – though not exclusive to them. Chen and colleagues (2014) discuss that the Chinese translation of the term dementia is a variant of the word for crazy. Prince and colleagues (2009: 337) report that in parts of India features of dementia are described as *'chinnan'* (childishness), *'nerva frakese'* (tired brain) and 'weak brain'. These understandings limit recognition and management of dementia as a condition that can attract help and services, and thus also limits provision of specialised training and funding and support for caregiving families (Prince et al, 2008).

Raising awareness of dementia can be targeted at the level of community (for example, through education), population (mass media) and healthcare/policy (ADI and DA, 2014; Chen et al, 2014). A randomised controlled trial in Asia found that brief exposure to information about dementia symptoms in the form of vignettes led to reduction in stigma (Batsch and Mittelman, 2012). Prince and colleagues (2008) emphasised the need to engage people in the media with evidence about dementia so that information can be related to populations in ways that have local relevance. Given the challenges for people living with dementia in LMICs cited earlier, appropriate infusion of factual evidence about dementia into traditional ways of life is an ongoing challenge, sometimes tackled alongside other parallel human rights vulnerabilities, including around gender and Indigenous rights (Parra et al, 2018).

Dementia fundamentally compromises a person's ability to protect their human rights (Prince et al, 2008). Developing countries have generally failed to prioritise comprehensive and effective systems of social protection (Prince et al, 2015). Further, even countries with growing national economies can have gross income distribution inequities, with older people among the least likely to benefit from a country's economic development (Prince et al, 2015). Rural areas of developing countries tend to be the last areas to be targeted for services and benefits.

Supporting people with dementia in under-resourced LMIC rural settings

In high-income countries, dementia care costs are shared relatively evenly across informal and formal social care, while in LMICs informal care costs are proportionately more often placed at community and family levels (ADI and DA, 2014; WHO, 2017b). As noted earlier, much care of those with dementia in rural settings of developing countries still lies with families and communities, but is subject to stigmatisation and, in contemporary times, to rural youth out-migration, leaving a 'social gap', with high concentrations of older people in rural communities. Prince and colleagues (2008) note that traditional intergenerational caring tends to prevail in LMICs, with scepticism about, and resistance to, other models. Carers, generally women, bear most of the burden. However, the increase in the numbers of women moving into mainstream workforces is likely to affect future care arrangements (Prince et al, 2007).

In traditional Chinese culture, as discussed by Wang and colleagues (2014), families are regarded as the caregivers for older family members, an expectation that is also enshrined in law. This assumption of family care, in turn, discourages development of other facilities and specialist carer roles. In rural China, for example, public health services are underdeveloped and lack of recognition of dementia as a health condition means that the pharmaceutical benefit scheme does not cover relevant drugs (Wang et al, 2014). Similarly, Prince and colleagues (2008) note that the Indian government passed a law in 2007 stating that families must provide care and financial support for older relatives. This is a response to a rapidly ageing population and fear of large costs to government if families start to move away from fulfilling obligations to care for relatives.

Often there is simply no support available other than families (ADI and DA, 2014; WHO, 2017a). Daily care responsibilities can be intensive and there is a lack of assistance for carers or perhaps even acknowledgement of the strains of this role (ADI and DA, 2014). WHO (2017a) resources have been developed to train community health workers to identify and reduce stress among carers, and to provide carers with training. However, even these efforts can be met with resistance. Chen and colleagues (2014) emphasise that models of dementia care in rural communities need to carefully align with local traditional cultures.

As noted, a crucial contemporary challenge to traditional family care for rural people with dementia is the massive demographic shift of rural people to urban areas. This is happening across the world and will leave larger proportions of older people behind in rural areas, with few young people to care for them. The prevalence of dementia is already considerably higher in rural than in urban areas due to these demographic effects, as in China for example (6.05 per cent versus 4.40 per cent; Jia et al, 2014), and will only continue to become more pronounced.

As primary healthcare, with its high level of community involvement, is particularly feasible and considered appropriate for rural places (Starfield, 1998; WONCA, 2014), the role of communities in dementia care is significant. In LMICs, community health workers with basic health training are often at the front line of local rural health services. Their role involves a variety of health, health literacy and promotion and navigation work (see WHO, 2017a). Focusing specifically on dementia, Benade (2012) discussed the awareness-raising role of an African community-based worker who visits families, community facilities and clinics, and runs staff training on dementia. As the likely first point of contact for families in rural communities in LMICs, community health workers must be prepared to observe and evaluate dementia symptoms so they can refer individuals to primary care physicians or nurses with mental health training for further assessment and services (WHO, 2017a). When discussing dementia, community workers are likely to need buy-in from community leaders. This can be additionally challenging as sometimes there is a lack of trust and belief in the skills of local practitioners, who may be perceived by locals as inexpert and 'just a neighbour' due to close relational knowledge of people in small rural communities.

The WHO (2017a) has developed a toolkit and a set of mental health resources – the WHO Mental Health Gap Action Programme (mhGAP) Intervention Guide – for community health workers with at least secondary level education. The toolkit comprises a community resources checklist, screening and detection tools, management and care tools, prevention and promotion activity lists, monitoring and evaluation tools, and a pocket guide for carers. It aims to support the development of 'dementia-friendly communities' to improve the autonomy, dignity and respect of people living with dementia, and to reduce costs for individuals, families and the community. The mhGAP resource also provides a set of evidence-based guidelines and tools for non-specialists, including primary healthcare workers, to engage with communities around collective decision making and resilience building (WHO, 2017a). It includes training materials relating to ten mental health conditions so that existing local health practitioners can gain skills in identification, treatment, care and prevention.

Advice from agencies such as Alzheimer's Disease International (ADI) and the WHO, increasingly backed by research evidence, has been to improve the quality of life of people living with dementia by providing community-level and community-wide awareness, education and skill development. This could be for and through schools and families, and for paid carers and community health workers, promoting the development of place-based, community health and care (Prince et al, 2009; Batsch and Mittelman, 2012).

Considering more highly qualified health worker roles, Mkhonto and Hanssen (2018) discussed the range of work done by nurses in dementia care in South African communities. In this context, nurses connect people with dementia and their carers with support and raise public awareness through clinics, churches and schools. To help with this work, Mkhonto and Hanssen identify a need to improve gerontology and geriatric care education among community nurses. They suggest that nursing curricula should include dementia as well as education about how to deal with local sociocultural attitudes and norms. This would assist with the acceptance of nurses in rural places and help workers to dispel any harmful aspects of cultural beliefs.

Regarding development of the overall workforce to deal with increasing numbers of people with dementia in developing countries, the human resource implications of dementia are staggering. The WHO and the World Bank estimate a need by 2030 for 40 million new health and social care jobs globally and about 18 million additional health workers, primarily in low-resource settings, in order to attain effective coverage (WHO, 2017b, 3). The WHO (2017b) *Global action plan on the public health response to dementia 2017–2025* identified key gaps in the supply of qualified and adequately trained workers to deliver evidence-based interventions and quality care.

Responding to the substantial gap between qualified workforce and rising community need, the WHO recognises the need for upskilling across communities. Beyond families and community health workers, this includes staff of businesses that provide healthcare products and assistive/health technologies; staff of NGOs, charities and volunteer groups; and other stakeholders (for example, emergency services workers, legal and transportation services) who can provide advocacy and/or support for people with dementia – in fact, potentially all community members (WHO, 2017a; WHO, 2018).

Other significant international organisations such as ADI and the Dementia Alliance (DA) suggest that training existing health specialists is also part of the equation (ADI and DA, 2014). For instance, staff of healthcare facilities and hospitals could be trained in identifying/ screening for risk, auditing physical spaces for safety, psychosocial interventions for behavioural/psychological symptoms, and the delivery of person-centred services such as end-of-life plans and palliative care. ADI and DA recommend teaching core dementia diagnostic, treatment and care competencies in undergraduate and graduate medical and paramedical training, with continuing training programmes for all health and social care professionals, in collaboration with regulatory bodies.

The problem for policy regarding improved care of people with dementia in rural areas of LMICs is the sheer competition for resources among many urgent issues. Mkhonto and Hanssen (2018) describe dementia as one of myriad health challenges in LMICs, where healthcare systems are already burdened by the range of acute health problems that come with economic hardship and political unrest, such as psychological and physical effects of trauma and violence, and high rates of communicable and chronic/non-communicable diseases. Strasser and colleagues (2016) discuss how healthcare in LMICs often takes the form of vertical programmes designed to target one key problem, often recently emergent, rather than the kind of ongoing, holistic patient- and family-centred care, services and support required for people with dementia.

As well as this, rural areas of LMICs are chronically depleted in terms of access to specialist facilities, including memory clinics and residential care (Patel and Prince, 2001) and the means of transportation or technology to reach these. Parra and colleagues (2018) report that in Mexico, only a third of rural people with dementia receive government support and very few can access specialist services. Dementia-friendly transport to health and social care facilities is rare, as is transport to deliver food and other resources for people with health conditions who remain living at home (Prince et al, 2008). In some places, residential care exists, but this tends to preclude people with dementia, due to lack of recognition of dementia as a medical condition, poor diagnostic capacity, or considering people with dementia as too challenging for the facility. Wu and colleagues (2016) conducted in-depth case studies of rural versus urban care in a Chinese region. One rural facility purported not to provide care for people with dementia, but the researchers found people with dementia living there who were not identified as such, and who did not have distinctive care provided. Lack of provision of specialised care and accommodation can go hand in hand with lack of recognition of dementia as a health condition and beliefs about carer roles, so any changes need to be aligned with local cultural beliefs and norms; for example, Wang and colleagues (2014) discuss that small, home-based, collective living options with financial incentives for village or peer support could be culturally congruent in rural Chinese settings, where large-scale institutionalised care would be unacceptable.

The Kyoto Declaration on minimum actions required for the care of people with dementia (cited in ADI and DA, 2014) recognises that countries vary in their capacity to develop a dementia workforce, and provides recommendations for low-, medium- and high-income countries (LICs, MICs and HICs) as follows:

- *LICs:* develop training and resource centres; initiate advanced training for primary healthcare workers in old age psychiatry and medicine;
- *MICs:* build a network of national training centres for physicians, psychiatrists, nurses, psychologists, occupational therapists and social workers;
- *HICs:* provide advanced treatment skills training for specialists; address workforce issues such as career development and remuneration across the health and aged care sectors.

The role of technology

Given the considerable challenges of connecting rural people with the range of services they need, one path to accessibility suggested is through information and communications technologies (ADI and DA,

2014). Technologies could provide access to knowledge, training and peer support for workers and community members through discussion forums, helplines, online bulletin boards and websites (ADI and DA, 2014). The WHO (2018) has developed iSupport for Dementia, an online training programme for informal carers about dementia, self-care, stress management and coping. However, for widespread effectiveness, country governments would have to collaborate with WHO to translate these tools into different local languages and dialects – an offer that, to date, few developing countries have taken up.

Platforms to track and evaluate the data of people with dementia in health and social care information systems have also been developed (WHO, 2017b). Ultimately, this will enable distribution of information on best practice (including prevention), knowledge exchange, and data for evidence-based resource and service planning, including policy and system development (WHO, 2017b). The WHO's data and knowledge exchange platform, Global Dementia Observatory (WHO, 2019), provides access to key dementia data and indicators, so progress in meeting global dementia targets can be benchmarked across countries consistently and longitudinally. Current lack of formal data-gathering systems in many LMICs currently presents a challenge for epidemiological studies and planning. Although international epidemiological studies confirm that dementia occurs globally, the results of studies vary due to differing research methods (WHO, 2018). For example, in countries where resources are low, researchers may leverage secondary data sources such as community health clinic or hospital records, death certificates, police reports and existing surveys to estimate prevalence rates. Widespread use of consistent indicators could make a significant impact on international efforts to promote funding for dementia at country and region levels.

Although technology could provide cost-effective solutions for rural and remote communities, practical challenges restrict the reach of such initiatives. Over 55 per cent of the world's population does not use the internet, with major gaps in access in developing countries (WEF, 2016); this is particularly acute in rural regions. Affordability, infrastructure, literacy, cultural acceptance and local adoption pose barriers to universal connectivity; indeed, 15 per cent of the global population does not have stable access to electricity (WEF, 2016). Much online content is only accessible in a limited range of languages (World Bank, 2014, cited in WEF, 2016). The World Economic Forum (WEF, 2016) recommends public, private and civil sector collaboration to tackle the digital divide. National dementia action plans could include measures to improve digital literacy and connectivity. Projects aimed at improving digital inclusion are already underway in countries such as Rwanda, Uganda, Kenya, South Sudan and Ethiopia, where more than two thirds of the total population have no internet access (WEF, 2016). In the meantime, Mkhonto and Hanssen (2018) suggest that existing technologies, such as television and news media, are tools for raising awareness and disseminating translated materials.

International efforts to influence dementia care

Given the range of challenges that particularly affect rural areas in LMICs, this section highlights three types of international efforts that could influence what develops on the ground: supra-national policy organisations, using the example of the WHO; civil society, considering the Dementia Alliance International (DAI); and the 10/66 Research Group. Here we aim to suggest their specific role and implications for rural places.

A number of principles are set out in the preamble to the WHO constitution, including:

> Unequal development in different countries in the promotion of health and control of diseases, especially communicable disease, is a common danger.

> We support Member States as they coordinate the efforts of multiple sectors of the government and partners – including bi- and multilaterals, funds and foundations, civil society organizations and private sector – to attain their health objectives and support their national health policies and strategies. (International Health Conference, 1946: 1)

For rural areas, we take this to imply that WHO is keenly concerned with addressing the kinds of within-country and between-countries inequality that can be observed for rural settings and that WHO has a role in stimulating action through collaborations of relevant partners.

Specifically, in relation to dementia, concerted global action over two decades led up to WHO's *Global action plan on the public response to dementia 2017–2025* (WHO, 2017b). The plan calls for a concerted approach and provides a toolkit to help all countries to develop their own contextually relevant strategies and programmes to address dementia. Guided by principles of multisectoral collaboration, equity, human rights, empowerment, prevention and service integration, the plan has seven action areas, with aligned targets for 2025:

- *dementia as a public health priority:* advocates support for governments to develop whole-of-government, multisector, multistakeholder approaches;
- *dementia awareness and friendliness:* recommends dementia-friendly initiatives and functioning public awareness campaigns;
- *dementia risk reduction:* provides a set of risk reduction targets;
- *dementia diagnosis, treatment, care and support:* advocates appropriate inputs across the spectrum of care for the dramatic increase in numbers of people recognised as having dementia, in more countries;
- *support for dementia carers:* recommends training and support for dementia carers in most countries;
- *information systems for dementia:* supports routine data collection in place, on core indicators;
- *dementia research and innovation:* recommends doubling global dementia research outputs.

Applying these principles equally, across rural regions within countries, will require navigating the issues outlined earlier in this chapter. While WHO declined to provide specific written input to this chapter, we did gain an interview with Katrin Seeher of WHO, in 2018, to inform the writing. Seeher (2018) explained that, for implementation, a country should synchronise its dementia plan with its own wider and existing national-level policy, systems and plans for change, and seek support from community-level leaders. As an example, the government of Togo created a Ministry of Ageing that is integrating dementia in the country's national non-communicable diseases plan and is considering a tobacco tax to support implementation of the plan. In addition, champions in Togo's rural and urban communities have been identified to act as local change agents. Elsewhere, Cuba's National Intervention Strategy for Alzheimer Disease and Dementia Syndromes, a response to WHO's call to make dementia a priority, provides another example. The strategy underpins Cuba's development of care guidelines, human rights education, research, and dementia prevention awareness. Cuban government plans include early detection, memory clinics, day centres and rehabilitation services (Bosch-Bayard et al, 2016).

To assist countries with planning how to implement dementia policy, WHO can provide support, but this first requires political commitment and an approach from a country's government to WHO. Once this has occurred, regional-level champions are established and encouraged to work collaboratively, both within and for their country, as well as across countries, facilitated by WHO. This strategy can help the different champions to share and learn effective strategies for implementation from each other at regional forum events. The WHO does not specifically address rural implementation issues; rather (as discussed in foregoing sections), it has developed a range of tools that can be adapted at individual country level, by countries in partnership with WHO, and could be particularly pertinent to rural places due to their emphasis on harnessing community and application for maximising use of resources in severely under-resourced environments.

Seeher (2018) from WHO noted that, alongside international organisations like ADI, which runs an Alzheimer University with regional hubs to raise awareness and offer support, the rise of civil society is a powerful force for countries to move to policy and action on dementia. To explore civil society, we turned, in 2018, to discussion with Kate Swaffer, a co-founder of DAI. DAI is a leading international civil society organisation providing advocacy and support for people with all forms of dementia.

Swaffer (2018) described the establishment of DAI in response to the need for a collective voice for people with dementia to demand inclusion, captured in its motto 'nothing about us, without us'. Starting with eight co-founders from the US, Canada and Australia, DAI now has members in 47 countries. Swaffer (2018) highlighted the unique role of DAI as the international voice of people with dementia (as opposed to health practitioners or carers). DAI campaigns for the human rights of people with dementia, and their inclusion in the disability policies of organisations such as WHO and the United Nations (UN), specifically and the 2006 Convention on the Rights of Persons with Disabilities.

DAI seeks to empower members to become self-advocates and to live with dementia more positively, rather than 'to go home and give up' (Swaffer, 2014). DAI members advocate using social media and cooperating to campaign on topics. Swaffer (2018) says hearing and seeing peers with dementia "empowers them, and seems to give them permission to be public about it". The internet has been a powerful tool for DAI's work and reach, enabling international membership, collaboration and planning. DAI provides educational webinars, online cafes, peer-to-peer support and mentoring for people with dementia. Many members do live in rural areas around the world, but internet access remains problematic in some regions, which limits the reach of DAI and its members.

Swaffer (2018) reports that government and non-governmental organisations in developing countries are keen to work with DAI but funding is a challenge. As such, DAI and ADI members work together to support the empowerment of new DAI members as self-advocates in developing countries specifically, with the idea of building local advocate groups.

Swaffer (2018) says there has been some positive change in attitudes to people with dementia since the first WHO Ministerial Conference on Global Action Against Dementia in March 2015, with increased attention to the human rights approach to dementia. People with dementia have increasingly been able to draw on existing rights frameworks, and there has been a rise in dementia rights charters (for example, Scottish Parliament, 2009) and public awareness campaigns (Prince et al, 2008; DAI, 2016; WHO, 2018). To date, Swaffer (2018) says that advocates are most active and vocal in developed countries. She believes that DAI is possibly the most significant agent for driving change in attitudes, in particular through the development of self-advocates and global human rights and disability activism.

Finally, regarding supra-national research efforts, until recently just 10 per cent of research focused on the two thirds of people with dementia living in LMICs (Prince et al, 2008). The aptly named 10/66 Research Group was developed in response to this research gap and includes 30 research teams in 20 countries including in Latin America, the Caribbean, India, Russia, China and South East Asia. Since its inception, the group has developed a culturally and educationally fair, community-level diagnostic tool for diagnosing people with little or no education, and has facilitated the collection of epidemiological data, enabling comparison across regions (Prince et al, 2003). The group also runs workshops in community settings, such as schools, following a social education model whereby people pass on awareness in families and communities (Prince et al, 2008).

International research organisations can stimulate the need for epidemiological, policy and health systems research in LMICs, including in and about rural areas, and support such research (Prince et al, 2008; ADI and DA, 2014; Shah et al, 2016). For example, international universities or research centres/institutes might partner with LMIC governments and organisations (WHO, 2018). Some LMIC regions are particularly under-researched, including Central Asia, Eastern Europe, southern Latin America, and eastern and southern Sub-Saharan Africa (Prince et al, 2015). Given our search for materials to inform this chapter, we also suggest a particular gap in specifically rural studies about experiences of dementia and new service implementation and evaluation in LMICs.

Conclusion

As highlighted by WHO (2018: 6), 'left unaddressed, dementia could represent a significant barrier to social and economic development'. This chapter has focused on the challenges for people living with dementia and their carers in LMICs and sought to specifically examine how this might affect rural places and rural people. Major challenges include attitudes to dementia, including stigmatisation of individuals living with the condition, and lack of access to supportive care for people with dementia, carers, families and communities. We have highlighted the currently vital role of the community and primary healthcare workers in rural areas that are essentially the front line of dementia care in LMICs, and the need for skill development and support. Global and policy-level responses are underway for all regions of all countries, with clear targets for 2025 that address dementia as a public health priority – though how this will play out in rural areas of LMICs is concerning. In these settings, we are talking about a poorly understood issue that is often culturally contested, and it affects people in the most resource-depleted areas of the world's most economically challenged countries. Simultaneously, these countries and areas are often having to deal with high-priority problems such as maternal and child health, communicable diseases, natural disaster and socioeconomic disruption due to globalisation. Thus, while there is some confidence that WHO strategies can reduce the worldwide burden of dementia substantially in the next 10 years, we suggest that particular attention should be given to developments in, and studies of, rural areas of LMICs (Shah et al, 2016).

A range of factors influence the scope of countries to respond to dementia. For developed countries, priorities include addressing service needs and system inefficiencies, while developing countries need knowledgeable workers and communities to address skills shortages and gaps in awareness (WHO, 2017b, 2018). WHO argues that disproportionate numbers of current and future cases of dementia in LMICs compared with HICs will exacerbate existing country/population inequalities (WHO, 2017b), underscoring the need to address skills shortages in LMICs through workforce training and development.

References

ADI (Alzheimer's Disease International) and DI (Dementia Australia) (2014) *Dementia in the Asia-Pacific region*, London: ADI.

Batsch, N.L. and Mittelman, M.S. (eds) (2012) *World Alzheimer's Report (2012): Overcoming the stigma of dementia*, London: World Alzheimer's Association.

Benade, S. (2012) 'Support services for people suffering from dementia in the rural areas of Kwa-Zulu Natal, South Africa', *Dementia*, 11(2): 275–7.

Bosch-Bayard, R.I., Borrego-Calzadilla, C., Moreno-Carbonell, C.R., Llibre-Rodriguez, J.J., Carrasco-Garcia, M.R., Reymond-Vasconcelos, A.G., Fernandez-Seco, A. and Zayas-Llerena, T. (2016) 'Cuba's Strategy for Alzheimer Disease and Dementia Syndromes', *International Journal of Cuban Health & Medicine*, 18(4): 9–13.

Chen, S., Boyle, L.L., Conwell, Y., Xiao, S. and Fung Kum Chiu, H. (2014) 'The challenges of dementia care in rural China', *International Psychogeriatrics*, 26(7): 1059–64.

DAI (Dementia Alliance International) (2016) *The human rights of people living with dementia: From rhetoric to reality*, Adelaide: DAI.

de Jager, C.A., Msemburi, W., Pepper, K. and Combrinck, M.I. (2017) 'Dementia prevalence in a rural region of South Africa: a cross-sectional community study', *Journal of Alzheimer's Disease*, 60(3): 1087–96.

Ferreira, M. and Kalula, S. (2009) 'Ageing, women and health: emerging caregiving needs in Sub-Saharan African countries', *Bold*, 19(4): 2–12.

Guerchet, M., Mayston, R., Lloyd-Sherlock, P., Prince, M., Aboderin, I., Akinyemi, R., Paddick, S.M., Wimo, A., Amoakoh-Coleman, M., Uwakwe, R. and Ezeah, P. (2017) *Dementia in sub-Saharan Africa: Challenges and opportunities*, London: Alzheimer's Disease International.

Gurayah, T. (2015) 'Caregiving for people with dementia in a rural context in South Africa', *South African Family Practice*, 57(3): 194–7.

Hari, J. (2009) 'Witch hunt: Africa's hidden war on women', *The Independent*, [online] 12 March. Available from: www.independent.co.uk/news/world/africa/witch-hunt-africas-hidden-war-on-women-1642907.html

Ingstad, B. (1990) 'Anthropological aspects of disability', Manuscript to oral presentation at Symposium on CBR, Uppsala, Sweden, 29 May.

International Health Conference (1946) *Constitution of the World Health Organization*. Available from: apps.who.int/gb/bd/PDF/bd47/EN/constitution-en.pdf

Jia, J., Wang, F., Wei, C., Zhou, A., Jia, X., Li, F., Tang, M., Chu, L., Zhou, Y., Zhou, C. and Cui, Y. (2014) 'The prevalence of dementia in urban and rural areas of China', *Alzheimer's & Dementia*, 10(1): 1–9.

Keynejad, R.C., Dua, T., Barbui, C. and Thornicroft, G. (2017) 'WHO Mental Health Gap Action Programme (mhGAP) Intervention Guide: a systematic review of evidence from low and middle-income countries', *Evidence-Based Mental Health*, 21(1): 30–4.

Maestre, G.E. (2012) 'Assessing dementia in resource poor regions', *Current Neurology & Neuroscience Reports*, 12(5): 511–19.

Mkhonto, F. and Hanssen, I. (2018) 'When people with dementia are perceived as witches: consequences for patients and nurse education in South Africa', *Journal of Clinical Nursing*, 27(1–2): e169–e76.

Parra, M.A., Baez, S., Allegri, R., Nitrini, R., Lopera, F., Slachevsky, A., Custodio, N., Lira, D., Piguet, O., Kumfor, F., Huepe, D., Cogram, P., Bak, T., Manes, F. and Ibanez, A. (2018) 'Dementia in Latin America: assessing the present and envisioning the future', *Neurology*, 90: 1–10.

Patel, V. and Prince, M. (2001) 'Ageing and mental health in a developing country: who cares? Qualitative studies from Goa, India', *Psychological Medicine*, 31(1): 29–38.

Prince, M., Acosta, D., Albanese, E., Arizaga, R., Ferri, C.P., Guerra, M., Huang, Y., Jacob, K.S., Jiminez-Velasquez, I.Z., Rodriguez, J.L., Sala, A., Sosa, A.L., Sousa, R., Uwakwe, R., van der Poel, R., Williams, J. and Wortmann, M. (2008) 'Ageing and dementia in low and middle income countries: using research to engage with public and policy makers', *International Review of Psychiatry*, 20(4): 332–43.

Prince, M.J., Acosta, D., Castro-Costa, E., Jackson, J. and Shaji, K.S. (2009) 'Packages of care for dementia in low- and middle-income countries', *PLoS Medicine*, 6(11): e1000176.

Prince, M., Acosta, D., Chiu, H., Scazufca, M. and Varghese, M. (2003) 'Dementia diagnosis in developing countries: a cross-cultural validation study', *The Lancet*, 361(9361): 909–17.

Prince, M., Acosta, D., Ferri, C.P., Huang, Y., Jacob, K.S., Llibre Rodriguez, J.J, Salas, A., Sosa, A.L., Williams, J.D. and Hall, K.S. (2011b) 'The 10/66 Research Group: a brief dementia screener suitable for use by non-specialists in resource poor settings – the cross-cultural derivation and validation of the Brief Community Screening Instrument for Dementia', *Geriatric Psychiatry*, 26(9): 899–907.

Prince, M., Bryce, R. and Ferri, C. (2011a) *World Alzheimer Report 2011: The benefits of early diagnosis and intervention*, London: Alzheimer's Disease International.

Prince, M., Ferri, C.P., Acosta, D., Albanese, E., Arizaga, R., Dewey, M., Gavrilova, S.I., Guerra, M., Huang, Y., Jacob, K.S. and Krishnamoorthy, E.S. (2007) 'The protocols for the 10/66 Dementia Research Group population-based research programme', *BMC Public Health*, 7(1): 165.

Prince, M., Wimo, A., Guerchet, M., Ali, G.C., Wu, Y.T. and Prina, M. (2015) *World Alzheimer Report 2015. The global impact of dementia: An analysis of prevalence, incidence, cost and trends*, London: Alzheimer's Disease International.

Salemink, K., Strijker, D. and Bosworth, G. (2017) 'Rural development in the digital age: a systematic literature review on unequal ICT availability, adoption and use in rural areas', *Journal of Rural Studies*, 54: 360–71.

Scottish Parliament (2009) *Charter of rights for people with dementia and their carers in Scotland*, Edinburgh: Scottish Parliament.

Seeher, K. (2018) Personal correspondence.

Shah, H., Albanese, E., Duggan, C., Rudan, I., Langa, K.M., Carrillo, M.C., Chan, K.Y., Joanette, Y., Prince, M., Rossor, M., Saxena, S., Snyder, H.M., Sperling, R., Varghese, M., Wang, H., Wortmann, M. and Dua, T. (2016) 'Research priorities to reduce the global burden of dementia by 2025', *The Lancet Neurology*, 15(12): 1285–94.

Sousa, R.M., Ferri, C.P., Acosta, D., Guerra, M., Huang, Y., Jacob, K.S., Jotheeswaran, A.T., Guerra Hernandez, M.A., Liu, Z., Rodriguez Pichardo, G., Llibre Rodriguez, J.J., Salas, A., Sosa, A.L., Williams, J., Zuniga, T. and Prince, M. (2010) 'The contribution of chronic diseases to the prevalence of dependence among older people in Latin America, China and India: a 10/66 Dementia Research Group population-based survey', *BMC Geriatrics*, 10: 53.

Starfield, B. (1998) *Primary care: Balancing health needs, services and technologies*, New York, NY: Oxford University Press.

Strasser, R. (2003) 'Rural health around the world: challenges and solutions', *Family Practice*, 20(4): 457–63.

Strasser, R., Kam, S.M. and Regalado, S.M. (2016) 'Rural health care access and policy in developing countries', *Annual Review of Public Health*, 37: 395–412.

Swaffer, K. (2014) 'Reinvesting in life is the best prescription', *Australian Journal of Dementia Care*, 3(6): 31–2. Available from: https://journalofdementiacare.com/reinvesting-in-life-is-the-best-prescription

Swaffer, K. (2018) Personal correspondence.

Wang, J., Xiao, L.D., He, G.P. and De Bellis, A. (2014) 'Family caregiver challenges in dementia care in a country with undeveloped dementia services', *Journal of Advanced Nursing*, 70(6): 1369–80.

WEF (World Economic Forum) (2016) *White Paper: Internet for all. A framework for accelerating access and adoption*, Cologny: WEF.

WHO (World Health Organization) (2017a) *Dementia: Toolkit for community workers in low- and middle-income countries. Guide for community-based management and care of people with dementia*, Manila: World Health Organization Regional Office for the Western Pacific.

WHO (2017b) *Global action plan on the public health response to dementia 2017–2025*, Geneva: WHO.

WHO (2018) *Towards a dementia plan: A WHO guide*, Geneva: WHO.

WHO (2019) 'Global Dementia Observatory', [online]. Available at: www.who.int/mental_health/neurology/dementia/Global_Observatory/en

WONCA (World Organization of Family Doctors) (2014) 'Gramado statement on rural health in developing countries – April, 2014', XII WONCA World Conference on Rural Health, Gramado, Brazil. Available from: www.acrrm.org.au/docs/default-source/documents/about-the-college/gramadostatement.pdf?sfvrsn=79c497eb_0

Wu, C., Gao, L., Chen, S. and Dong, H. (2016) 'Care services for elderly people with dementia in rural China: a case study', *Bulletin of the World Health Organization*, 94(3): 167–73.

3

Addressing dementia needs in Australia

Irene Blackberry, Clare Wilding, Michael Bauer,
Margaret Winbolt and Hilary Davis

Introduction

Of 23 million Australians, there were 436,366 people living with a diagnosis of dementia in 2018 (Dementia Australia, 2018a). Dementia Australia estimates that close to 600,000 people will be living with dementia in the next decade and by 2058, the number will rise to over a million (Dementia Australia, 2018a). Dementia is the second leading cause of death for Australians (AIHW, 2016) and the single greatest cause of disability in older Australians (aged 65 years or older) (AIHW, 2012).

By 2025, the annual cost of dementia, to Australia, is projected to be around A\$18.7 billion and A\$36.8 billion by 2056. Unpaid family carers play a critical role in providing care for Australians living with dementia; informal carers are estimated to provide approximately A\$60.3 billion of unpaid services annually, which translates to over A\$1 billion per week (Deloitte Access Economics, 2015).

People of Aboriginal and Torres Strait Islander background have up to five times higher risk of developing dementia, compared with the general population (NATSEM, 2017) and Indigenous people tend to be affected by dementia at an earlier age than other Australians. Around 20 per cent of Australians with dementia come from a culturally or linguistically diverse (that is, non-White English-speaking) background.

Australian Government policy relating to dementia

Australia's current policy approach is guided by the National Framework for Action on Dementia 2015–2019 (Department of Health, 2015) and aims to 'Improve the quality of life for people living with dementia and their support networks' (p 2) by 'drawing on current evidence to promote dementia friendly societies and delivery of consumer-focused care' (p 1).

The priority areas of the framework comprise:

- a commitment to increasing awareness and reducing risk;
- timely diagnosis;
- access to care and support following diagnosis;
- access to ongoing care and support;
- access to care and support during and after hospital care;
- access to end-of-life and palliative care; and
- promotion of, and support for, research.

Driven by these priorities, the objectives of the framework are supported through a complex network of health and aged care services delivered variously through funding and services from Commonwealth (that is, national federal) government, state and territory governments, and local governments as well as private and not-for profit service providers. Specifically, services provided for older people with dementia include: primary healthcare led by general medical practitioners; specialist memory clinics; personal and nursing care in the home; Home Support Programme and Home Care Package Programme (home care packages are delivered through a Consumer Directed Care model, meaning that the client controls a package of funds and can directly purchase services); residential care; home care, personal care; and carer respite and support services. Some of these services are provided directly by different levels of government, some via contracts with private or non-governmental organisation providers, and some via consumer-directed care. Because availability differs by state and also by what is available locally or in different service centres and cities, navigating this fragmented service landscape is notoriously complex.

As well as these general services for older people, there are a series of dementia-specific offerings. For example, there is a series of Commonwealth-funded programmes aimed at improving 'awareness and understanding about dementia and [to] increase the skills and confidence of people living with dementia, their carers, families, health professionals, volunteers and community contacts' (Department of Health, 2018). These supplemental services include: the National Disability Insurance Scheme (NDIS), which provides care and support to assist people with younger onset dementia (those under the age of 65); and the National Dementia Support Program, which includes access to:

- a national website (www.fightdementia.org.au);
- the National Dementia Helpline and Referral Service;
- one-to-one and small-group counselling, access to support groups and information, and recommendations and referrals;
- early intervention programmes (for example, Living With Dementia);
- non-accredited training for professionals, carers and communities; and
- advice and support services delivered by advocacy group Dementia Australia.

The Commonwealth government also funds: the Younger Onset Dementia Key Worker Program (through the NDIS), which provides people with younger onset dementia, their families and carers with a key contact person for advice and support; the Dementia Education and Training for Carers programme – which provides information, education and training to informal, family carers to increase their skills and confidence in caring for a person with dementia; and Dementia Support Australia, which provides client-specific support and advice to service providers and informal carers about managing challenging behaviours of people living with dementia.

In efforts to ease access to these services, the Australian Government has developed an online portal – My Aged Care (www.myagedcare. gov.au) – which aims to provide a nationwide means of accessing information and guidance. Assessment and approval processes to access services is also managed via this portal, by Regional Assessment Services and Aged Care Assessment Teams. The Commonwealth government subsidises the cost of aged care services to the individual; however, service users must contribute to the cost where they are assessed as financially able. Theoretically, a person would, from diagnosis, be guided by using My Aged Care along a cohesive pathway, being referred to and receiving, relevant services in accordance with their needs as these change.

In 2012, the Australian Government announced its Living Longer Living Better reforms, aimed at building an improved and equitable aged care system (AIHW, 2012). Funds of A$268 million over five years were allocated to address issues relevant to health and care services, informal services, and managing dementia in the community. This included: expanding the Dementia Behaviour Management Advisory Service into acute care; providing support for older Australians experiencing severe dementia with challenging behaviours in residential care, including training, guidelines and procedures to ensure best practice by aged care providers; the introduction of the Dementia

Supplement to offset the higher costs for caring for older Australians with dementia; enhancing coordination across care services for people with dementia; and providing coordinated support for people with younger onset dementia.

In the same year, the national government declared dementia as a National Health Priority Area (AIHW, 2012), which was a significant move critical to facilitating a unified agenda. In collaboration with non-government agencies, service providers and consumers, actions for addressing dementia at national, local and state and territory government levels were planned for delivery.

To boost research, in 2015, a targeted A$200 million fund for Australian dementia research was announced. This fund targeted the development of new researchers, encouraged study of key challenges, stimulated research translation, and invested in dementia research infrastructure. The National Institute of Dementia Research was also launched, to ensure coordination and engagement of people living with dementia and relevant stakeholders.

Dementia and rural Australia

According to the Australian Bureau of Statistics (ABS, 2016a), there are five categories of geographical regions in Australia: major cities, inner regional areas, outer regional areas, remote areas and very remote areas. Remoteness is defined by combining measures of road distance to the nearest urban centre and population density (ABS, 2016a). Approximately a third of Australians live in regional, rural and remote areas (AIHW, 2017). Of these, 18 per cent live in inner regional areas, 8.9 per cent live in outer regional areas, and 2.3 per cent live in remote or very remote areas (AIHW, 2017). Around 21 per cent of Indigenous Australians live in remote areas. People who live in rural Australia face distinct challenges related to health and wellbeing, compared with people living in urban areas. Most notable are higher rates of chronic disease and mortality, the presence of behaviours associated with poorer health outcomes, and reduced access to health services (AIHW, 2018). Although there is a lower actual number of older people living in regional, rural and remote areas, compared with metropolitan areas, older people in the rural and remote population is proportionately higher. Two of every five people with dementia live outside metropolitan areas (NATSEM, 2017) and this proportion is expected to rise over the next four decades (NATSEM, 2017). Risk factors for dementia are more prevalent among people living in regional, rural and remote areas (AIHW, 2016).

There is evidence of lack of awareness of dementia among rural community members (Orpin et al, 2014) and there is a workforce shortage, particularly for general practitioners and geriatricians, which affects timely diagnosis, early intervention and ongoing condition management. Support services in remote and rural communities are minimal due to dispersed populations, distances from service centres, lack of access to transport, and long travel times. Despite these significant challenges, people living with dementia and their carers prefer to stay in their local communities following a dementia diagnosis, and some report high levels of satisfaction with rural life (Orpin et al, 2014).

A study by Saunders (2013) showed that stigma about dementia means that some rural Australians do not seek support. Reluctance to acknowledge the possible presence of dementia may also result in lack of a timely diagnosis (Saunders, 2013). A limitation of research on dementia in rural and remote Australian communities is that studies may have small numbers of participants and, coupled with a lack of robust comparative data with urban or other types of settings, this may prohibit generalisability of findings and transfer of innovations across communities.

Dementia and the rural workforce

There is a workforce of paid carers that supports family carers and people with dementia to continue to live at home. There is also a paid carer workforce providing social and nursing care to people living in residential aged care. Most of this formal workforce comprises personal care workers, whose role is to assist with meeting daily personal care needs. Health professionals such as nurses and allied health practitioners deliver the more specialist services of clinical assessments, clinical care and case management, in community and residential settings.

A skilled and knowledgeable workforce is needed if people living with dementia are to receive optimal levels of care and support. Education and training therefore play a vital role in upskilling the workforce and promoting high-quality, evidence-based dementia care. Education is provided by a variety of organisations, including through government funded programmes, Dementia Australia, service providers, and private training organisations, including a Commonwealth-funded national training programme delivered by Dementia Training Australia – a consortium of five universities, Dementia Australia and the Wicking Dementia Research and Education Centre.

Organisations delivering home and residential care services to people with dementia in rural areas face challenges including staff recruitment, but this is often offset by a low staff turnover rate and high staff retention levels (Savy et al, 2017). Staff are usually drawn from the local community and therefore may have longstanding relationships with those in their care, which can support a person-centred approach. Service providers experience challenges in access to training, especially if there is a requirement to travel, and low staff numbers make it difficult to release staff to attend training. Training can be costly and although online access is an option, there can be problems with poor internet connectivity in rural areas. If training is provided on site in a rural area, there may only be small numbers of staff who can attend the training, therefore making it less economically viable and less attractive for external training providers who may need to travel from a major city to provide the training on location in a rural town.

Dementia and rural family carers

Family carers provide a significant amount of care for people living with dementia and although caring has many positive aspects, it can also place substantial emotional, psychological and physical demands on carers (Dementia Australia, 2018b). A survey by Ervin and colleagues (2015) examining wellbeing and carer distress in relation to the behavioural and psychological symptoms of dementia in a rural region in northern Victoria found that 58 per cent of carers reported moderate to severe levels of stress, 38 per cent described moderate to severe depression, and 26 per cent experienced moderate to severe anxiety. This finding is consistent with other Australian research (Brodaty et al, 2003; Pallant and Reid, 2013). The requirements of caregiving can result in disengaging socially and becoming more isolated (Schulz and Martire, 2004; Papastavrou et al, 2015). Carers are, in general, more likely to have smaller social networks than non-carers, and carers' social support often decreases over time (Orpin et al, 2014). The demands of caring, including loss of sleep, can result in carer exhaustion (Ervin et al, 2015).

While these challenging issues may be experienced by all carers irrespective of geography, they can become amplified in rural and remote regions where people with dementia and their carers are often disadvantaged in terms of access to health and other supports that meet their needs (Ervin et al, 2015). Providing appropriate and timely services and supports is therefore a crucial strategy to help allay rural family carer stress and burden.

In 2007, Alzheimer's Australia conducted a survey and interviews with 173 people with dementia and their carers and 74 service providers in four Australian states. They identified needs that were specific to

Table 3.1: Rural dementia carers' support and service needs from 2018 study

• Better and timely access to appropriate dementia services including less travel and reduced waiting time for appointments;
• Assistance to find information about what dementia services and other help is available to carers and how to access these;
• More training for health professionals to help them understand the experience of living with dementia, what it's like to be a carer and the importance of sharing of information about current best practice;
• Improving early diagnosis of dementia so that services and appropriate information can be accessed;
• More community awareness and education about dementia and living with dementia to reduce stigma in the community and increase awareness of the support needs of carers;
• More memory support nurses to provide care;
• More day care and respite care options such as extended times and evening care;
• More support for carers and someone to talk to and share experiences about fears, loneliness, struggles, health and wellbeing, and care strategies;
• Training for carers about how to care for someone with dementia and manage issues that arise;
• More training of health professionals so that they acknowledge carers' role in decision making and as partners in care;
• A greater role for volunteers to help carers; and
• Better care coordination to keep services involved and up to date with the needs of the person with dementia.

people living in rural and remote areas, including emotional and social support; education and awareness about use of technology-based information channels; travel and transport options for people with dementia; ways to alleviate the apparent higher financial burden experienced by people with dementia and their carers living in remote and regional areas; and need for consultation with Indigenous people with dementia and their carers and families living in remote and regional areas. Improvements were also desired in identifying dementia support-related needs, priorities and recommendations; local community service access; diagnosis, assessment and medical management; and flexible respite and residential care options. More recently, a study focusing on one rural region confirmed similar needs for rural carers of people with dementia living in the community (Bauer et al, 2019). Table 3.1 summarises the findings.

The findings of these two studies are similar, but rural communities are not homogenous, and specific priorities vary by rural place. Differences between rural communities mean that communities can face varying and sometimes even unique challenges. Evidence from the state of South Australia highlighted a need for a better navigation process to identify and access local support services (Saunders, 2013). However, participants in a study in the state of Tasmania reported no major concerns about the availability of, or their access to, formal support services, although some participants were not satisfied with respite services and the knowledge and expertise of general practitioners (Orpin et al, 2014). It appears that the Tasmanian community may have been more willing than the South Australian one to accept the available services, and that the Tasmanian community's expectations could be lower than those of the South Australians.

Despite their relative satisfaction with services, carers in Orpin and colleagues' (2014) study of rural Tasmania reported feeling ill equipped for their carer role and they sought assistance from health professionals in building skills, knowledge, capacity and confidence. To understand the needs of carers requires a deep, sophisticated and multidimensional understanding of their role and experiences (Orpin et al, 2014).

Innovative approaches to dementia services in rural Australia

A number of different initiatives and approaches are emergent throughout Australia to try to improve accessibility of care for rural and remote residents living with dementia. The following examples are primarily based on the work and knowledge of the author team who are all located in the state of Victoria.

Example 1: training rural dementia volunteers

The first initiative was run in two rural local government areas, with the idea of providing basic training for local volunteers in helping rural people with dementia and their carers to navigate services and to be a 'listening ear' for carers. We first provide a quick snapshot to give some feel for the context of the two rural communities covered, in Victoria where the initiative took place, and then describe some features of the initiative itself.

The small township of Edenhope is 395 km west (for example, about five hours' driving distance) from Melbourne (the capital city of Victoria) and 30 km from the South Australian border. The township was established through colonisation around 1860 and sits on the shores of Lake Wallace, a fishing and water sports destination. The local hospital serves the 4,250 people of West Wimmera Shire (local government area) (approximately 9,000 km^2). Most local residents are White English-speaking Australians (89.4 per cent) and 0.7 per cent are Indigenous Australians. There are a small number of people from other ethnic and cultural backgrounds present. The wider area features small towns, many with declining populations, a high proportion of ageing people and high levels of chronic disease. Based on national data about deprivation, the West Wimmera Shire area where Edenhope is located has higher socioeconomic disadvantage than the state and the rural parts of the state averages. Recent demographic changes are of population decline and service centralisation (West Wimmera Shire area population declined by 475 people during 2001–11) (Wimmera Primary Care Partnership, 2013).

The primary local employment is in agriculture, forestry, fishing, construction, retail, education and healthcare. Significant local issues include securing water supplies and updating road and service infrastructure. Unemployment was 5.5 per cent in March 2016 (national unemployment rate = 5.8 per cent). Voluntary groups are active, including church groups, Rotary, Lions Club and others. The community is culturally active with well-preserved old buildings such as the courthouse open to the public. There are also sports groups, an annual Gourmet Food and Wine Day, the Lake Wallace Festival and Lake Charlegrark Country Music Marathon.

The other town in the pilot project is Warracknabeal, which is a larger town. Rural Northwest Health provides services for the area of Yarriambiack Shire including to Warracknabeal (population 2,438) (ABS, 2016b) and the townships of Hopetoun (541) (ABS, 2016c) and Beulah (329) (ABS, 2016d). Warracknabeal is 342 km from Melbourne, Victoria. Yarriambiack Shire presents a very similar demographic, employment and cultural picture to West Wimmera Shire depicted previously.

The initiative we implemented was funded by a philanthropic organisation called the Foundation for Rural and Regional Renewal. The purpose of the initiative, called HelpDem, was to train volunteers to meet five key needs that were identified by a study carried out in the local area (Bauer et al, 2019). The research identified services that would enhance quality of life for carers of people with dementia living in the community. Carers and health staff suggested that volunteers could work in a person–centred and integrated manner with trained healthcare providers to enhance local services (Bauer et al, 2019). Five primary areas of need that carers and healthcare staff thought could be fulfilled by volunteers were: providing information about available local and state-level services and how to navigate them; being available to talk to carers; advising local businesses and services about how to interact with people with dementia in the community; finding and accessing transport; and providing respite for carers.

Volunteers were recruited from Edenhope and Warracknabeal. Evidence-based, localised training was developed and tested by a local volunteer advocacy organisation. Volunteers attended a one-day training course that included material on understanding dementia and carers' challenges and needs, navigating local and state services, connecting with local services, understanding the scope of volunteering practice including familiarisation with referral procedures, and how to practise as a volunteer with people with dementia and their carers. Training also included information about accessing the My Aged Care website.

Most significantly, the volunteers developed through this initiative helped carers to navigate local and distant services through understanding local people's needs, the local context and how people live and operate in the rural townships. Additionally, volunteers had a role in advising local services and businesses about dementia and how to engage with people with dementia to reduce stigma and help to keep people included in local life. This emphasis on local contexts is especially important for rural communities because service delivery and organisation can be very different from one rural community to the next and also markedly different from that of metropolitan settings.

Example 2: Wattle House, a rural hospital dementia unit

Wattle House is a residential care programme for people living with dementia. Wattle House is managed by Rural Northwest Health in Warracknabeal. Nurses and carers at the unit have co-developed a capability model of care, and apply techniques developed from the Montessori training method. The four main principles of the capability model are: recognising a resident's capability and ability; knowing each resident's background; leadership; and continually improving and adapting the environment to the residents' needs.

Prior to the programme, many residents spent much of their time in sedentary positions, generally sitting and watching television. Medication was also used extensively. After the introduction of the new programme, residents were actively engaged in performing useful, everyday tasks based on their personal histories and likes and dislikes. For example, residents set places at the dining table, made their beds, and watered plants in the garden. In addition, they engaged in activities that helped to maintain, and in some cases to restore, physical function.

For example, one resident who had a stroke was able to return to independently feeding himself.

The focus of staff is to have a resident actively engaged beside them as they work. Staff resist completing tasks for residents, and rather they aim to maximise residents' capabilities while giving support and encouragement to participate. Risk assessments are in place to help enhance the safety of residents. Activities are fun and engaging and help to maintain residents' sense of self-worth. A YouTube video showcasing the programme at Wattle House is available (Rural Northwest Health, 2013). The Wattle House model is equally appropriate for use in rural and urban settings; however, it is mentioned here as an example of best-practice residential care for people living with dementia that has been implemented in a small rural town very distant from metropolitan settings – showing the quality of care that can be achieved in rural contexts. Although lack of services often characterises rural experiences, in this example a small rural community is providing leadership in best-practice care.

Example 3: SENDER and Verily Connect: apps to help navigate the service landscape

Here we discuss applications ('apps') we designed to address some specific challenges experienced by rural people living with dementia, and their carers and families, including a lack of services in small communities with a low population, the need to travel long distances to receive services and support, and concern about lack of privacy in small rural communities.

With the development of cheaper and more accessible internet access, there are novel solutions to rural challenges that may be afforded though utilising digital technologies. Two projects that have trialled the use of technology to increase support for rural carers of people living with dementia are Service Navigation and Networking for Dementia in Rural Communities (SENDER) and Virtual Dementia Friendly Rural Communities (Verily Connect).

SENDER was a project that piloted a prototype mobile app for Android technology users in two small rural communities in the state of Victoria – Warracknabeal and Heathcote. The SENDER app's main features were information provision about locally available dementia care services (including direct email, telephone, and Worldwide Web access to these services, and navigation to the services using Google Maps) and a chat function for connecting carers to other carers and to service providers. As a pilot, the number of participants in this project was 17 in total: nine carers and eight service providers. Qualitative feedback provided by the participants indicated that the app was promising regarding its potential to assist carers with attaining easy and ready access to services and they liked the idea of better connection with other carers. However, uptake of the app was hampered by the users' general lack of experience in using mobile technology and their subsequent lack of confidence with this type of information provision and communication.

Using learning from the SENDER project, a subsequent study was designed and the project received funding from the Australian Government Department of Health. The Verily Connect project is currently (2019–20) undertaking a national trial using a whole-of-community action research approach and a stepped-wedge cluster randomised trial design to test strategies to increase support for carers of people living with memory loss and dementia in 12 rural communities across three Australian states. The communities varied in population size from less than 1,000 to over 40,000. While Australia is becoming a much more multicultural society, in many rural communities the majority of population remains Anglo-Celtic or English-speaking. Out of 12 participating communities, only one featured a high percentage (60 per cent) of culturally or linguistically diverse residents.

Verily Connect builds on the work of the earlier SENDER app project. The app functionality was expanded; in addition to information and connection to locally available dementia care services, there is also brief information about dementia, about ways that carers can maintain their wellbeing, and an overview of the types of services and supports available for people living with dementia and their carers. Three main strategies are being implemented in the Verily Connect project: an app with functions of information provision and connection; video-conferenced peer support groups for carers; and support in using technology, from local volunteers. The information provided is packaged into 12 topics that are designed to provide easily manageable, small amounts of information, with links to further information and resources for more in-depth exploration. This feature was provided in response to feedback that although information was wanted, many of the available sources were overwhelmingly dense and information-rich. Qualitative findings, to date, from the project confirm that the objective of making information more accessible and useable was achieved, as illustrated by the following quote from a carer participant: "Sometimes we've got the information, but there is too much information…. The simplicity of Verily probably is a positive, because you're not getting bombarded with too much information".

Opportunities for connection with other carers were increased in the Verily Connect project by supplementing the previously available text chat with the addition of real-time videoconference meetings. This feature is likely to be especially useful for communities with no existing face-to-face carer peer support group, which is the case for approximately half of the 12 communities involved in Verily Connect. Also, Verily Connect participants have reported that the online meetings are convenient, as carers can participate in the meetings wherever they happen to be and do not need to undertake travel to a specific location. During recent meetings, carers logged on from their homes, from places of work, and while visiting with relatives living in a metropolitan area.

The addition of the strategy of having local volunteers from each participating community to support carers in using online technologies was created in response to feedback from SENDER participants. Most of the carer participants in SENDER were novices at using smartphones and tablets; they needed more face-to-face assistance when using these technologies. Clearly, for online support technologies to be effective, they need to be used, and the local volunteers, who receive training as part of Verily Connect, are there to make using the technology easier. Participants in Verily Connect reported that volunteers assisted them to utilise technology: "She [the volunteer] had a lot of computer skills that I didn't have…. I thought that she was a very nice person. I felt instantly that she was there to help…. She was very positive".

Example 4: improving rural dementia care pathways

The Webster Rural and Regional Dementia Care project is a three-year research initiative (2018–2020) targeting carers of people living with dementia in Bendigo, a regional city (population approximately 100,000) in the state of Victoria and its surrounding rural areas. The project aims to improve dementia care pathways, with a specific emphasis on developing innovative and sustainable care for residents of Bendigo and surrounding regions.

In Australia, Dementia Service Pathways were developed for the commonwealth government Department of Health and Ageing to assist with service planning to improve dementia services along the continuum of care for people living with dementia and their carers. Pathways are provided for four key stages of dementia management: awareness, recognition and referral; initial assessment and diagnosis, and post-diagnosis support; management, care, support and review; and end of life (KPMG, 2011).

Figure 3.1: The Webster project outline in Bendigo, Victoria, Australia

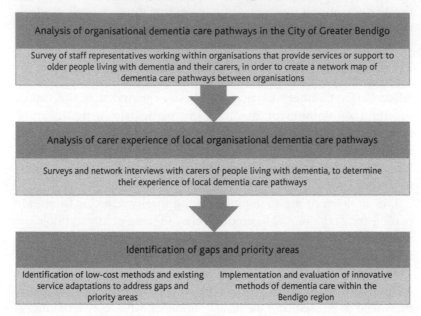

The Webster project builds on previous work by Ollerenshaw and colleagues (2017), who created an online Dementia Pathways tool that included a decision tree and region-specific dementia services for primary health practitioners (Ollerenshaw et al, 2017). Ollerenshaw and colleagues (2017) trialled their tool in regional Victoria and found that general practitioners and nurses experienced improvements in their knowledge, skills and confidence in providing dementia care when they used the Dementia Pathways tool.

The Webster project is being conducted using a mixed-method study design in partnership with local health, community and aged care providers, and people living with dementia and their carers. The project maps services in the greater Bendigo region and explores experiences of rural carers and providers in accessing services. Findings will inform the development of the co-designed Bendigo Dementia Friendly Community initiative. Figure 3.1 shows the main stages of the project.

Example 5: Let's CHAT: an ageing well initiative for Aboriginal and Torres Strait Islander peoples

As mentioned at the start of this chapter, Aboriginal and Torres Strait Islander peoples are disproportionately affected by dementia and there is a tendency for this group to experience the development of dementia at an earlier age than in the general Australian population. According to the Australian Institute of Health and Welfare (AIHW, 2015), the number of Aboriginal and Torres Strait Islander people aged 55 years and over will more than double between 2011 and 2026, and given this increase in older Aboriginal people there is a need for strategies to promote the concept of 'ageing well' for Indigenous older people.

The Let's CHAT (Community Health Approaches To) dementia initiative in Aboriginal and Torres Strait Islander communities focuses on identifying and supporting older people who attend Aboriginal primary healthcare services and who have cognitive impairment or dementia. Let's CHAT is a large cluster randomised controlled trial, funded by a National Health and Medical Research Council Boosting Dementia grant over three years. Twelve Aboriginal and Torres Strait Islander communities located in urban, rural and remote areas in four Australian states are participating to implement and evaluate a new model of care centred within Aboriginal Community Controlled Health Services (primary care services). Inclusion of, and engagement with, local services is critical to ensure the model of care meets the needs of Aboriginal people living with dementia in rural and remote settings.

The project aims to improve the timely detection and ongoing management of older Aboriginal people living with dementia or cognitive impairment. This project will use a community-wide approach and engages community members and Aboriginal health professionals. Outcomes of this project will include culturally adapted Medicare Benefit Schedule (MBS) 715 screening, support for adapting locally used software, training programmes and a best-practice guide. The MBS is a fee-for-service scheme under the Australian national public health funding scheme. The 715 item covers 'Professional attendance by a general practitioner at consulting rooms or in another place other than a hospital or residential aged care facility, for a health assessment of a patient who is of Aboriginal or Torres Strait Islander descent-not more than once in a 9-month period' (Australian Government Department of Health, 2018). Training packages and best-practice guidelines will be developed, primarily for Aboriginal health professionals and general practitioners. Local Ageing Well Champions will spearhead a programme to raise community awareness.

Future initiatives

Technology may be a key solution to enhance service delivery in rural communities. Overall, uptake of technology as a solution to rural service delivery challenges in Australia has been slow, due to unavailability of internet access in some remote areas, low digital literacy levels, reluctance among health practitioners and the fragmented service landscape (Moffatt and Eley, 2011; Bradford et al, 2016). In addition, people living with dementia and their carers often state that they prefer face-to-face rather than online care. Despite these preferences, a recent study evaluating the effectiveness of telemedicine in dementia care compared with face-to-face care found that changes in annual Mini-Mental State Examination scores were similar over time (Kim et al, 2017). The Verily Connect project discussed previously provides an example of using technology to augment support for carers of people living with dementia.

Technology shows promise for providing easier access to specialised services, reducing the need to travel long distances (with concurrent benefits of saving time, energy, and money for the people who previously travelled), augmenting face-to-face services, and increasing access to services and supports that may otherwise be lacking in rural and remote areas. There is also potential for technology to improve support for culturally and linguistically diverse peoples living in rural areas: technology can shrink geographical distance and increase access to resources. Technology can bring diverse languages and cultures into a person's home and can enable people to reach out and connect with other language and cultural groups across the globe. However, there are ongoing challenges around supporting people to appropriately use technology, increasing peoples' confidence in using technology and designing technologies that are empathetic to peoples' needs and learning stages (Berkowsky et al, 2017; Vaportzis et al, 2017).

Conclusion

Despite being geographically large, Australia has a relatively small population and most of those people are located in major cities. Access to care in rural areas is limited by a host of challenges, including access to a skilled workforce and the very long distances involved for travel. The Australian healthcare system is regarded as among the most comprehensive in the world. However, given the magnitude of the number of Australians affected by dementia, and despite the apparent proliferation of different types of services, the bulk of support and care for people living with dementia in rural communities still tends to rest largely with informal carers, most often family members, neighbours and community members. Government policy therefore needs to recognise the essential role played by providers of informal support and care to people living with dementia. Key non-governmental organisations, including Dementia Australia and Carers Australia, are critical in providing information, guidance and support to people living with dementia and their caregivers. Technology can bridge the geographical barrier in the delivery of care and services for people living with dementia in rural Australia, but there is still much research needed to understand how this can work effectively. The lack of internet connectivity, infrastructure and digital literacy presents challenges in providing timely diagnosis, optimum management of dementia and support for those with dementia and their many community supporters. Ultimately, as with many issues in rural communities, the innovation and sustainability of rural dementia care in Australia relies on active participation of the whole rural community. Future initiatives need to further build on, and acknowledge, the role of community in designing approaches that combine the best of technology, local communities and more distantly based services working collaboratively together.

References

ABS (Australian Bureau of Statistics) (2016a) 'Australian Statistical Geography Standard (ASGS): Volume 5 – Remoteness structure, July 2016. Defining remoteness areas', [online]. Available from: www.abs.gov.au/ausstats/abs@.nsf/Latestproducts/1270.0.55.005Main%20Features15July%202016?opendocument&tabname=Summary&prodno=1270.0.55.005&issue=July%202016&num−&view [Accessed 19 December 2018].

ABS (2016b) 'Census quickstats: Warracknbeal', [online]. Available from: https://quickstats.censusdata.abs.gov.au/census_services/getproduct/census/2016/quickstat/SSC22684 [Accessed 24 October 2019].

ABS (2016c) 'Census quickstats: Hopetoun', [online]. Available from: https://quickstats.censusdata.abs.gov.au/census_services/getproduct/census/2016/quickstat/UCL221035?opendocument [Accessed 24 October 2019]

ABS (2016d) 'Census quickstats: Beulah', [online]. Available from: https://quickstats.censusdata.abs.gov.au/census_services/getproduct/census/2016/quickstat/SSC20230?opendocument [Accessed 24 October 2019].

AIHW (Australian Institute of Health and Welfare) (2012) *Dementia in Australia*, Canberra: AIHW.

AIHW (2015) *The health and welfare of Australia's Aboriginal and Torres Strait Islander peoples: 2015*, Canberra: AIHW.

AIHW (2016) *Australia's health 2016*, Canberra: AIHW.

AIHW (2017) 'Rural & remote Australians', [online]. Available from: www.aihw.gov.au/rural-health-rrma-classification [Accessed 19 December 2018].

AIHW (2018) 'Rural & remote Australians: overview', [online]. Available from: www.aihw.gov.au/reports-data/population-groups/rural-remote-australians/overview [Accessed 19 December 2018].

Alzheimer's Australia (2007) 'Support needs of people living with dementia in rural and remote Australia: report of findings', [online]. Available from: www.dementia.org.au/files/20070200_Nat_SUB_SuppNeedsPplLivDemRurRemAus.pdf [Accessed 24 October 2019].

Australian Government Department of Health (2018) Medical Benefits Scheme (MBS) [online]. Available from: www9.health.gov.au/mbs/fullDisplay.cfm?type=item&q=715&qt=ItemID

Bauer, M., Farmer, J., Fetherstonhaugh, D., Wilding, C. and Blackberry, I. (2019) 'Identifying support needs to improve rural dementia services for people with dementia and their carers: a consultation study in Victoria', *Australian Journal of Rural Health*, 27: 22–7.

Berkowsky, R.W., Sharit, J. and Czaja, S.J. (2017) 'Factors predicting decisions about technology adoption among older adults', *Innovation in Aging,* 1(3): igy002.

Bradford, N.K., Caffery, L.J. and Smith, A.C. (2016) 'Telehealth services in rural and remote Australia: a systematic review of models of care and factors influencing success and sustainability', *Rural Remote Health*, 16(4): 4268.

Brodaty, H., Draper, B.M. and Low, L.F. (2003) 'Behavioural and psychological symptoms of dementia: a seven-tiered model of service delivery', *Medical Journal Australia,* 178(5): 231–4.

Deloitte Access Economics (2015) *The economic value of informal care in Australia in 2015*, Canberra: Deloitte Access Economics.

Dementia Australia (2018a) *Dementia Prevalence Data 2018–2058*, Canberra: NATSEM, University of Canberra.

Dementia Australia (2018b) 'Dementia statistics: key facts and statistics', [online]. Available from: www.dementia.org.au/statistics [Accessed 19 December 2018].

Department of Health (2015) *National Framework for Action on Dementia 2015–2019*, Canberra: Department of Health, Australian Government. Available from: https://agedcare.health.gov.au/ageing-and-aged-care-older-people-their-families-and-carers-dementia/national-framework-for-action-on-dementia-2015-2019 [Accessed 19 August 2019].

Department of Health (2018) *'Australian Government programs to support people living with dementia, and their support networks'*, Canberra: Australian Government Department of Health, [online]. Available from: https://agedcare.health.gov.au/funding/dementia-and-aged-care-services-fund-dacs/dementia/australian-government-programs-to-support-people-living-with-dementia-and-their-support-networks [Accessed 19 December 2018].

Ervin, K., Pallant, J. and Reid, C. (2015) 'Caregiver distress in dementia in rural Victoria', *Australasian Journal on Ageing*, 34(4): 235–40.

Kim, H., Jhoo, J.H. and Jang, J.W. (2017) 'The effect of telemedicine on cognitive decline in patients with dementia', *Journal of Telemedicine & Telecare*, 23(1): 149–54.

KPMG (2011) Dementia services pathways: an essential guide to effective services planning. Available from: www.wimmerapcp.org.au/wp-gidbox/uploads/2014/04/KPMG-2011-Dementia-Services-Pathways.pdf

Moffatt, J.J. and Eley, D.S. (2011) 'Barriers to the up-take of telemedicine in Australia – a view from providers', *Rural Remote Health*, 11(2): 1581.

NATSEM (National Centre for Social and Economic Modelling) (2017) *Economic cost of dementia In Australia 2016–2056*, Canberra: NATSEM at the Institute for Governance and Policy Analysis, University of Canberra.

Ollerenshaw, A., Wong Shee, A. and Yates, M. (2017) 'Towards good dementia care: awareness and uptake of an online Dementia Pathways tool for rural and regional primary health practitioners', *Australian Journal of Rural Health*, 26: 112–18.

Orpin, P., Stirling, C., Hetherington, S. and Robinson, A. (2014) 'Rural dementia carers: formal and informal sources of support', *Ageing & Society*, 34(2): 185–208.

Pallant, J. and Reid, C. (2013) 'Measuring the positive and negative aspects of the caring role in community versus aged care setting', *Australasian Journal on Ageing*, 33(4): 244–9.

Papastavrou, E., Andreou, P., Middleton, N., Tsangari, H. and Papacostas, S. (2015) 'Dementia caregiver burden association with community participation aspect of social capital', *Journal of Advanced Nursing*, 71(12): 2898–910.

Rural Northwest Health (2013) 'Wattle's innovative program for people living with dementia – Australia', [online]. Available from: www.youtube.com/watch?v=1LCRrcxlrXE [Accessed 20 December 2018].

Saunders, P. (2013) 'Living with dementia in country South Australia', Paper presented at the 12th National Rural Health Conference, Adelaide, 7–10 April.

Savy, P., Warburton, J. and Hodgkin, S. (2017) 'Challenges to the provision of community aged care services across rural Australia: perceptions of service managers', *Rural & Remote Health*, *17*(2). Available from: https://pdfs.semanticscholar.org/2c7c/30393d09bfe3db3696a4aaa60b36b5d8e2a9.pdf

Schulz, R. and Martire, L. (2004) 'Family caregiving of persons with dementia: prevalence, health effects, and support strategies', *The American Journal of Geriatric Psychiatry*, 12(3): 240–9.

Vaportzis, E., Clausen, M.G. and Gow, A.J. (2017) 'Older adults perceptions of technology and barriers to interacting with tablet computers: a focus group study', *Frontiers in Psychology*, 8: 1687.

Wimmera Primary Care Partnership (2013) *Population health and wellbeing profile*, Horsham: Wimmera Primary Care Partnership. Available from: www.wimmerapcp.org.au/wp-gidbox/uploads/2014/02/Population-Health-Wellbeing-Profile.pdf [Accessed 24 October 2019].

4

Norwegian remote and rural dementia care

Oyvind Kirkevold and Kari Midtbo Kristiansen

Introduction

Norway is a sovereign state in north-west Europe with a population of 5.3 million. It is sparsely populated with a landmass of 323,803 km² stretching nearly 1,800 km from north to south. The majority of inhabitants live in the south-eastern part of the country. Just under two million live in the eight largest cities with more than 70,000 inhabitants each; 2.2 million people live in smaller towns and communities and more than one million Norwegians live in rural areas.

Norway has 422 municipalities; more than half have less than 5,000 inhabitants who live dispersed over a large area. In 2018, 158 of the municipalities had less than 3,000 inhabitants and 29 had less than 1,000 inhabitants.

An increase in the proportion of older people in the population is anticipated over the next 40 years. Statistics Norway has calculated that the proportion of people over the age of 70 will increase from the current 12 per cent to 21 per cent by 2060 (Leknes et al, 2018). The population over the age of 80 will triple in the same period. This pattern is even more dramatic in Norway's rural areas due to migration to urban areas, within the country. Younger people are moving to more central urban areas and older people remain in the rural municipalities. It is expected that in some remote municipalities more than one in three inhabitants will be over the age of 70 by 2040 (Leknes et al, 2018).

Figures from 2018 indicate that there are approximately 80,000 people with dementia in Norway; 1.5 per cent of the total population. By applying the prevalence rates calculated by Prince and colleagues (2013) to the Norwegian population, the number of people with dementia in Norway is projected to be 130,000 by 2050. The largest growth will be over the next decade, with an increase of about 30,000 to more than 110,000 by 2030. Accurate Norwegian population studies about dementia prevalence are lacking. The Norwegian Dementia Plan 2020 will provide more nuanced and detailed information regarding the prevalence of dementia in Norway. This is based on an ongoing study of a representative selection of 10,000 people over the age of 60.

Norway has a publicly funded health and social care system. Hospitals and specialist health services are run by national government-owned health trusts, while the municipalities have the responsibility to provide primary healthcare for the inhabitants. All inhabitants have a 'primary physician' (general practitioner [GP]) who is usually the entry point to the healthcare system. All Norwegian municipalities have the obligation to provide home care services and residential care for those who need it, including for older people.

The funding for the municipal services comes mainly from two sources: direct municipal tax and funding from the government. The amount of government funding depends on the size of the population, age structure, distances and other factors that may influence the cost of municipal services. This means that rural municipalities most often receive more funding per capita compared with metropolitan municipalities.

In Norway, the employer must pay employer's national insurance contributions, which are taxes for their employees as part of the financing of the national insurance scheme. The level of this tax depends on residence in one of five geographical zones, meaning that employers in rural municipalities pay lower tax than those in metropolitan areas. For 2019, this tax was 14 per cent (zone 1) for the largest metropolitan areas and 0 per cent for the municipalities in the far north (zone 5). To stimulate the recruitment of professionals in zone 5, those who work in the most rural municipalities receive a reduction in their student loans, with up to Kr25,000 (€2,500) for each year they stay working in rural municipalities. This is an important stimulation for activities in the most rural areas of Norway.

Services for people with dementia

The diagnosis and follow-up of people with dementia takes place in the municipalities. Most municipalities have a memory team or a dementia coordinator who can assist GPs in assessing dementia. General practitioners refer patients for additional services such as memory clinics, x-rays or neurology if needed. Especially challenging diagnoses, for example in younger people (less than 65 years) or other complicated cases, are referred to a memory clinic, a neurological clinic or a clinic for old-age psychiatry in the specialist healthcare system.

In-home care is provided by district nurses and home helpers employed directly by the municipalities, or by private companies contracted by the municipalities. A person with dementia requiring help for activities of daily living is offered nursing services (such as administration of medication, personal hygiene and support of family carers) and practical, home help services (such as housework, cleaning, food preparation and grocery shopping).

Recent public funding to municipalities has promoted the introduction of day-care services especially adapted for people with dementia. These services have two main aims. The first aim is to provide personalised activities and stimulation to participants, with meaningful activities to help slow down functional decline. Regular structured activities become a valued part of the weekly routine, providing structure for the rest of the week. The second aim of day care services is to give respite to the family carers. It is assumed that this can postpone nursing home placement, although there is no research evidence to confirm this.

As at 2018, over 70 per cent of Norwegian municipalities offer day care services specially adapted for people with dementia. However, services are not meeting demand as only one in six people with dementia living at home receives day care services, and this is generally limited to two or three days a week.

Most day care services are located in or near to a residential care home and are only open during office hours from Monday to Friday. There are some alternative day-care models, and the municipalities are encouraged to develop flexible day care services that can also offer flexible respite services. Day care services in the evenings and weekends are not common, but they are highly desired by carers and family members.

Residential care, mainly at nursing homes, is available for people severely affected by dementia. All Norwegian municipalities have nursing homes, and about 90 per cent of the municipalities have special care units for people with dementia, constituting about 25 per cent of the total number of beds in nursing homes. Another residential care service available for appropriate recipients in Norway is sheltered living collectives. These are small living units, with separate bedrooms and a common living room and kitchen, and with 24-hour staffing cover. Although nursing homes and sheltered collectives involve quite different services covered by different legislation, they are referred to by the umbrella term 'residential care' in this chapter.

Residential care is usually long term and for the remainder of the person's life. In addition, most municipalities have wards or reserved beds in residential care for short stays of up to 60 days for respite care or rehabilitation. This is often delivered as a two-week stay in residential care followed by a short-term period of in-home support. This is beneficial for both the carer and the person with dementia. It enables people to remain in their homes for longer periods of time and assists with transition if long-term care becomes necessary. It also relieves pressure on long-term care bed places.

Policy drivers

Over the past ten years, the main policy drivers for the diagnosis, treatment, follow-up and care of people with dementia, have been the two national dementia plans: Dementia Plan 2015 (Norwegian Ministry of Health and Care Services, 2011); and Dementia Plan 2020 (Norwegian Ministry of Health and Care Services, 2015). These plans informed the development of the *National professional guidelines on dementia*, launched in August 2017 (Directorate of Health, 2017). All three documents are important for the development of healthcare services for people with dementia in Norway.

Another significant policy driver is the different funding systems that are at play within the country. While each is intended to stimulate certain activities, they can inadvertently function as a barrier for some services. For example, municipalities can apply for funding for educational programmes for family members and carers, for day-care services and for building nursing homes. They also get funding and support for establishing 'ABC groups' (Dementia ABC being the national dementia educational programme for staff, discussed later in the chapter). However, as funding for programmes such as day-care services only covers 30 per cent of the real costs, there remains a wider challenge as to how to establish sufficient flexible day care services in line with community expectations.

Legislation

In planning and delivering health services, municipalities are bound by legislation regulating the healthcare system in Norway. Four laws, discussed in the following sections, are crucial for the treatment and care of people with dementia.

Patients' Rights Act

The Patients' Rights Act (1999) (PRA) stipulates the right to become a patient and receive necessary treatment, as well as several procedural rights. The PRA covers three main rights: health services access; participation and information; and consent to healthcare. The right to consent to care also covers situations where the patient lacks the capacity to consent to somatic health care, a matter significant to dementia care.

Health and Care Services Act

The Health and Care Services Act (2011) (HCSA) is a comprehensive Act that applies to health and care services provided within a municipality either by the municipality or a private enterprise contracted by the municipality to deliver services on its behalf.

Under the HCSA, municipalities are obliged to offer health promoting and preventive services, including:

- pregnancy and post-natal care services;
- assistance in the event of accident and other acute situations;
- assessment, diagnosis and treatment, including the regular GP scheme;
- social, psychosocial and therapies and rehabilitation;
- other health and care services, including health services at home such as personal assistance, practical assistance and a contact person for leisure activities;
- places in institutions, including nursing homes, and respite measures.

The HCSA includes requirements for professional conduct, patient safety and quality. It states that health and care services offered or provided by law must be sound and that the municipality shall organise services such that the individual patient or user is given a comprehensive and coordinated health and care service offer, and valuable useful services, and that the health and care services and personnel performing the services are able to comply with their statutory duties and have sufficient professional competence to provide services.

Special Health Services Act

The Special Health Services Act (1999) applies to specialist services provided by both public and private providers. The state has the overall responsibility to ensure that the population is provided with necessary specialist health services. Government-owned regional health trusts are responsible for specialist health services planning and provision. These health trusts run nearly all the hospitals in Norway. They are required to provide access to in-patient and out-patient specialist services for all permanent residents within the health region.

Health Care Personnel Act

The Health Personnel Act (1999) regulates the registration and conduct of health professionals. It covers matters such as authorisation, obligations, professional conduct, duty of confidentiality and the right of disclosure. This Act provides for independent scrutiny of the soundness and quality of health professionals' work, and also covers individual employment agreements.

National Dementia Plan 2015

The Norwegian government was a world leader with its 2007 commitment to developing a national dementia plan. The first plan, Dementia Plan 2015 (Norwegian Ministry of Health and Care Services, 2011) identified five care challenges: quality development, research and planning; capacity growth and raising skills and knowledge; improving collaboration among professions and medical follow-up; active care; and partnership with families and local communities. The Dementia Plan 2015 had three main foci, which were to develop day programmes (discussed later in this chapter); living facilities better adapted for people with dementia; and increased knowledge and skills.

More than 80 per cent of people living in nursing homes in Norway have dementia and require adequate and appropriate quality of residential care. From the perspective of the person with dementia, small residential groups and person-centred care that facilitates autonomy are the most important factors when it comes to quality of living conditions. Thus, this was one of the main features for educational programmes and funding in the Dementia Plan 2015.

Several programmes were launched following the Dementia Plan 2015, aimed at increasing the knowledge and skills of the workforce. There was a programme to develop person-centred care in residential care, and a significant expansion of the Dementia ABC educational programme for staff support and development.

The Dementia ABC programme is an interdisciplinary educational programme based on the values that all health and social care workers contributing to the life of the person with dementia are of equal importance regardless of their education or experience. The programme aims to increase workers' awareness of their own values and approaches to people with dementia. The programme has three main components: a series of study booklets presenting information about dementia; local (in the residential care facility or at the level of the in-home nursing district) discussion groups, with six to eight participants in each group (groups meet regularly to reflect on the topics presented in the booklets, relating content to their own care practice); and two annual workshops run by resource workers recruited from the network of regional centres for development and education in dementia care. The costs associated with the workshops are covered by the Dementia Plan 2015. The municipalities cover the costs of the learning materials. The work time used by staff to participate in the group meetings and costs for necessary substitute carers during group meetings are also covered by the municipality (Rokstad et al, 2017).

The Dementia ABC programme is well suited for use in rural areas. The model enhances cooperation between different units in the municipality and makes workers aware of local priorities and opportunities. When the local context is more transparent, as it often is in rural areas, the opportunities for workers to apply new knowledge directly in their own local practice are greater. The programme stimulates workers to undertake tasks such as investigating how their community has solved a certain care issue, or how they can use aspects of their local context in activities and services for people with dementia.

The Dementia ABC programme also provides a pathway for experienced care workers without any formal education to become a registered auxiliary nurse. In these cases, the candidate is evaluated according to prior education and experience to determine their 'learning gap' to meet registration requirements. By participating in the Dementia ABC programme, distance education, workplace supervision and a final exam, participants may qualify for registration. This is a significant feature of this programme for rural areas, where workers would otherwise face long travelling distances to access adult learning programmes.

At the municipal level, a local dementia sub-plan for the healthcare sector can be a useful means for putting future healthcare challenges, such as those relating to dementia, on the agenda of municipal planning. These plans require the support of local politicians who allocate resources for the full range of health services so they can both understand dementia as a priority and comprehend how plans for dementia services fit with other aspects of the health service. According to national surveys, those municipalities that include in their plans information on the needs of people with dementia can be seen to offer specific services targeted at people with dementia. This has been observed particularly in relation to small municipalities (Gjøra et al,

2015). Small municipalities need to deal specifically with dementia in their local plans and do so by placing it explicitly on the agenda so as to elicit commitment both from the top down and across all aspects of services where possible. Information about dementia is less observable in plans for larger municipalities, perhaps due to the large number of people affected, making it a much more obvious issue that does not need explanation or specific highlighting.

In a summary by Gjøra (2016), exploring the measures taken under Dementia Plan 2015, some of the results from implementing the five main strategies for meeting the future care challenges in dementia are described. These strategies are: quality development, research and planning; workforce capacity growth and raising skills and knowledge; improving collaboration among professions and medical follow-up; active care; and partnerships with families and local communities. For all strategies, there was significant activity at the national and local level during the time period covered by the plan. Models and learning materials were developed that have been implemented in rural municipalities.

Three surveys (including Eek and Kirkevold, 2011; Gjora et al, 2015) conducted about the services in the municipalities showed a marked increase in several of the services available for people with dementia and their families during the plan period. Research into dementia increased considerably during the plan period, and a process was begun to develop national guidelines on the assessment of dementia and follow-up of people with dementia and their families. This implies a substantial step towards more equal services across every municipality, regardless of its population size or rurality.

During the plan period, a total of 95 per cent of all the municipalities in Norway were involved in Dementia ABC education, with a total of 22,000 employees registered for training.

As Norwegian municipalities vary greatly in size and organisation, it is difficult to recommend a single model for the provision of dementia assessment. However, the establishment of a dementia team has proven to be an appropriate way to organise in order to ensure the assessment and follow-up of people with dementia. It is possible to establish dementia teams in small, medium-sized and large municipalities. They can also be organised in conjunction with municipalities (Gjøra, 2016).

National Dementia Plan 2020

The goal for the Dementia Plan 2020 is to build a dementia-friendly society, where people with dementia are cared for and integrated into the community (Norwegian Ministry of Health and Care Services, 2015). The plan has been developed in close cooperation with people with dementia and their families, together with voluntary workers, employees and researchers. The plan builds on the previous Dementia Plan 2015. The Dementia Plan 2020 identifies six main challenges:

- Insufficient attention is paid to the risk factors that may lead to dementia.
- There is a lack of knowledge and expertise on dementia in society at large, among personnel in the health and care services and among people with dementia themselves and their families.
- Diagnosis can occur too late to gain comprehensive support and amelioration strategies, and post-diagnostic support can be inadequate.
- There is little provision of adequate, meaningful activities for people with dementia, and of respite for carers.
- General health and care services are not sufficiently adaptive to people with dementia.
- People with dementia and their families need to be more closely involved in decisions that affect them.

From these six challenges, the Ministry of Health and Care Services has derived six strategies or principles for developing flexible, high-quality services tailored to the needs of people with dementia and their families: self-determination, involvement and participation; prevention – what's good for your heart is good for your brain; timely diagnosis and post-diagnostic follow-up; activity, coping and respite care; a patient care pathway with systematic follow-up; and tailored services.

The Dementia Plan 2020 retains several of the initiatives from the Dementia Plan 2015. This includes funding for day care services, funding for building nursing homes, and the Dementia ABC educational programme for staff and memory teams in the municipalities. New initiatives include educational sessions or 'schools' for people with dementia and their carers; post-diagnostic support programmes; adapted home-based services for people with dementia; and educational programmes for end-of-life care.

National guidelines for dementia diagnostics and care

In 2017 The Norwegian Directorate of Health launched the first national guidelines for dementia diagnostics and care (Directorate of

Health, 2017). They are consistent with health legislation outlined earlier and serve as a good-practice guide for the operationalisation of the legislation. The main purpose of the guidelines is to provide knowledge-based recommendations on the assessment, treatment and follow-up of people with dementia and their relatives. The guidelines establish a common professional national standard to enhance the quality of services for people with dementia and their relatives, regardless of where they live.

The guidelines are comprehensive, with different themes – 19 chapters and 58 recommendations. The policy is written and published in digital format in a separate application, which makes it easy to use and to update, and accessible for people in all locations across the country.

The guidelines state that when it is suspected that a person may have dementia, the basic diagnostic work is to be conducted by the patient's GP. The investigation and collection of relevant information is done in cooperation with healthcare staff in the municipality, mainly with the memory team. Models for the evaluation and diagnosis of people with dementia were developed and tested during the implementation of the Dementia Plan 2015. At the same time, about 80 per cent of municipalities established memory teams or a dementia coordinator role. As a part of this, a tool for use in dementia evaluation in the municipalities was developed (Engedal et al, 2011). This tool is now recommended by the Norwegian Directorate of Health.

Patients requiring complicated medical evaluations beyond the capacity and resources of the municipal health and care services are referred to the specialist health service. This can include specialist examinations with computed tomography (CT) x-ray, specialist neurologist examinations or the completed diagnostic work could be taken over by the specialist health service such as a memory clinic. Once specialist services are provided, patient care returns to the municipal health and care provider.

The main challenge for people with early stage dementia is receiving a dementia diagnosis rather than support and health services (Gjøra, 2016). This issue is being addressed in the Dementia Plan 2020 and as a result 15 municipalities are developing and testing different models for following up people with dementia at an early stage.

Services for rural people early in their dementia journey

Even though the intention is to offer the whole population services of comparable quality regardless of where they live, there are some challenges with living in rural areas regarding diagnosis and follow-up.

Small municipalities have relatively few new cases of dementia each year; that is, in a municipality with 3,000 inhabitants, there are an estimated five new cases per year. Such low numbers allocated to the three or four GPs in the municipality results in each individual GP having limited experience in the diagnosis of dementia. The majority of dementia cases involve people aged 80 years or older with uncomplicated symptoms. Presentations from younger people and people with unusual disease profiles are rare. This can result in a lack of experience and knowledge among rural GPs in dealing with the ways that dementia can present. A study among people over the age of 70 who received municipal health and/or social services in 2015 showed that only one of five with dementia was actually diagnosed as having dementia (Wergeland et al, 2015). If there are few diagnosed clients, the memory team and/or dementia coordinator will also have little experience in collecting information to support GPs.

GP recruitment is a particular challenge in some areas of the country, especially in remote municipalities. To cover for GP shortages, municipalities hire substitute or locum GPs from agencies for periods of up to three months. The substitutes are often not Norwegian, but Swedish or Danish. This is problematic for people with dementia when the GP does not know the patient and must rely on information from others, with patients or their next of kin often required to tell the same story several times to different GPs. Communication problems also arise from the challenge of conversing in different Scandinavian languages and with different dialects.

Information from other parts of the healthcare system indicates an underuse of some examinations or treatments for people living long distances from these services compared with those who live closer (for example, underuse of radiation therapy in cancer). While there is a lack of evidence about whether this applies for dementia, it is reasonable to believe that when deciding whether or not to refer a person to – for example – a CT examination, the burden of long-distance travel and the need to stay multiple days or nights in the treatment location, is taken into consideration by health practitioners and might make them more reluctant to advise such activities.

As mentioned earlier, when a person with dementia needs help to perform different daily tasks, they are offered help either from nursing services or social services (home help). The amount of help offered will vary depending on the need of the person with dementia. It can be anything from a weekly visit to deliver a medication pack, to visits several times a day to help with personal hygiene, meals or orientation, or to 'keep an eye' on a person's overall wellbeing. One challenge in all municipalities (not simply in rural areas) is that this often involves a lot of different people who come into the home of the person with dementia. Some municipalities have tried to reduce the number of people who contact the person with dementia by establishing 'dementia work groups'. These are formed by allocating a group of staff in the home nursing district to focus on dementia patients, leaving the patients that receive home nursing for other reasons to the rest of the staff. This leads to fewer people in contact with the individuals with dementia and thus more stability in the services they experience. The dementia work groups have also inspired groups in other fields, such as cancer/palliative care and diabetes. The organisation of these groups provides career opportunities for nurse specialisation and recruitment of staff with special interests.

One initiative of the Dementia Plan 2015 was to increase the number of people with dementia who are offered a day-activity programme. This is mainly day-care services adapted for people with dementia and including tailored, meaningful activities. Under the Dementia Plan 2015, separate funding for day-activity programmes was introduced to stimulate development of these services. The funding system continues under the Dementia Plan 2020.

As a result of this funding, a number of different models of day care have emerged. One model in rural areas is known as 'green care' and provides day care services located at a farm. By January 2017, a total of 34 farms throughout Norway were offering day care services to people with dementia (Ibsen et al, 2018). They are often tailored for people with young onset dementia, who are more physically fit than older people with dementia, and benefit from physical farming and outdoor activities. Some green day care services are also provided for the main cohort of dementia patients, who tend to be older and less physically capable. These people can take part in ordinary indoor farm activities modified to their abilities, such as making traditional foods or handcrafting. In relation to green care, there are health benefits from the natural outdoor setting and close contact with animals on the farm.

There are also rural examples of 'blue care', where some of the activities take place in a fishing boat. In one of the municipalities with Indigenous Sami people in the northern part of Norway, there is a day care service established around Sami culture and tradition. In other areas, day care services are located in the local museum or sometimes as an ambulant service based in the home of the person with dementia. The diversity of models for day care services provides opportunities for people with dementia to have different experiences that suit them. By responding to the environment and its impact on culture and daily life, the services become an important part of person–centred care for people with dementia. In rural areas, such services can also play a part in the local community, providing a meeting point for more than those with dementia, for example by hosting educational programmes for family members, carers and the wider community.

It is a challenge in rural areas to operate specialised work groups for in–home care, mainly due to long distances that carers are required to travel. Long distances for people travelling to day care centres, as well as low numbers of people with dementia, can make it difficult to maintain rural day care centres. While one might expect the green care model to be embraced in rural municipalities, it is a challenge to recruit new farms to this programme, and there are currently less than 40 such services.

Services for rural people with more advanced dementia

More than half of people who die in Norway do so in nursing homes; for older people, this proportion is even higher (Norwegian Institute of Public Health, 2018). This indicates that even though the mandatory system for in–home care and home help in all the municipalities is well established, when the need for help is extensive, most people find themselves in a residential care facility. The four main predictors for placement in residential care are old age, dementia, challenging behaviour and extensive need for help in activities for daily living (Wergeland et al, 2015). More than 80 per cent of residents in Norwegian nursing homes have dementia. As early as the 1990s, the Norwegian Directorate of Health recommended that municipalities build or rebuild nursing homes into small units especially adapted for people with dementia, known as Special Care Units (SCUs). The proportion of beds in nursing homes that are in SCUs increased from 13 per cent in 1996 to 24 per cent in 2011, and further increased to about 26 per cent in 2014 (Eek and Kirkevold, 2011; Gjøra et al, 2015).

As with diagnosis and in–home services, discussed previously, it can be challenging for the less populated municipalities to provide specialised services for different groups. A report from 2015 (Gjøra et al, 2015) shows that counties with the most dispersed populations have the lowest proportions of SCUs in their municipalities compared with the more central counties.

However, many of the smallest municipalities have small nursing homes in a multifunctional site collocated with the health centre, mother–child centre and rehabilitation services. These small nursing home facilities function in ways more similar to a SCU than to a larger nursing home facility.

Conclusion

With around one in five of Norwegians living in rural areas, policy to stimulate these areas is not dementia-specific, but applicable to all kinds of activities both public and private (as described in the introduction), and the main 'tool' for this is the system for funding and taxes.

As described previously in this chapter, while there are several challenges in taking care of people with dementia in the rural districts of Norway, there are benefits from living in small communities or sparsely populated areas. In these cases, benefits derive from local relationships, flexible service provision and local knowledge.

'Everybody knows everybody', and in rural districts, there is a stable workforce where care practitioners know the users of the services, their families, carers and communities. In addition, health and care practitioners know each other, and can capitalise on personal knowledge between employees in different services. The smaller scale of organisations and management structures makes it easier for staff to communicate when a change in the situation for a person with dementia perhaps demands new or different services. Smaller services can be more flexible, being tailored to a person's individual needs rather than being fixed to home care, day care or nursing homes.

The main challenges in rural settings are the stability of the GP workforce, the recruitment of skilled care staff and distances to specialist examinations. In some small municipalities, lack of training due to few cases also may influence the ability to give optimal services. An additional challenge for rural areas is that demographic changes are occurring at a more rapid and dramatic rate than in the metropolitan areas of Norway.

References

Directorate of Health (2017) *Nasjonal faglig retningslinje om demens* [National professional guidelines on dementia]. Oslo: Helsedirektoratet. Available from: https://helsedirektoratet.no/retningslinjer/nasjonal-faglig-retningslinje-om-demens

Eek, A. and Kirkevold, Ø. (2011) *Nasjonal kartlegging av tilbudet til personer med demens 2010–2011: Demensplan 2015* [National survey of services for people with dementia 2010–2011; Dementia Plan 2015], Tønsberg: Aldring og helse. Available from: https://omsorgsforskning.brage.unit.no/omsorgsforskning-xmlui/handle/11250/2394627

Engedal, K., Brækhus, A., Lillesveen, B., Breien, A.T., Gausdal, M., Gjøra, L., Haugen, P.K. and Strobel, C. (2011) *Utredningsverktøy til bruk for helsepersonell* [Assessment tool for health professionals]. Norwegian Health Directorate. Available from: https://aldring-og-helse-edia. s3.amazonaws.com/documents/Utredningsverkt%C3%B8y_ helsepers.pdf

Gjøra, L. (2016) *Aim wide and hit straight: A summary of the measures taken under Dementia Plan 2015*, Tønsberg: Norwegian National Advisory Unit on Ageing and Health. Available from: https://butikk. aldringoghelse.no/ViewFile.aspx?ItemID=8486

Gjøra, L., Eek, A. and Kirkevold, Ø. (2015) *Nasjonal kartlegging av tilbudet til personer med demens – 2014: Demensplan 2015* [National survey of services for people with dementia – 2014: Dementia plan 2015], Tønsberg: Aldring og helse. Available from: www. akademika.no/nasjonal-kartlegging-av-tilbudet-til-personer-med-demens-2014/gjora-linda/eek-arnfinn/kirkevold

Ibsen, T.L., Eriksen, S. and Patil, G.G. (2018) 'Farm-based day care in Norway: a complementary service for people with dementia', *Journal of Multidisciplinary Healthcare*, 11: 349–58.

Leknes, S., Løkken, S., Syse, A. and Tønnessen, M. (2018) *Befolkningsframskrivingene 2018: Modeller, forutsetninger og resultater* [Population projections 2018: models, assumptions and results], Oslo: Statistics Norway. Available from: www.ssb.no/befolkning/ artikler-og-publikasjoner/_attachment/354129?_ts=1643ab45088

Norwegian Institute of Public Health (2018) 'De fleste dør på sykehjem, få dør hjemme' [Most people die in nursing homes, few die at home], [online]. Available from: www.fhi.no/nyheter/2018/ de-fleste-dor-pa-sykehjem

Norwegian Ministry of Health and Care Services (2011) *Dementia Plan 2015: Subplan of care plan 2015*, Oslo: Norwegian Ministry of Health and Care Services.

Norwegian Ministry of Health and Care Services (2015) *Dementia Plan 2020: A more dementia-friendly society*, Oslo: Norwegian Ministry of Health and Care Services. Available from: www.regjeringen.no/ contentassets/3bbec72c19a04af88fa78ffb02a203da/dementia_-plan_ 2020_long.pdf

Prince, M., Bryce, R., Albanese, E., Wimo, A., Ribeiro, W. and Ferri, C.P. (2013) 'The global prevalence of dementia: a systematic review and metaanalysis', *Alzheimer's & Dementia*, 9(1): 63–75 e2.

Rokstad, A.M.M., Doble, B.S., Engedal, K., Kirkevold, O., Benth, J.S. and Selbaek, G. (2017) 'The impact of the Dementia ABC educational programme on competence in person-centred dementia care and job satisfaction of care staff', *International Journal of Older People Nursing*, 12(2).

Wergeland, J.N., Selbaek, G., Bergh, S., Soederhamn, U. and Kirkevold, O. (2015) 'Predictors for nursing home admission and death among community-dwelling people 70 years and older who receive domiciliary care', *Dementia and Geriatric Cognitive Disorders Extra*, 5(3): 320–9.

PART II

Research evidence

This section of the book focuses on research evidence from Canada, Austria and Ireland. However, the chapters in section 3 of this book are also informed by research evidence in relation to practice innovations. Research can throw light on areas that require policy support and practice developments to improve the lives of those with dementia. Research also often focuses on neglected areas of policy and practice concern, and rural dementia care has characteristically been a relatively neglected area for both rurality researchers and dementia researchers. As such this section provides a showcase for the models of care that have been developed in one area of Canada and one area of Austria that provide an evidence base to shape and inform practice developments and also to influence policy. The contribution from our Irish authors in this section demonstrates the need to collate evidence that illuminates policy and practice differences within a country and how this may lead to social exclusion and as such impacts on the lived experience of dementia. Research is a vital component of a change agenda, and the chapters in this section clearly demonstrate this.

5

Rural dementia research in Canada

Debra Morgan, Julie Kosteniuk, Megan E. O'Connell,
Norma Stewart and Andrew Kirk

Introduction

Canada, like other countries around the world, has an ageing population and growing numbers of people with dementia. Although rural Canada makes up 95 per cent of the country's land mass (Moazzami, 2014), Canada is becoming increasingly urbanised as cities grow and the proportion of people living in rural areas has declined and aged (Statistics Canada, 2017a). These changes have socioeconomic impacts on rural communities, including ability to deliver health and social services for ageing rural populations. The challenges of ageing in rural communities, such as disparities in access to services (Keating et al, 2011) are compounded when living with dementia. This chapter reviews the Canadian dementia care context, issues and challenges in rural dementia care, and Canadian research addressing these issues. The chapter provides an overview of the Rural Dementia Action Research (RaDAR) programme based in Saskatchewan, Canada, which has focused on rural dementia care for over 20 years.

Dementia in Canada

The number of people over age 65 in Canada is projected to increase from 17 per cent in 2017 to 23 per cent by 2031 (Statistics Canada, 2017a). The number of people with dementia is also projected to increase, from 564,000 in 2016 to around one million by 2033 (ASC, 2016). A number of Canadian initiatives have been implemented to address growing dementia care needs. Most of the ten provinces in Canada have established dementia strategies, some as early as 2002, and a national dementia strategy was released in 2019 (Public Health Agency of Canada). A 2016 report by the Senate of Canada included 29 recommendations to inform development of the national strategy (Senate of Canada, 2016). The Alzheimer Society of Canada has published several studies of projected prevalence and monetary costs using different data sources and intervention scenarios (ASC, 2010, 2016). The Canadian Institutes of Health Research Dementia Research Strategy included C$32 million in federal funding over five years for Phase I of the Canadian Consortium on Neurodegeneration in Aging (CCNA) and C$46 million for Phase 2 (2019–24). This network of 20 research teams involves over 350 researchers conducting research in dementia prevention, treatment and quality of life (CCNA, 2019). The Canadian Chronic Disease Surveillance System was expanded to include dementia in 2011, creating national data on dementia incidence and prevalence to support planning and evaluation of policies and services (Public Health Agency of Canada, 2017; CIHI, 2018).

Rural dementia care in Canada

Dementia care is of particular interest in rural and remote Canada where ageing populations mean more people at risk for dementia, but where there is often less capacity to provide specialised dementia services. The proportion of Canadian seniors living in rural areas (those outside centres of 10,000 or more population) is higher than in urban settings (20 per cent rural versus 16 per cent urban) (Statistics Canada, 2017b). This trend of ageing rural communities is the result of in-migration of older residents to rural communities, out-migration of younger people, and immigration settlement in cities (Moazzami, 2014; Hanlon et al, 2016). The 2016 Senate report (Senate of Canada, 2016) on dementia identified limited access to health and social services for dementia in Indigenous and rural and remote communities and recommended that the future Canadian dementia strategy include the assessment and promotion of specific models of dementia care for rural and remote communities. Several provincial dementia strategies have also identified the unique challenges of meeting the needs of people with dementia in rural communities (Department of Health and Wellness, Nova Scotia, 2015; Government of Alberta, 2017). As described in Chapter 11, Canada's Indigenous population is young but ageing (Statistics Canada, 2017c), and age-related dementias are a growing concern (Jacklin et al, 2013).

Aging in rural Canada (Keating, 1991) was one of the first books to highlight issues in rural ageing in Canada. Since then, Canadian researchers have advanced the state of knowledge in this area (for example, Keefe, 2011; Skinner and Hanlon, 2016), and a 2011 review of rural ageing research in Canada provides an analysis of 20 years of research (Keating et al, 2011). Research in rural dementia care in

Canada has also developed, exploring issues such as barriers to accessing and implementing dementia best-practice information by rural home care providers (Forbes et al, 2015; Bayly et al, 2018); rural long-term care (Brassolotto et al, 2019); the role of social networks and informal social support in northern rural communities (Wiersma and Denton, 2016; Herron and Rosenberg, 2017); the dementia journey in northern communities from the perspective of people with dementia, caregivers, community members and healthcare providers (Di Gregorio et al, 2015); experiences of voluntary service organisations such as Alzheimer societies in providing service in rural communities (Herron et al, 2016); and rural family physicians' challenges in providing dementia care (Constantinescu et al, 2018). Research conducted by the RaDAR team has identified gaps in rural dementia care, including delays in diagnosis (Morgan et al, 2014c); barriers to use of formal services (Morgan et al, 2002); limited diagnostic and post-diagnostic services, and low public and healthcare provider knowledge of dementia (Morgan et al, 2012); low availability of dementia-specific services (Morgan et al, 2015); low levels of formal dementia training among home care staff (Kosteniuk et al, 2016a); and lack of access to services for caregivers of individuals with atypical and young onset dementias (O'Connell et al, 2014b).

RaDAR research programme

Since 1997, members of the interdisciplinary RaDAR team have collaborated with community partners in the western Canadian province of Saskatchewan to improve health service delivery for people with dementia and their caregivers in rural and remote settings. The province covers an area of 652,000 km^2, which, to provide perspective, is over five times the size of England. The population of Saskatchewan has been fairly stable at about one million people for almost 100 years. Compared with other parts of Canada, Saskatchewan has a higher proportion of people living in rural areas of less than 10,000 population (19 per cent versus 39 per cent) (Moazzami, 2014). Almost half the population lives in the two major cities. The rural population is older, with seniors aged 65 and over making up 18 per cent of the population compared with 14 per cent in urban centres (Statistics Canada, 2017b). The average population density is 1.8 people per km^2 but is much lower in the sparsely populated north (Statistics Canada, 2017d). The economy is driven by resource-based industries, including agriculture, mining, oil and gas, and forestry. Over time, the province has transitioned from 30 health regions, to 12 regional health authorities, to a single provincial health authority that is responsible for delivery of health services, with medically necessary health services covered by the public health care insurance plan.

When first established over two decades ago, the RaDAR team recognised the importance of using a community-based participatory research approach (Morgan et al, 2014a), beginning with meetings with all 30 health region boards in the province at that time and a priority-setting workshop to establish collaborative relationships and research priorities. RaDAR projects have continued to involve stakeholders in the research process. For example, to develop the Rural and Remote Memory Clinic, which we implemented and evaluated as a research demonstration project in 2004 and continue to operate, the team travelled over 7,000 km to consult with healthcare professionals. This engagement approach led to changes in the proposed clinic format and evaluation that resulted in improved fit with community needs, better buy-in, and improved feasibility and sustainability of the intervention (Morgan et al, 2009). In 2008, we established a 27-member Decision-Maker Advisory Council, which has evolved into the Knowledge Network in Rural and Remote Dementia, which engages over 100 people with dementia, families, healthcare providers and policy makers from across the province and beyond. Since 2008, the network has met annually at the RaDAR Rural Dementia Summit, to share emerging best practices in rural dementia care and inform new and ongoing RaDAR research projects. The summit, which engages stakeholders in the larger RaDAR programme, and the individual stakeholder engagement strategies linked with specific RaDAR projects, provide an integrated approach to research-informed practice and practice-informed research.

The format for the Rural Dementia Summit is an informal, interactive, evening research poster session, followed by a full-day knowledge exchange meeting. Sessions include a national or international keynote speaker, small-group work related to RaDAR research planning, educational sessions, community service provider presentations on local innovations in service delivery, and panel discussions. To improve accessibility to rural participants, we do not have a registration fee and travel costs are covered for some participants who would not otherwise be able to attend. Impacts of this embedded knowledge translation and exchange platform include sustaining RaDAR innovations, supporting local dementia initiatives, accelerating application of research to policy and practice, and advancing new research directions. The RaDAR website and newsletters also facilitate communication with network members. Over the evolution of our programme (Morgan et al, 2014a), we have seen the impact of our community-based approach on the quality, relevance and application of our research, and become even more committed to involving community partners in all phases of the research.

The RaDAR research programme has had continuous research funding from the Canadian Institutes of Health Research, the main federal health research funding organisation, and from the provincial health research funding body, for 20 years. Since 2014, the RaDAR team has been one of the 20 research teams making up the CCNA. As the only team focused specifically on rural dementia care issues, our involvement has helped to raise awareness of rural dementia care nationally, and facilitated collaborations with other teams investigating issues such as driving, technology and primary healthcare in dementia. RaDAR team members and trainees have published close to 90 peer-reviewed papers to date (see link to RaDAR website in reference list). In this chapter, we focus on two of the major research streams in the RaDAR programme: the clinical and health service delivery research linked to the Rural and Remote Memory Clinic, and development of primary healthcare models for dementia in rural settings.

Rural and Remote Memory Clinic

To mitigate the rural–urban disparity in access to specialist services in Saskatchewan, Morgan and colleagues (2009) implemented the one-stop diagnostic Rural and Remote Memory Clinic (RRMC) in 2004 as a demonstration project funded by the Canadian Institutes of Health Research. The RRMC changed from a research-based mandate, for example with random assignment to in-person versus telehealth follow-up assessments (Morgan et al, 2011) and follow-up assessments for all families, to a clinical mandate with research as a secondary aim in 2009. The RRMC is now a sustained provincial government-funded clinical resource. The RRMC model was devised to reduce travel burden for rural and remote residents of the province; consequently, the model includes a single full-day assessment with diagnosis provided by the end of day. Follow-up occurs as needed, and is provided by the neurologist using telehealth. At one year after initial assessment, all families return to the RRMC for a half-day assessment by neuropsychology and physical therapy; further assessment and feedback of the in-person assessments is provided by telehealth with the neurologist. In-person assessments after the one-year follow-up are provided only for a sub-set of patients: those whose diagnosis remains ambiguous; those who are diagnosed with mild cognitive impairment;

and those whose presentation of dementia is atypical. Most families agree to have their data entered into a de-identified database, which is the current research platform. Nevertheless, the change from a research to clinical mandate means that use of the database for longitudinal research is limited after the one-year follow-up, because not all patients are followed beyond one year.

Since its inception, the RRMC has been an interprofessional clinic with a neuropsychology team, a neurologist, a nurse, physical therapist, and a registered dietitian when available. To achieve the aim of providing a diagnosis to families by the end of the day, numerous changes were required to the typical practices of these healthcare professionals. Foremost, the clinic nurse sends each family requisitions for blood work to rule out potential medical causes of the cognitive impairment and an electrocardiogram to assess for potential contraindications for anticholinesterase medications. Ideally, these results are obtained before the one-day, in-person assessment, but in cases where appointments have arisen via cancellations these procedures are completed on the day of the in-person assessment. Consistent with best practice in the diagnosis of dementia, family members are encouraged to attend the assessment to provide collateral information. In the rare circumstances where patients attend alone, the team attempts to interview a collateral informant by telephone. When families attend the RRMC in person, they complete consent procedures, a medical history and a medication review with the clinic nurse. This information is provided to the interprofessional team, which subsequently joins the family for an interprofessional joint interview (neurology, neuropsychology and physical therapy). This has the advantage of being time-efficient, and also allows families to share their stories only once and allows all team members to hear the clinical history.

After the joint interview, the patient completes a neurological exam while the family stays with the rest of the team. The patient then attends a neuropsychological assessment, or 'battery', which lasts for approximately two hours and assesses the domains of premorbid cognitive status, suboptimal effort, language, visuospatial processing, attention, speed of mental processing, semantic memory, episodic memory, executive function, and social cognition. Neuropsychological batteries are adapted according to clinical needs, for example in cases of potential mild frontal dysfunction requiring a more in-depth assessment of prefrontal function, or for people for whom English is not a first language and for those with very few years of formal education. During at least two breaks in the neuropsychological battery, the testing materials are left outside the testing room for a psychometrist to score concurrent with testing. This procedure allows for the results from the two-hour neuropsychological battery to be rapidly available to the supervising neuropsychologist.

Concurrent with the neuropsychological battery, family members (many of whom are caregivers) complete standardised scales of informant reports relating to the patient's instrumental and basic activities of daily living, health status and health-related habits (such as alcohol use), neuropsychiatric symptoms and sleep patterns. Family members also report on their own perceived burden, psychological distress and quality of life. After completing the reports, family members are interviewed by the neuropsychology team. This process has the advantage of allowing the family members to freely discuss the patient without the patient present, but with knowledge of the limits of confidentiality. After a lunch break, the patients participate in a physical therapy assessment. Depending on the status of the patient, some of the physical therapy-related information is obtained from family members (for example, falls history). In addition, the patient completes a physical therapy examination and standardised scales relating to physical functioning (such as physical activity and exercise). When the physical therapy assessment is completed, patients receive a head scan. Families then have some unscheduled time, during which patients complete standardised scales of depressed mood.

Finally, the team meets and discusses the profession-specific findings (the neurologist interprets the head scan and blood work), and the neurologist and neuropsychologist come to a consensus diagnosis. The team members contribute to an interprofessional letter with recommendations, and the physical therapist might include an additional personalised letter. The neurologist and neuropsychologist meet with the family and communicate the diagnosis, recommendations, and plan for management and follow-up. The neurologist and neuropsychologist then write reports for the patient's primary care provider. This process occurs for two families on clinic day: the intake and feedback interviews are staggered, and while one family is performing the neuropsychology assessment, the other family is receiving the physical therapy assessment. The in-person, follow-up procedure is similar, but the neuropsychological battery lasts for only one hour, as does the physical therapy assessment. If the neurologist needs to repeat the neurological exam, families travel into Saskatoon; otherwise neurological follow-up occurs by telehealth. Use of telehealth was studied during the first four years after implementation of the RRMC. Morgan and colleagues (2011) found that satisfaction with telehealth and in-person follow-up appointments was similar, but telehealth was rated as significantly more convenient and reduced travel by 426 km per round trip on average. As a result, telehealth was adopted for all follow-up appointments in the first year after initial assessment.

Training and capacity building

The RRMC is also used for training and capacity building. Part of capacity building includes use of the data platform for research mentorship, with 28 trainee publications to date. In addition, the RRMC increases clinical capacity for the diagnosis and management of dementia. The RRMC includes an opportunity for clinical psychology graduate students to receive supervision over the course of eight to ten months. Students learn about dementia and related conditions, and how to administer the neuropsychological battery, perform an interprofessional interview and conduct the family interview. Medical students and residents in neurology and other specialties frequently attend for one-day or half-day observations. The RRMC specialists are also involved in capacity building for rural primary care providers, including by observation (rural primary healthcare providers and international visitors have visited). We have provided lectures to rural primary healthcare providers by telehealth, but are aware of the limitations of this method for capacity building for dementia in primary healthcare (Aminzadeh et al, 2012). We are in the process of implementing a method of remote capacity building that leverages case-based learning with an app-based, retrieval-practice method. We are also implementing methods of remote case-based support. We investigated use of a computerised neuropsychological battery, but discovered that this approach was not feasible.

We propose using the RRMC resources to remotely deliver a telephone-administered neuropsychological assessment to the patients of rural primary healthcare providers as part of our rural model of dementia care (Morgan et al, 2019). The RRMC neuropsychologist has been involved with the Canadian Longitudinal Study on Aging and was on the team that created normative data for the telephone battery given to over 21,000 Canadians aged 45 years and older. The neuropsychologist is developing an interpretive algorithm summarising cognitive impairment versus no impairment from this brief neuropsychological battery that can be provided to rural primary healthcare providers as additional evidence for use in the diagnostic assessment process.

RRMC patient and caregiver database

The longitudinal, interdisciplinary RRMC database is a rich resource for RaDAR investigators and trainees (39 publications to date), with baseline and follow-up data from 650 patient–caregiver dyads to date. These studies reflect the interaction between research and practice, with many of the studies initiated in response to issues or questions emerging from the clinic practice, and results informing practices in the RRMC. Although too numerous to detail here, they include studies on medication use (Saleh et al, 2013; Verity et al, 2016); trajectories of cognitive decline (Hager et al, 2016); trajectories of depressive symptoms (Kosteniuk et al, 2016b); predictors of functional impairment (Burton et al, 2018); characteristics of patients with subjective cognitive impairment (Verity et al, 2018); predictors of caregiver burden (Branger et al, 2017); caregiver coping (Branger et al, 2016); models of caregiver burden (Stewart et al, 2016); caregiver reactions to the memory clinic (Morgan et al, 2014c); issues related to neuropsychological assessment (O'Connell et al, 2014b; Burton et al, 2015; Enright et al, 2015; Jodouin et al, 2017; O'Connell et al, 2018); and other fundamental measurement issues (Morgan et al, 2014b; Branger et al, 2016). The RRMC patient and caregiver population has also been the recruiting base for additional studies, including for the creation of a novel telehealth support group co-developed with spouses of RRMC patients diagnosed with frontotemporal dementia (O'Connell et al, 2014a); for a telehealth physical activity trial (Dal Bello-Haas et al, 2014); for understanding physical activity and exercise in patients and caregivers (O'Connell et al, 2015); for understanding goals for cognitive rehabilitation (Burton et al, 2016); and for understanding the positive aspects of the caregiving experience (Branger et al, 2018).

Future research in RRMC

The RRMC has been a success (Morgan et al, 2009) and is a sustainable, province-wide clinical resource, but the benefits are predominantly for diagnosis. We are in the preliminary stages of implementing a suite of healthcare interventions, called the RRMCi (short for RRMC interventions). This involves a novel model of distributed healthcare, where a highly trained RRMC clinician delivers a suite of province-wide interventions via technology. Remote healthcare has the additional advantage of providing access to specialist interventions for those who reside in urban and in rural locations. There is generally a lack of highly trained clinicians, and where clinicians do exist they tend to be located in urban centres. This geographic maldistribution of highly trained clinicians is mitigated by use of technology for remote healthcare.

Our approach to these remote interventions is to focus on people with mild cognitive impairment or dementia and their caregivers. We have had experience of delivering telehealth-based interventions since 2009. The neuropsychologist began a monthly support group lasting for one-and-a-half hours and comprising RRMC spousal caregivers of people diagnosed with atypical and young onset dementias (O'Connell et al, 2014a). We found that emotional connection related to common experiences (that is, universality) was key to therapeutic benefits for spouses of people with young onset dementias. In 2013, the neuropsychologist began co-facilitating a similar group for spouses with frontotemporal dementia (FTD) with the Alzheimer Society of Saskatchewan, which was open to spouses from across the province. This collaboration continued until 2017 when the Alzheimer Society had sufficient capacity to continue this intervention model alone. There are currently multiple telehealth FTD support groups hosted by the Alzheimer Society for spouses from across the province, based on the model developed by RaDAR. The original group facilitated by the neuropsychologist persists, but they have requested we move from telehealth to an asynchronous model (via secure mobile app). We plan to co-develop this RuralCARE app intervention by modifying an existing mental wellness app developed in collaboration with local industry, which will then serve as the model for the Alzheimer Society of Saskatchewan support groups province-wide. This study is another example of the interaction between research and practice.

Two main additional telehealth intervention plans for the RRMCi are cognitive rehabilitation and treatment for insomnia targeted at people with dementia or mild cognitive impairment and their caregivers. Cognitive impairment, core to dementia and mild cognitive impairment, is the target of cognitive rehabilitation, and although cognition cannot be restored, cognitive rehabilitation can help people with mild cognitive impairment and dementia achieve personally meaningful goals (Bahar-Fuchs et al, 2013). Burton and O'Connell (2018) demonstrated with a randomised controlled trial that cognitive rehabilitation can be delivered by telehealth. The second main intervention project is cognitive behavioural therapy for insomnia (CBTi). There is robust evidence for remote delivery of talk-based psychological interventions (reviews by Bee et al, 2008; Backhaus et al, 2012) such as psychological interventions for insomnia

(Lichstein et al, 2013; Holmqvist et al, 2014). A quarter to one-half of adults with dementia experience sleep disruptions (Deschenes and McCurry, 2009; Shub et al, 2009; Rongve et al, 2010; Rose, 2010; Guarnieri et al, 2012), and sleep disruptions in people with dementia negatively affect caregivers (McCurry et al, 2009; Rongve et al, 2010; Rose, 2010; Terum et al, 2017). CBTi is a well-supported treatment of insomnia (Brasure et al, 2016), and is recommended as the first-line treatment rather than medications for insomnia (clinical practice guidelines by Qaseem et al, 2016). CBTi has been successfully used with people with cognitive impairment (Ouellet and Morin, 2007; Nguyen et al, 2017).

Rural primary healthcare research

The RaDAR team's research focus on rural primary healthcare evolved from our clinical work and research linked to the Rural and Remote Memory Clinic, where we observed the challenges of dementia diagnosis and management from the perspective of patients, families and healthcare providers.

Need for model of rural primary healthcare for dementia

Worldwide, studies have reported low diagnostic rates for dementia (Aminzadeh et al, 2012; WHO, 2012; Lang et al, 2017). Alzheimer's Disease International (ADI, 2016) has recommended that primary healthcare (PHC) professionals assume more responsibility for diagnosis and management, and that specialists shift their role from patient care to capacity building and support of PHC professionals. Although the view that PHC professionals should assume more responsibility is supported by Canadian consensus guidelines (Moore et al, 2014), many primary care physicians are not comfortable with dementia diagnosis and management, and cite barriers to this role that lead to delays in diagnosis and more referrals to specialists services (Massoud et al, 2010; Constantinescu et al, 2018). The referral of relatively uncomplicated patients to memory clinics creates long waiting lists and reduces access for complicated cases (Massoud et al, 2010).

There is a particular need for rural PHC professionals in Saskatchewan to take on responsibility for all but the most complex cases of dementia care that require specialist support. First, Saskatchewan has a lower specialist-to-population ratio for sub-specialists in dementia care (geriatricians, neurologists and psychiatrists) compared with Canada overall (0.1–7.4 versus 0.8–13.2 per 100,000 population) (CIHI,

2017; CMA, 2018). Second, only 0.7 per cent of all specialists in Saskatchewan practice in rural communities compared with 2.3 per cent in the rest of rural Canada (CIHI, 2017).

Our research indicates that there is room to increase the capacity of rural PHC professionals in Saskatchewan, which in turn may allow the RRMC to focus on patients with atypical or complex presentations. Since implementing the RRMC in 2004, 61 per cent of all RRMC diagnoses have been for either Alzheimer's disease dementia (38 per cent) or no cognitive impairment (23 per cent). Our research with caregivers indicates that it took approximately two years from the time signs and symptoms were first noticed to the time a diagnosis was received in the RRMC, including an 11-month wait for an RRMC appointment (Morgan et al, 2014c). Some caregivers characterised themselves as anxious, frustrated and distressed during this period, and patients experienced declining health.

Stakeholder planning session on priorities in rural dementia care

In 2011, RaDAR held a one-day planning session with researchers and stakeholders from across the province of Saskatchewan to identify important issues for people with dementia living in rural and remote areas (Morgan et al, 2012). In terms of service issues, planning session participants noted problems associated with the accessibility, availability and timeliness of diagnostic services, particularly in the early stages of the condition. Post-diagnostic services were also reported to be unavailable, inaccessible or inappropriate across the continuum of care. Day care and respite services to support ageing in place were observed to be lacking, as were local nursing and personal care homes that would allow individuals to remain in their community close to family and friends. Low levels of public awareness and healthcare professional knowledge were also recognised as shortcomings.

Recommendations for action included introducing dementia case managers and standards of dementia care into the provincial healthcare system; establishing guidelines for dementia prevention, early detection and diagnosis; providing training to improve the knowledge base of healthcare professionals; and supporting a provincial and national strategy for dementia. Participants were particularly interested in improving early symptom recognition and diagnosis as a way to mitigate the crises associated with later-stage help seeking. These findings influenced the direction of the RaDAR team's rural primary healthcare research programme, including a clinical intervention to improve healthcare professionals' knowledge and access to guidelines, and support early detection and diagnosis.

Provincial environmental scan

RaDAR conducted a provincial environmental scan in 2013 to learn more about the availability of dementia-related services and resources across Saskatchewan and how the available services aligned with six PHC principles (Morgan et al, 2015). Only one in three respondents agreed that the services and resources available in rural communities were adequate to allow individuals to remain at home for as long as possible. Themes identified in respondents' comments focused on limited dementia-related service options in rural communities resulting in waiting lists and referrals to urban-based services, limited staffing and funding creating reliance on informal support, inadequate services leading to community displacement, and service referrals occurring late in the disease stage and during times of crisis.

Partnership with Sun Country Health Region

Prior to 2017, Saskatchewan had 13 health regions that governed healthcare decision making and budgeting, which are now amalgamated into one health authority. In 2013, RaDAR and the former Sun Country Health Region in south-eastern Saskatchewan partnered on a five-year research intervention programme (2014–19) as part of the Canadian Consortium on Neurodegeneration in Aging. The region, which is located approximately 400 km from the University of Saskatchewan, is predominantly rural (68 per cent, population density 1.8 people per km^2), covering 33,239 km^2 with a population of 58,644 (Sun Country Regional Health Authority, 2014). Individuals aged 65 years and older account for 16 per cent of the regional population. The regional Dementia Steering Committee was created in 2013 to support the five-year research programme and to connect dementia-related services across healthcare sectors. The committee consists of health region managers (PHC, home care, long-term care, social work, chronic disease management and mental health), Alzheimer Society of Saskatchewan staff and the RaDAR team.

The committee's first initiative was an assessment of the dementia-specific work activities, competence and learning needs of home care staff in the region (Morgan et al, 2016). The assessment indicated that home care staff were least likely to discuss legal issues such as power of attorney with patients or families (35 per cent), evaluate cognitive status with a standardised test (28 per cent) and recognise differences between causes of dementia (18 per cent). Staff also reported the lowest perceived competence related to performing these three activities. All home care staff demonstrated the greatest interest in learning more about recognising differences between causes of dementia, detecting early symptoms, and talking to families about changes to expect during disease progression and strategies to manage behavioural symptoms (Morgan et al, 2016).

Development and implementation of a rural PHC model for dementia

The main goal of our research collaboration with the Sun Country Health Region was to create an effective and sustainable model of rural PHC for dementia diagnosis and management. In 2015, we conducted a regional needs assessment of strengths and challenges in dementia care (Morgan et al, 2019). PHC team members rated their teams highest on interprofessional team care, moderately on access to decision support tools, and lowest on access to specialist-to -provider support. Subsequently, we used a five-step approach informed by frameworks for adapting interventions to local settings (McKleroy et al, 2006; Lee et al, 2008; Cabassa et al, 2014; Jansen et al, 2014) to develop and operationalise a rural PHC model for dementia (Morgan et al, 2019). This project was undertaken in collaboration with a rural PHC team in one initial site and scaled up to two other rural PHC teams in the health region. The model integrates three components – interprofessional care, remote specialist-to-provider support and decision support tools – informed by seven principles of effective primary care for individuals with dementia associated with positive outcomes for healthcare providers, individuals with dementia and caregivers (Aminzadeh et al, 2012).

Step 1 of the five-step process involved building relationships with Sun Country Health Region directors and managers, as well as with members of PHC Team 1, whose practice served as the site for operationalising and pilot testing the model. Team 1 was newly established at the time of the study and consisted of three family physicians, a nurse practitioner, an occupational therapist, and two home care nurses. Located in a small community (1,000 population), Team 1 also served surrounding towns, villages and farms. As part of Step 2, a needs assessment of Team 1 found that patients were generally identified with dementia in the later disease stages, which led to crises and earlier long-term care placement. Late diagnosis was partly attributed to the team's low access to standardised tools and guidelines for dementia care and partly to patient resistance to help seeking due to stigma. Team 1 also had many strengths, including multiple professions working together, a shared electronic medical record (EMR), and a local Alzheimer Society First Link Coordinator who was keen to support Team 1.

In Step 3, RaDAR adapted the Primary Care Assessment and Treatment Algorithm (PC-DATA™) to become the main decision support element in the model. PC-DATA™ is a suite of decision support tools based on Canadian consensus guidelines that consists of point-of-care visit flow sheets, decision algorithms and education materials (Seitz, 2019). In Step 4, we collaborated with Team 1 over a three-year period (2015–18) to operationalise the seven principles of the model in its practice (Table 5.1).

To operationalise interprofessional care, we ensured that the EMR visit flow sheet reflected the involvement of all Team 1 members in the initial evaluation process, which had not been the case before the intervention. We integrated the Alzheimer Society First Link Coordinator within the team to provide education and support to patients and caregivers, and introduced case conferences between the team and patient/family. To facilitate remote specialist-to-provider support, the RaDAR specialists and the PC-DATA™ developer mentored team members and delivered education sessions on topics identified by Team 1. Some Team 1 members also travelled to the University of Saskatchewan for a one-day observation in the RRMC and have referred atypical and complex cases to the RRMC. To operationalise decision support tools, we collaborated with Team 1 to adapt the PC-DATA™ visit flow sheets for its interprofessional team by determining which team members would complete which sections and reorganising the flow sheets by team member. The adapted version was added to the team's EMR system, which is accessible by most team members. Team 1 also created a handbook of decision support tools, including scripts for discussing the diagnosis and driving with patients and families.

To alleviate delay between assessments by individual team members and the burden of repeated travel on patients and families, Team 1 transitioned the sequential rural PHC model for dementia to a one-day memory clinic model similar to the RRMC. On clinic day, the team first meets to discuss the patients to be seen that day, then the full team meets with the first patient and family before the patient is assessed by team members individually. Once testing is complete, the full team reviews the results together before a final case conference

Table 5.1: RaDAR primary healthcare model for dementia

Interprofessional care	Remote specialist-to-provider Support	Decision support tools
Multidisciplinary team • Family physician or nurse practitioner • Home care nurses • Occupational therapist • Others such as office staff, PHC facilitator	**Access to dementia specialists** • Referral – to Rural and Remote Memory Clinic • Consultation – with RaDAR specialists, PC-DATA™ developer • Team 1 nurse practitioner, occupational therapist, and home care nurse observed Rural and Remote Memory Clinic team functioning	**Standard tools and guidelines** • PC-DATA™ tools, including visit flow sheets, education manual, and care pathways/algorithms (the three visit flow sheets have been adapted and added to the regional EMR system as a single-visit flow sheet with a separate section for each provider) • Work standards to guide the use of the EMR visit flow sheet and dementia case conferences have been developed by Team 1 • Scripts for driving and communicating a diagnosis were developed by Team 1
Care management • Team coordination has been built into EMR visit flow sheet • Dementia case conferences implemented (between team and patient/family)	**Education sessions** • PC-DATA™ info session • PC-DATA™ education sessions • Differential diagnosis • Capacity and competency • Driving and dementia	**Access to IT resources** • All Team 1 members have access to work standards • All Team 1 members have access to EMR visit flow sheets
Education/support for patient and caregiver • Alzheimer Society First Link Coordinator is included in case conferences • A link to Alzheimer Society referral form added to EMR visit flow sheet		

Source: Morgan et al, 2019, Cambridge University Press 2019.

with the patient and family. A follow-up appointment with the patient is scheduled at this time.

As part of the final step, we scaled up and adapted the one-day rural PHC memory clinic model to two additional teams in the Sun Country Health Region while sustaining the model in Team 1. Team 2 serves a small city of 11,000 plus surrounding communities and Team 3 consists of healthcare providers who travel one to two days each week to three different communities located approximately 65 km apart. Whereas Teams 2 and 3 include family physicians, a nurse practitioner, an occupational therapist, a physical therapist and home care staff, only Team 2 also includes social workers. Additionally, the same occupational therapist and physical therapist serve both Teams 2 and 3. The EMR flow sheets developed by Team 1 were adapted to accommodate the different configurations of team members, to create a single standardised version across teams.

Process evaluation

We intend to further scale up the rural PHC memory clinic model to other PHC teams in Saskatchewan. A process evaluation analysed the strengths and challenges involved in the implementation of the model in Team 1. The five domains of the Consolidated Framework for Implementation Research provided the structure for analysis, namely innovation characteristics, outer setting, inner setting, individual characteristics and process (Damschroder et al, 2009). Using the domain themes as codes for the focus group and one-to-one interview data, all themes were considered as either implementation strengths or challenges. Factors that supported implementation included leadership engagement at all stages, presence of champions and opinion leaders, and presence of a shared EMR system accessible by most team members. Challenges included scheduling team meetings, changing established practice patterns, and turnover of team members.

Future RaDAR research directions

The RaDAR research programme demonstrates the inter-relationship of PHC and specialist services in the diagnosis and management of dementia. While the RRMC has proven to be a feasible and effective strategy for improving access to specialist diagnosis of complex, atypical dementias in rural settings, with current resources it is not able to meet the demand for service, so waiting times are long and diagnoses are not made in a timely way. Some referrals to RRMC are for more typical dementias that could be diagnosed in PHC if more supports were in place for PHC providers, and some referrals are for issues that may not require the full-day assessment (for example, help with treatment and management decisions). To address these issues, we plan to use telephone assessment of cognition and function to remotely triage patients to the current one-day interdisciplinary specialist RRMC, for diagnosis of possible cases of young onset or atypical dementia;

RRMC interventions (RRMCi) to deliver interventions directly (from specialists in RRMC) to patients and caregivers (for example, sleep, cognitive rehabilitation and driving cessation psychological support); and a collaborative care model where RRMC specialists remotely provide assessment results and support to primary care providers to facilitate diagnosis of typically presenting or moderately advanced dementia.

Second, we aim to continue our PHC model research to build capacity for dementia diagnosis and management in rural PHC, and focus on components of the model that are currently less well developed, particularly strategies for delivering education and case-based support to rural PHC providers via technology. To extend the team-based assessment to caregivers, we plan to develop an EMR-based flow sheet for PHC teams to monitor caregiver wellbeing. Related projects are underway to understand patient and family experiences of the rural PHC model (one-day clinic) and to explore the processes of interdisciplinary team-based care before and after the PHC model intervention. Our goal is to continue to spread the PHC model geographically, and focus on policy change to sustain the intervention in the healthcare system.

Alzheimer's Disease International (ADI, 2016) proposed that a global action plan should be aimed at supporting people with dementia to stay in the community for as long as possible (including the use of technology to extend services into rural areas) and strengthening PHC as a key part of the health system. The RaDAR programme focuses on identifying evidence-based based practices for delivering both comprehensive PHC and specialist dementia services that fit the needs and resources of rural people and communities, and are adaptable, scalable and sustainable across diverse, low-resource rural settings. This research will help to address gaps in dementia care best practices for PHC in rural settings, and address recommendations for improving rural dementia care in Canada and internationally.

References

ADI (Alzheimer's Disease International) (2016) *World Alzheimer Report 2016. Improving healthcare for people living with dementia: Coverage, quality and costs now and in the future*, London: ADI. Available from: www.alz.co.uk/research/world-report-2016 [Accessed 14 September 2018].

Aminzadeh, F., Molnar, F., Dalziel, W. and Ayotte, D. (2012) 'A review of barriers and enablers to diagnosis and management of persons with dementia in primary care', *Canadian Geriatrics Journal*, 15: 85–94.

ASC (Alzheimer Society of Canada) (2010) *Rising tide: The impact of dementia on Canadian society*, Toronto: ASC. Available from: https:// alzheimer.ca/sites/default/files/files/national/advocacy/asc_rising_ tide_full_report_e.pdf [Accessed 9 January 2020].

ASC (2016) *Prevalence and monetary costs of dementia in Canada*, Toronto: ASC. Available from: http://alzheimer.ca/sites/default/ files/files/national/statistics/prevalenceandcostsofdementia_en.pdf [Accessed 21 August 2018].

Backhaus, A., Agha, Z., Maglione, M.L., Repp, A., Ross, B., Zuest, D., Rice-Thorp, N.M., Lohr, J. and Thorp, S.R. (2012) 'Videoconferencing psychotherapy: a systematic review', *Psychological Services*, 9(2): 111–31.

Bahar-Fuchs, A., Clare, L. and Woods, B. (2013) 'Cognitive training and cognitive rehabilitation for persons with mild to moderate dementia of the Alzheimer's or vascular type: a review', *Alzheimer's Research & Therapy*, 5(4): 35.

Bayly, M., Forbes, D., Blake, C., Peacock, S. and Morgan, D. (2018) 'The development and implementation of dementia-related integrated knowledge translation strategies in rural home care', *Online Journal of Rural Nursing and Health Care*, 18(2): 29–64.

Bee, P.E., Bower, P., Lovell, K., Gilbody, S., Richards, D., Gask, L. and Roach, P. (2008) 'Psychotherapy mediated by remote communication technologies: a meta-analytic review', *BMC Psychiatry*, 8(1): 60.

Branger, C., Enright, J., O'Connell, M.E. and Morgan, D. (2017) 'Variance in caregiver burden predicted by patient behaviors versus neuropsychological profile', *Applied Neuropsychology: Adult*, 25(5): 441–7.

Branger, C., O'Connell, M.E. and Morgan, D. (2016) 'Factor analysis of the 12-item Zarit Burden Interview in caregivers of persons diagnosed with dementia', *Journal of Applied Gerontology*, 35(5): 489–507.

Branger, C., O'Connell, M.E. and Peacock, S. (2018) 'Protocol for meta-integration: positive aspects of caregiving in dementia', *BMJ Open*, 8(7): e021215.

Brassolotto, J., Haney, C., Hallstrom, L. and Scott, D. (2019) 'Continuing care in rural Alberta: a scoping review', *The Canadian Geographer*, 63(1): 159–70.

Brasure, M., Fuchs, E., MacDonald, R., Nelson, V.A., Koffel, E., Olson, C.M., Khawaja, I.S., Diem, S., Carlyle, M., Wilt, T.J., Ouellette, J., Butler, M. and Kane, R.L. (2016) 'Psychological and behavioral interventions for managing insomnia disorder: an evidence report for a clinical practice guideline by the American College of Physicians', *Annals of Internal Medicine*, 165(2): 113–24.

Burton, R. and O'Connell, M.E. (2018) 'Telehealth rehabilitation for cognitive impairment: randomized controlled feasibility trial', *Journal of Medical Internet Research Protocols*, 7(2): e43.

Burton, R., Enright, J., O'Connell, M.E., Lanting, S. and Morgan, D. (2015) 'RBANS embedded measures of suboptimal effort in dementia: effort scale has a lower failure rate than the effort index', *Archives of Clinical Neuropsychology*, 30(1): 1–6.

Burton, R., O'Connell, M.E. and Morgan, D. (2016) 'Exploring interest and goals for videoconferencing delivered cognitive rehabilitation with rural individuals with mild cognitive impairment or dementia', *NeuroRehabilitation*, 39(2): 329–42.

Burton, R., O'Connell, M.E. and Morgan, D. (2018) 'Cognitive and neuropsychiatric correlates of functional impairment across the continuum of no cognitive impairment to dementia', *Archives of Clinical Neuropsychology,* 33(7): 795–807.

Cabassa, L., Gomes, A., Meyreles, Q., Capitelli, L., Younge, R., Dragatsi, D., Alvarez, J., Manrique, Y. and Lewis-Fernández, R. (2014) 'Using the collaborative intervention planning framework to adapt a health-care manager intervention to a new population & provider group to improve the health of people with serious mental illness', *Implementation Science*, 9: 178. doi: 10.1186/s13012-014-0178-9.

CCNA (Canadian Consortium on Neurodegeneration in Aging) (2019) http://ccna-ccnv.ca [Accessed 18 August 2019].

CIHI (Canadian Institute for Health Information) (2017) 'Data tables: supply, distribution and migration of physicians in Canada, 2016', [online]. Available from: www.cihi.ca/en/data-tables-supply-distribution-and-migration-of-physicians-in-canada-2016 [Accessed 14 September 2018].

CIHI (2018) 'Dementia in Canada' [online]. Available from: www.cihi.ca/en/dementia-in-Canada?utm_medium=email&utm_source=crm&utm_campaign=dementia-2017&utm_term=26-06-2018&utm_content=en-public [Accessed 21 August 2018].

CMA (Canadian Medical Association) (2018) 'Canadian specialty profiles', [online]. Available from: www.cma.ca/canadian-specialty-profiles [Accessed 14 September 2018].

Constantinescu, A., Li, H., Yu, J., Hoggard, C. and Holroyd-Leduc, J. (2018) 'Exploring rural family physicians' challenges in providing dementia care: a qualitative study', *Canadian Journal of Aging*, 37(4): 390–9.

Dal Bello-Haas, V., Cammer, A., Morgan, D., Stewart, N. and Kosteniuk, J. (2014) 'Rural and remote dementia care challenges and needs: perspectives of formal and informal care providers residing in Saskatchewan', *Canada Rural and Remote Health*, 14: 2747.

Damschroder, L.J., Aron, D.C., Keith, R.E., Kirsh, S.R., Alexander, J.A. and Lowery, J.C. (2009) 'Fostering implementation of health services research findings into practice: a consolidated framework for advancing implementation science', *Implementation Science*, 4: 50.

Deschenes, C.L. and McCurry, S.M. (2009) 'Current treatments for sleep disturbances in individuals with dementia', *Current Psychiatry Report*, 11(1): 20–6.

Department of Health and Wellness, Nova Scotia (2015) *Towards understanding: A Dementia Strategy for Nova Scotia*. Halifax: Department of Health and Wellness, Nova Scotia. Available from: http://novascotia.ca/dhw/dementia/Dementia-Report-2015.pdf [Accessed 21 August 2018].

Di Gregorio, D., Ferguson, S. and Wiersma, E. (2015) 'From beginning to end: perspectives of the dementia journey in Northern Ontario', *Canadian Journal on Aging*, 34(1): 100–12.

Enright, J., O'Connell, M.E., MacKinnon, S. and Morgan, D. (2015) 'Predictors of completion of executive functioning tasks in a memory clinic dementia sample', *Applied Neuropsychology: Adult*, 22(6): 459–64.

Forbes, D., Strain, L., Blake, C., Peacock, S., Harrison, W., Woytkiw, T., Hawranik, P., Thiessen, E., Woolf, A., Morgan, D., Innes, A. and Gibson, M. (2015) 'Dementia care evidence: contextual factors that influence use in northern home care centres', *Online Journal of Rural Nursing and Health Care*, 15(1): 117–49.

Government of Alberta (2017) *Alberta Dementia Strategy and Action Plan*, Edmonton: Government of Alberta. Available from: www.alberta.ca/alberta-dementia-strategy-and-action-plan.aspx [Accessed 9 January 2020].

Guarnieri, B., Adorni, F., Musicco, M., Appollonio, I., Bonanni, E., Caffarra, P., Caltagirone, C., Cerroni, G., Concari, L., Cosentino, F.I.I., Ferrara, S., Fermi, S., Ferri, R., Gelosa, G., Lombardi, G., Mazzei, D., Mearelli, S., Morrone, E., Murri, L., Nobili, F.M., Passero, S., Perri, R., Rocchi, R., Sucapane, P., Tognoni, G., Zabberoni, S. and Sorbi, S. (2012) 'Prevalence of sleep disturbances in mild cognitive impairment and dementing disorders: a multicenter Italian clinical cross-sectional study on 431 patients', *Dementia and Geriatric Cognitive Disorders*, 33(1): 50–8.

Hager, D., Kirk, A., Morgan, D., Karunanayake, C. and O'Connell, M.E. (2016) 'Predictors of cognitive decline in a rural and remote Saskatchewan population with Alzheimer's disease', *American Journal of Alzheimer's Disease & Other Dementias*, 31(8): 643–9.

Hanlon, N., Skinner, M., Joseph, A., Ryser, L. and Halseth, G. (2016) 'New frontiers of rural ageing: resource hinterlands', in M. Skinner and N. Hanlon (eds) *Ageing resource communities: New frontiers of rural population change, community development and voluntarism*, New York, NY and London: Routledge, pp 11–23.

Herron, R.V. and Rosenberg, M.W. (2017) '"Not there yet": examining community support from the perspective of people with dementia and their partners in care', *Social Science & Medicine*, 173: 81–7.

Herron, R.V., Rosenberg, M.W. and Skinner, M.W. (2016) 'The dynamics of voluntarism in rural dementia care', *Health & Place*, 41: 34–41.

Holmqvist, M., Vincent, N. and Walsh, K. (2014) 'Web- vs telehealth-based delivery of cognitive behavioral therapy for insomnia: a randomized controlled trial', *Sleep Medicine*, 15(2): 187–95.

Jacklin, K., Walker, J. and Shawande, M. (2013) 'The emergence of dementia as a health concern among First Nations populations in Alberta, Canada', *Canadian Journal of Public Health*, 104(1): e39–e44.

Jansen, S., Haveman-Nies, A., Duijzer, G., Beek, J., Hiddink, G. and Feskens, E. (2014) 'Adapting the SLIM diabetes prevention intervention to a Dutch real-life setting: joint decision making by science and practice', *BMC Public Health*, 13: 457.

Jodouin, K., O'Connell, M.E. and Morgan, D. (2017) 'RBANS Memory Percentage Retention: no evidence of incremental validity beyond RBANS scores for diagnostic classification of mild cognitive impairment and dementia and for prediction of daily function', *Applied Neuropsychology: Adult*, 24(5): 420–8.

Keating, N. (1991) *Aging in rural Canada*, Toronto: Butterworths.

Keating, N., Swindle, J. and Fletcher, S. (2011) 'Aging in rural Canada: a retrospective and review', *Canadian Journal on Aging*, 30(3): 323–38.

Keefe, J. (2011) *Supporting caregivers and caregiving in an aging Canada*, Institute for Research in Public Policy Study No. 23, Montreal: IRPP. Available from: https://irpp.org/wp-content/uploads/assets/research/faces-of-aging/supporting-caregivers-and-caregiving-in-an-aging-canada/IRPP-Study-no23.pdf [Accessed 21 August 2018].

Kosteniuk, J., Morgan, D., O'Connell, M.E., Dal Bello-Haas, V. and Stewart, N. (2016a) 'Focus on dementia care: continuing education preferences, challenges, and catalysts among rural home care providers', *Educational Gerontology*, 42(9): 608–20.

Kosteniuk, J., Morgan, D., O'Connell, M.E., Kirk, A., Crossley, M., Stewart, N. and Karunanayake, C. (2016b) 'Trajectories of depressive symptomatology in rural memory clinic patients between baseline diagnosis and 1-year follow-up', *Dementia and Geriatric Cognitive Disorders Extra*, 6(2): 161–75.

Lang, L., Clifford, A., Wei, L., Zhang, D., Leung, D., Augustine, G., Danat, I., Zhou, W., Copeland, J., Anstey, K. and Chen, R. (2017) 'Prevalence and determinants of undetected dementia in the community: a systematic literature review and a meta-analysis', *BMJ Open*, 7:e011146.

Lee, S., Altschul, I. and Mowbray, C. (2008) 'Using planned adaptation to implement evidence-based programs with new populations', *American Journal of Community Psychology*, 41: 290–303.

Lichstein, K.L., Scogin, F., Thomas, S.J., DiNapoli, E.A., Dillon, H.R. and McFadden, A. (2013) 'Telehealth cognitive behavior therapy for co-occurring insomnia and depression symptoms in older adults', *Journal of Clinical Psychology*, 69(10): 1056–65.

Massoud, F., Lysy, P. and Bergman, H. (2010) 'Care of dementia in Canada: a collaborative care approach with a central role for the primary care physician', *Journal of Nutrition, Health & Aging*, 14(2): 105–6.

McCurry, S.M., Gibbons, L.E., Logsdon, R.G., Vitiello, M.V. and Teri, L. (2009) 'Insomnia in caregivers with dementia: who is at risk and what can be done about it?', *Sleep in Medical Clinics*, 4: 519–26.

McKleroy, V., Galbraith, J., Cummings, B., Jones, P., Harshbarger, C., Collins, C., Gelaude, D., Carey, J. and the ADAPT team (2006) 'Adapting evidence-based behavioural interventions for new settings and target populations', *AIDS Education and Prevention*, 18: 59–73.

Moore, A., Patterson, C., Lee, L., Vedel, I. and Bergman, H. (2014) 'Fourth Canadian Consensus Conference on the Diagnosis and Treatment of Dementia: recommendations for family physicians', *Canadian Family Physician*, 60: 433–8.

Morgan, D., Crossley, M., Kirk, A., D'Arcy, C., Stewart, N.J., Biem, J. and McBain, L. (2009) 'Improving access to dementia care: development and evaluation of a rural and remote memory clinic', *Aging and Mental Health*, 13(1): 17–30.

Morgan, D., Crossley, M., Kirk, A., McBain, L., Stewart, N., D'Arcy, C., Forbes, D., Harder, S., Dal Bello-Haas, V. and Basran, J., (2011) 'Evaluation of telehealth for pre-clinic assessment and follow-up in an interprofessional rural and remote memory clinic', *Journal of Applied Gerontology*, 30: 304–31.

Morgan, D., Crossley, M., Stewart, N., Kirk, A., Forbes, D., D'Arcy, C., Dal Bello-Haas, V., McBain, L., O'Connell, M.E., Bracken, J., Kosteniuk, J. and Cammer, A. (2014a) 'Evolution of a community-based participatory approach in a rural and remote dementia care research program', *Progress in Community Health Partnerships: Research, Education, and Action*, 8(3): 337–45.

Morgan, D., Kosteniuk, J., Crossley, M., Kirk, A., O'Connell, M.E., Stewart, N., Forbes, D., Dal Bello-Haas, V., Innes, A., Keady, J., Vaitheswaran, S. and Murdoch, A. (2012) *Planning for the rising tide: New models of rural primary healthcare for persons with dementia. Community-Based Primary Healthcare Team Grant Planning Session, October 17, 2011 Report*, Saskatoon: University of Saskatchewan.

Morgan, D., Kosteniuk, J., O'Connell, M.E., Dal Bello-Haas, V., Stewart, N. and Karunanayake, C. (2016) 'Dementia-related work activities of home care nurses and aides: frequency, perceived competence, and continuing education priorities', *Educational Gerontology*, 42(2): 120–35.

Morgan, D., Kosteniuk, J., Seitz, D., O'Connell, M.E., Kirk, A., Stewart, N., Holroyd-Leduc, J., Daku, J., Hack, T., Hoium, F., Kennett-Russill, D. and Sauter, K. (2019) 'A 5-step approach for developing and implementing a rural primary health care model for dementia: a community-academic partnership', *Primary Health Care Research and Development*, 20(e29): 1–11.

Morgan, D., Kosteniuk, J., Stewart, N., O'Connell, M.E., Karunanyake, C. and Beever, R. (2014b) 'The Telehealth Satisfaction Scale (TeSS): reliability, validity, and satisfaction with telehealth in a rural memory clinic population', *Journal of Telemedicine and e-Health*, 20(11): 997–1003.

Morgan, D., Kosteniuk, J., Stewart, N., O'Connell, M.E., Kirk, A., Crossley, M., Dal Bello-Haas, V., Forbes, D. and Innes, A. (2015) 'Availability and primary health care orientation of dementia-related services in rural Saskatchewan, Canada', *Home Health Care Services Quarterly*, 34(3–4): 137–58.

Morgan, D., Semchuk, K., Stewart, N. and D'Arcy, C. (2002) 'Rural families caring for a relative with dementia: barriers to use of formal services', *Social Science & Medicine*, 55(7): 1129–42.

Morgan, D., Walls-Ingram, S., Cammer, A., O'Connell, M.E., Crossley, M., Dal Bello-Haas, V., Forbes, D., Innes, A., Kirk, A. and Stewart, N. (2014c) 'Informal caregivers' hopes and expectations of a referral to a memory clinic', *Social Science and Medicine*, 102: 111–18.

Moazzami, B. (2014) *Strengthening rural Canada: Fewer & older: Population and demographic crossroads in rural Saskatchewan*, Strengthening Rural Canada, [online]. Available from: http://strengtheningruralcanada. ca/file/Strengthening-Rural-Canada-Fewer-and-Older-Population-and-Demographic-Crossroads-in-Saskatchewan.pdf [Accessed 21 August 2018].

Nguyen, S., McKenzie, D., McKay, A., Wong, D., Rajaratnam, S.M., Spitz, G., Williams, G., Mansfield, M. and Ponsford, J. (2017) 'Exploring predictors of treatment outcome in cognitive behavior therapy for sleep disturbance following acquired brain injury', *Disability and Rehabilitation*, 40(16): 1906–13.

O'Connell, M.E., Crossley, M., Cammer, A., Morgan, D., Allingham, W., Cheavin, B., Dalziel, D., Lemire, M., Mitchell, S. and Morgan, E. (2014a) 'Development and evaluation of a telehealth videoconferenced support group for rural spouses of persons diagnosed with atypical early-onset dementias', *Dementia*, 13(3): 382–95.

O'Connell, M.E., Dal Bello-Haas, V., Crossley, M. and Morgan, D. (2014b) 'Clinical correlates of awareness for balance, function, and memory: evidence for the modality specificity of awareness', *Journal of Aging Research*, doi: 10.1155/2014/674716.

O'Connell, M.E., Dal Bello-Haas, V., Crossley, M. and Morgan, D. (2015) 'Attitudes toward physical activity and exercise: comparison of memory clinic patients and their caregivers and prediction of activity levels', *Journal of Aging and Physical Activity*, 23(1): 112–19.

O'Connell, M.E., Gould, B., Ursenbach, J., Enright, J. and Morgan, D. (2018) 'Reliable change and minimum clinically important difference (MCID) of the Repeatable Battery for the Assessment of Neuropsychology Status (RBANS) in a heterogeneous dementia sample: support for reliable change methods but not the MCID', *Applied Neuropsychology: Adult*, 26(43): 1–7. doi: 10.1080/ 23279095.2017.1413575

Public Health Agency of Canada (2019) 'A dementia strategy for Canada'. Available from: https://www.canada.ca/en/public-health/ services/publications/diseases-conditions/dementia-strategy.html. [Accessed 9 January 2020].

Ouellet, M.C. and Morin, C.M. (2007) 'Efficacy of cognitive-behavioral therapy for insomnia associated with traumatic brain injury: a single-case experimental design', *Archives of Physical Medicine and Rehabilitation*, 88(12): 1581–92.

Qaseem, A., Kansagara, D., Forciea, M.A., Cooke, M. and Denberg, T.D. (2016) 'Management of chronic insomnia disorder in adults: a clinical practice guideline from the American College of Physicians', *Annals of Internal Medicine*, 165(2): 125–33.

RaDAR team website https://cchsa-ccssma.usask.ca/ruraldementiacare/ [Accessed 9 January 2020].

Rongve, A., Boeve, B.F. and Aarsland, D. (2010) 'Frequency and correlates of caregiver-reported sleep disturbances in a sample of persons with early dementia', *Journal of the American Geriatrics Society*, 58(3): 480–6.

Rose, K.M. (2010) 'Sleep disturbances in dementia: what they are and what to do', *Journal of Gerontological Nursing*, 36(5): 9–14.

Saleh, S., Kirk, A., Morgan, D. and Karunanayake, C. (2013) 'Less education predicts anticholinesterase discontinuation in dementia patients' *Canadian Journal of Neurological Science*, 40(5): 684–90.

Seitz, D. (2019) 'PC-DATA: Supporting people affected by Alzheimer's disease and related dementias'. Available at: www.pcdata.ca [Accessed 9 January 2020].

Senate of Canada (2016) 'Dementia in Canada: A national strategy for dementia friendly communities'. Available at: https://sencanada.ca/content/sen/committee/421/SOCI/Reports/SOCI_6thReport_DementiaInCanada-WEB_e.pdf. [Accessed 9 January 2020].

Shub, D., Darvishi, R. and Kunik, M.E., (2009) 'Non-pharmacologic treatment of insomnia in persons with dementia', *Geriatrics*, 64(2): 22–6. Available from: www.ncbi.nlm.nih.gov/pubmed/19256583 [Accessed 21 August 2018].

Skinner, M. and Hanlon, N. (2016) 'Introduction to ageing resource communities', in M. Skinner and N. Hanlon (eds) *Ageing resource communities: New frontiers of rural population change, community development and voluntarism*, London and New York, NY: Routledge, pp 106–18.

Statistics Canada (2017a) 'Age and sex, and type of dwelling data: key results from the 2016 Census', [online], Ottawa: Government of Canada. Available from: https://www150.statcan.gc.ca/n1/daily-quotidien/170503/dq170503a-eng.htm [Accessed 9 January 2020].

Statistics Canada (2017b) 'Age and sex highlight tables, 2016 Census. Population by broad age groups and sex, Canada, by Statistical Area Classification, 2016 Census – 100% data', [online], Ottawa: Government of Canada. Available from: www12. statcan.gc.ca/census-recensement/2016/dp-pd/hlt-fst/as/Table. cfm?Lang=E&T=21 [Accessed 21 August 2018].

Statistics Canada (2017c) 'Aboriginal peoples in Canada: key results from the 2016 Census', [online], Ottawa: Government of Canada. Available from: http://www150.statcan.gc.ca/n1/daily-quotidien/ 171025/dq171025a-eng.htm [Accessed 21 August 2018].

Statistics Canada (2017d) 'Focus on Geography Series, 2016 Census', [online], Ottawa: Government of Canada. Available from: www12. statcan.gc.ca/census-recensement/2016/as-sa/fogs-spg/Facts-pr-eng.cfm?Lang=Eng&GK=PR&GC=47&TOPIC=1 [Accessed 21 August 2018].

Stewart, N., Morgan, D., Karunanayake, C., Wickenhauser, J., Cammer, A., Minish, D., O'Connell, M.E. and Hayduk, L. (2016) 'Rural caregivers for a family member with dementia: models of burden and distress differ for women and men', *Journal of Applied Gerontology*, 35(2): 150–78.

Sun Country Regional Health Authority (2014) *Sun Country Health Region Annual Report 2013-14*, Weyburn: Saskatchewan. Available from: www.suncountry.sk.ca/gsCMSDisplayPluginNewsletter/show/ id/158/menu_id/31/year/2014/pN/annual-reports [Accessed 14 September 2018].

Terum, T.M., Anderson, J.R., Rongve, A., Aarsland, D., Svendsboe, E.J. and Testad, I. (2017) 'The relationship of specific items on the Neuropsychiatric Inventory to caregiver burden in dementia: a systematic review', *International Journal of Geriatric Psychiatry*, 32(7): 703–17.

Verity, R., Kirk, A., Morgan, D. and Karunanayake, C. (2016) 'Trends in medication use over eleven years in patients presenting to a rural and remote memory clinic', *Canadian Journal of Neurological Sciences*, 43(6): 815–18.

Verity, R., Kirk, A., O'Connell, M.E., Karunanayake, C. and Morgan, D. (2018) 'The Worried Well?: characteristics of cognitively normal patients presenting to a rural and remote memory clinic', *Canadian Journal of Neurological Sciences*, 45(2): 158–67.

WHO (World Health Organization) (2012) *Dementia: A public health priority*, Geneva: WHO. Available from: www.who.int/mental_health/publications/dementia_report_2012/en [Accessed 21 August 2018].

Wiersma, E. and Denton, X. (2016) 'From social network to safety net: dementia-friendly communities in rural northern Ontario', *Dementia*, 15(1): 51–68.

6

Timely diagnosis of dementia in rural areas in Austria: the Dementia Service Centre model

Stefanie Auer, Paulina Ratajczak, Edith Span and Margit Höfler

Introduction

Seventy-eight per cent of the 8.7 million Austrians live in rural areas with limited or reduced access to specialised medical and psychosocial support services as compared with urban areas. With respect to dementia, Alzheimer Europe has estimated that approximately 145,431 people were living with dementia in Austria in 2013 (Alzheimer Europe, 2013) and according to Alzheimer's Disease International (ADI, 2015) it is estimated that the number of affected people will double every 20 years worldwide. Care cost attributed to dementia in Austria is estimated to be about €5 billion per year and will rise to €9 billion per year by 2050 (Gleichweit and Rossa, 2009). The economic strain placed on the healthcare systems by these high numbers is in large part caused by the high institutionalisation rates associated with dementia (ADI, 2015). Studies suggest that early diagnosis (Koch and Iliffe, 2010) and psychosocial interventions (Olazaran et al, 2010; Logsdon et al, 2007) for people with dementia and their caregivers could not only help to improve the quality of life of people with dementia, but also delay institutionalisation (Mittelman et al, 1996). Therefore, early or timely diagnosis could reduce the financial burden on the healthcare system.

Approximately 20 to 30 per cent of affected people in Austria receive a medical diagnosis during their illness. The highest diagnosis rate was found in the main cities (Gleichweit and Rossa, 2009). This diagnosis rate is comparable to that of other European countries (Barth et al, 2018). Interestingly, the Organisation for Economic Co-operation and Development (OECD, 2018) points out that only 40 per cent of OECD countries can provide information on their detection rate and that under-detection of dementia is high globally (Lang et al, 2017).

Consequently, studies in different international environments have investigated hurdles to early detection of dementia. The overriding hurdle of low diagnosis rates in urban and rural environments is the general stigma of dementia within societies and stigmatisation by healthcare professionals (Vernooij-Dassen et al, 2005; Morgan et al, 2014). Rural areas in addition are even more difficult to serve. Here, problems are compounded by a shortage of professionals and the difficulty of reaching services due to transportation cost and distance (Szymczynska, et al, 2011). In rural areas of Austria, delays in diagnosis are often due to long waiting lists at specialist doctors' offices, limited access to diagnostic services in specialised clinics and a lack of pre-diagnostic counselling services. In rural areas of Austria in particular, the fear of being stigmatised as a family in the event of a dementia diagnosis is still an issue. The results from focus group discussions with caregivers and people with dementia as well as our clinical observations revealed that integrated, community-based services close to home are preferred over centralised and highly specialised services that might be beneficial for other medical conditions (Cowan et al, 2016). International literature supports this observation (Morgan et al, 2015). Traditional medical and social services in Austria are currently not prepared for the challenge of addressing the complex needs of families affected by dementia, especially in the early phases. In Austria, 'community care before nursing home care policy' is in place, but for families affected by dementia, few specialised services providing early detection, information and support are offered throughout the country. The Austrian Dementia Strategy issued by the Federal Ministry of Labour, Social Affairs and Consumer Protection (Bundesministerium für Arbeit, Soziales und Konsumentenschutz) and the Federal Ministry of Health (Bundesministerium für Gesundheit) in 2015, called for evidence-based care models to guide the political decision-making process and to verify the efficacy of different treatments and interventions for people with dementia. This chapter provides a description of the Dementia Service Centres (DSC) model, a service model specifically developed to provide early detection and training for people with dementia as well as support for family caregivers living in rural areas. Funded by several research grants, in which focus group interviews were organised for the assessment of needs of people with dementia and their caregivers, a longitudinal database was founded providing information on the assessed population. A randomised controlled trial at the beginning of the model development was also conducted. Based on these studies, the Dementia Service Centres model was developed into a practice concept. An anonymous satisfaction questionnaire for family caregivers provided important insights into the needs of family caregivers and pointed to the deficits of the service.

This chapter reports on the following points: the development of the Dementia Service Centres model; the ways in which a Dementia Service Centre works; whether the Dementia Service Centre is fit for early detection; current development and implementation status of the Dementia Service Centres; and the future outlook for Dementia Service Centres.

Development of the Dementia Service Centres model

The development of the Dementia Service Centres (DSC) model started in 2001 with a research grant exploring services for the rural population of Upper Austria, one of the nine regions in Austria. Austria has about 8.8 million inhabitants in an area of 83,879 km². Upper Austria in contrast has a population of about 1.5 million people in an area of 11,980 km² (Statistik Austria, 2017). Currently, six DSCs are operating in Upper Austria (see Figure 6.1). All centres are located in rural areas of the county with about 4,000 to 6,000 inhabitants, also serving the surrounding rural areas. In comparison, the capital city of Upper Austria, Linz, has about 203,000 inhabitants at present. In 2017, there were 177 medical doctors in Upper Austria, specialising in neurology and/or psychiatry (Statistik Austria, 2017). These doctors are mainly located in urban centres and rural communities have reduced access to their services.

To gain insight into the needs of people with dementia and their families, especially in the early phases, focus groups with affected people and with family members were organised. The main barriers identified to early medical diagnosis were lack of public awareness, shortage of medical specialists (neurology and psychiatry), specialists located too far away from the communities to be reached easily, and insufficient knowledge and awareness of dementia among general practitioners. Participants of the focus groups (people with dementia as well as support providers) were more specifically concerned and insecure about the best time for receiving a medical diagnosis. This insecurity mainly originated from the fear of 'being stigmatised' when diagnosed too early. Simultaneously experiencing (person with dementia) and observing symptoms (family) without being certain (no medical diagnosis) was described as creating a 'field of tension' within the family system that was difficult to handle. Support providers voiced the urgent need for information and early support. They asked for instructions on how to deal with difficult situations at home and how to cope with observing

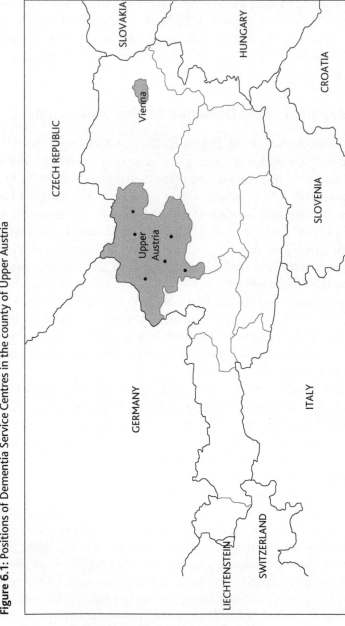

Figure 6.1: Positions of Dementia Service Centres in the county of Upper Austria

a loved-one's decline, and associated sorrow, without being able to do anything about it. Most caregivers clearly indicated that placement in a nursing home was only an option as a last resort. Their motivation for keeping the person at home was high and openly voiced. We concluded that the services developed for this population needed to be specifically tailored and that general social counselling was not sufficient. It also became clear in the focus groups that people with dementia and their support providers, especially as the dementia progresses, do not have the strength to coordinate support services from different organisations by themselves. Furthermore, it became clear that most of them were not even aware that these services existed. Some of the focus group participants voiced shame at accepting financial state help (in the form of 'care money'), which they felt was further stigmatising. We realised that the needs of different families were diverse, but that responding to these needs in a service was important to acceptance of the services being developed. From our observations in the focus groups, we also concluded that all services needed to be stage-specific since needs in the different stages of dementia are fundamentally different.

Goals and basic definitions

Based on our observations in the focus groups in the first project phase, we developed the service elements of the DSCs. In particular, we defined the function of a DSC as a multicomponent, low-threshold, 'one-stop shop', psychosocial support model, specifically addressing the needs of people with dementia and their family carers and support providers (Auer et al, 2015). The main goals of the DSC care model are timely detection of dementia; delaying the institutionalisation of people with dementia; and reducing the burden of support providers. Features identified to support these outcomes are depicted in Table 6.1. To reach these goals in rural areas is a particular challenge mainly because of long travelling time and the lack of medical and other specialised personnel. Whereas in urban areas many different services are readily available, in rural areas the diversity of social services that meet the needs of people with dementia is often absent.

Dementia specificity

People with dementia progress from a normal state of cognitive functioning to severe disability. To counsel and guide people with dementia and their support providers following diagnosis, profound knowledge with respect to the stages of dementia is paramount.

Table 6.1: Features of a Dementia Service Centre

Feature	Description
1. **Dementia specificity**	Services should be specifically designed to address the needs of persons with dementia and their support providers
2. **Pre-diagnosis counselling**	Developing a life perspective before the medical diagnosis, support during the diagnosis
3. **Long-term support**	Right service at the right time
4. **Easy, low-threshold access**	Low-threshold access without administrative hurdles, acceptable travel time
5. **Spirit of encouragement**	Developing a positive life concept despite dementia
6. **One-stop shop**	Centralised and bundled service and information
7. **Public relations**	Fighting stigma
8. **Research**	To improve the services

Understanding the individual needs of the person with dementia and the support provider and translating them into meaningful support services is the goal of the counselling process. Understanding and reacting to changes in needs is also part of the specific expertise of a DSC. The DSC was therefore developed as a highly specialised centre. This was especially difficult to negotiate with the different stakeholders in rural areas, since they were in favour of general social counselling centres. In rural areas, where different specialised medical and counselling expertise is not readily available, this dementia specificity seems especially important for success.

Pre-diagnostic counselling

A medical dementia diagnosis is still highly stigmatising for affected people and their families, especially in rural areas where community members know each other well and meet frequently. Preparatory counselling and awareness building within rural communities may therefore be even more important than in urban communities. Analysis of our database revealed that 58.4 per cent of assessed individuals did not have a medical diagnosis at baseline (see Table 6.4). We identified the importance of counselling activities for a timely diagnosis, and termed this activity 'pre-diagnostic counselling'. Without pre-diagnostic counselling, a diagnosis might be substantially delayed. We recently found that in rural nursing homes, a large proportion of tested residents had symptoms of dementia but no medical diagnosis of dementia (Auer et al, 2018). Without pre-diagnostic counselling, people with dementia may become hopeless and depression may occur as a reaction to the medical diagnosis of dementia. Preparatory counselling for people with significant memory problems and no medical dementia diagnosis currently takes a central role in the DSC model. People coming forward with their fears and complaints of memory loss are supported, the advantages of receiving a medical diagnosis are explained, and a positive life perspective after a diagnosis is developed. Training of cognitive functions is introduced and an active lifestyle reinforced. Diagnostic procedures are tailored to individual needs, and are discussed until a medical diagnosis can be accepted. The DSC model promotes a positive outlook on life despite a dementia diagnosis, and encourages discussion of life plans from the present onwards.

Long-term support

Dementia usually has a long duration and due to the progressive nature of the disease, needs are constantly changing. The relationship between the person with dementia and the support provider as well as the entire family is planned for the long term. Our research confirmed that families on average remain in the DSC for two years with a maximum stay of 11 years (Auer et al, 2015). Regular check-ups are therefore carried out so that the care can be adapted according to need. As to introducing the right services at the right time, a long-term, integrated support system has been conceptualised. The active role of the social worker in the DSC model seems to be particularly important for rural areas, since rural communities have limited access to counselling specialists.

Easy, low-threshold access

Many people living with symptoms of memory decline and their families often feel insecure about where to turn for help, especially in rural areas, where the only point of reference for medical problems is usually the family physician. If, however, the family physician does not specialise in dementia care, and does not refer the family to specialised services, the needs of the family are not appropriately met. Many questions arise about the consequences of a possible diagnosis, and the consequences of loss of dignity are feared. Some people do not think that their symptoms are serious enough yet to seek medical attention and are insecure about the timing of a diagnosis. In this situation, many months and sometimes years may pass and create difficult situations and conflicts within families and partnerships. Focus group participants had already voiced such problems in the developmental phase of the project as well as in the support groups. Here, the DSC takes a low-threshold approach, with the team being easily accessible, discreet and ready to act without bureaucracy. Also in times of crisis, those affected by dementia and/or their support providers appreciate being able to turn without delay to a person they already know and trust. The team is readily available for telephone and personal counselling without long waiting times. DSCs are, moreover, within easy reach and involve little travel time for community members.

Spirit of encouragement

Dementia progression varies according to the individual, but may last up to 15 years (Reisberg and Franssen, 2010). This is a substantial part of a human lifetime and as such should be used productively. The DSC model supports the development of a positive outlook on life despite dementia. Patients are offered an alternative to the nihilistic perspective of 'losing everything', and are encouraged to adopt a positive outlook on the future. The aim is to implement meaningful activities that can be performed without pressure in order to achieve personal growth and improved quality of life during this phase. People with dementia and their support providers are encouraged to find multiple ways in which to enrich their environment. Within this positive spirit, a medical diagnosis might be easier to accept since a life plan after diagnosis has already been conceptualised. Optimising health and fostering a healthy lifestyle are fundamental building blocks of this approach. Ideally, the well-informed person complaining of a memory problem should decide on the right time for seeking a diagnosis. It is the task of DSC staff to support the person in developing successful coping strategies for this challenging phase of their life. Encouraging people with dementia to work on their life situation also allows for reconciliation (for example, with family members). An early diagnosis might be relevant for an entire family, since common plans for the future can be made and a learning process initiated early.

One-stop shop

People with dementia and their support providers usually do not have the capacity to search for all the available services that are appropriate for their situation and that may be long distances apart, especially in rural areas. Different institutions provide different services and all of them should be available to all families if they are appropriate for a given situation. The DSC staff collaborate closely with different care professionals (general practitioners, hospitals, specialist doctors and care organisations) in order to help families access appropriate services and support, including financial support such as 'care money'.

Public relations

Extensive public relations efforts are made to increase awareness of dementia within all layers of society and all age groups locally (around the DSCs) and nationally (within Austria). The DSCs organise events that are open to the general public in order to promote social solidarity and social inclusion of people with dementia and their support providers. Newspaper articles, television programmes and books provide insights into the world of people with dementia, and encourage them to share their challenges and struggles in daily life. In one project, an e-learning tool was developed for police officers, who are often the first point of contact of a person with dementia in a crisis situation. The programme consists of three training modules and a certification process, whereby police officers learn about dementia and the principles of communication as well as problem-solving strategies in difficult situations. Around 7,000 officers have been trained nationally so far, and more than one hundred police stations around Austria have been certified as 'dementia-friendly'.

Research

In 2001, a database was established with the goal to providing evidence for the support model. Furthermore, research projects, including a randomised controlled trial, were conducted.

How does a Dementia Service Centre work?

Case example: Mr H

Mr H calls the social worker in the DSC. He reports that he has seen a flyer for the DSC in his doctor's office. His memory has declined in the past few months and he said that he is extremely worried about this. The social worker listens carefully and suggests a personal meeting. She explains that a psychologist will perform a 'memory check' and that Mr H may bring his wife to this meeting, which he declines at this moment. At the first meeting, the memory check reveals deficits described as 'mild cognitive impairment'. The meaning of this finding is explained, and a thorough medical examination is suggested. Mr H is also invited to regular meetings with a training group in order to prevent further decline. The social worker suggests inviting Mr H's wife to the next meeting. Mr H is relieved and agrees to discuss the issue with his wife. Some written information is provided to Mr H and he agrees to be further contacted by the DSC staff. Some days later, Mr H calls to arrange another meeting together with his wife and the social worker arranges an appointment at the nearby memory clinic. At the next meeting, there is a discussion about the results of the diagnosis of 'mild cognitive impairment' confirmed by a medical specialist. Meanwhile, Mr H is well established in his training group. Mrs H is invited to the training modules for family members. Mrs H is very worried about her husband and she schedules individual counselling sessions with the psychologist.

The support pathway of a Dementia Service Centre

Figure 6.2 depicts the main support elements of a DSC.

Figure 6.2: Overview of the support pathway in a Dementia Service Centre

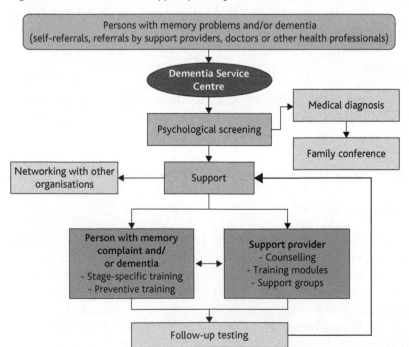

Sources of referral and recruitment

People who are concerned about their memory, or their support providers, can easily initiate contact with a DSC by telephoning (the usual approach, as in the case of Mr H) or walking into the centre. Patients can be also referred by a doctor in private practice or in a hospital, or by any other health professional (for example, from a care organisation). There is an extensive homepage, describing all the services and activities, and these services are also described in community newspapers on a regular basis. The first contact is crucial and the team needs to be reachable. If no one is available to take a call, individuals can leave a message and their call will be returned as soon as possible.

Psychological screening

A clinical psychologist performs a one-hour 'memory check' with the person complaining of memory problems. The history of memory problems is taken, and medications and illnesses are recorded. The psychologist performs memory tests, which are embedded in a clinical interview. The goal is to estimate the intensity of the memory problem and to measure the intensity on the Global Deterioration Scale (Reisberg et al, 1982). The clinical psychologist screens the medical records provided for any medical diagnosis of dementia. In cases where there is a significant memory problem evident from the psychological screening and no medical diagnosis, the affected person is prompted to accept a referral to a medical specialist. Written informed consent is signed by the person with memory problems and the support provider. Both agree that their data are stored and used anonymously for research purposes. For people participating in the stage-specific training, the assessment is repeated once a year. Those not participating in a stage-specific training are followed up with regular telephone interviews with the social worker, who performs an interview using the Functional Assessment Staging (Reisberg, 1988). If the person with memory complaints is accompanied by a support provider, this person is interviewed by the social worker. The person with the memory complaint needs to consent to this interview as well.

From the time of the initial research project in 2001 leading to the development of the DSC model, the same protocol – consisting of internationally well-known clinical instruments and different clinical and sociodemographic information on the person with memory complaints and their support provider – has been used. Some scales have been added later such as the assessment of life quality. For assessing cognition, the Mini Mental State Examination (MMSE) (Folstein et al, 1975) and the Brief Cognitive Rating Scale (Reisberg and Ferris, 1988) are used. To assess limitations in activities of daily living, the Functional Assessment Staging Test (FAST) (Reisberg, 1988) is utilised. Behavioural symptoms are assessed with the Behavioural Pathology in Alzheimer's Disease Frequency Weighted Severity Scale (BEHAVE-AD) (Reisberg et al, 1987) and the Empirical Behavioural Pathology in Alzheimer's Disease Rating Scale (E-BEHAVE-AD) (Auer et al, 1996). The stage of dementia is assessed with the Global Deterioration Scale (GDS) (Reisberg et al, 1982). The GDS distinguishes seven clinical distinct stages. Furthermore, three pre-stages (GDS stages 1–3) are defined, describing the development from a stage of no cognitive deficit (stage 1) to a subjective stage of cognitive deficit (stage 2) and finally to mild cognitive impairment (stage 3). From stage 4 onwards, a medical diagnosis of dementia can be given by a specialist medical doctor. Stages 5, 6 and 7 describe clinical conditions of moderate, severe and very severe dementia. Quality of life of people with dementia is assessed with the Quality of Life in Alzheimer's Disease (QOL-AD) scale (Logsdon et al, 1999) from the point of view of the person with dementia (QOL-AD participant version) as well as from that of the support provider (QOL-AD family version). To assess depression and the level of burden in support providers, the Zarit Burden Interview (Zarit Burden short version) (Bedard et al, 2001) and the Geriatric Depression Scale (Yesavage et al, 1982) are used.

Currently the data are stored in a secure, open-source technology database. The database structure has been continuously reworked in order to improve data entry, storage and retrieval. Social workers enter contact data and sociodemographic data, as well as information on psychosocial support measures and stage-specific training. Cognitive test data and medical data are entered by the psychologists. Most data are entered after the baseline and regular follow-up visits. Social workers also enter data between regular follow-up visits if any changes occur in the clients' or support providers' status. Data on psychosocial support, stage-specific training, and changes in contact data are entered and updated on a regular basis in order to guarantee timeliness.

Stage-specific retrogenetic training

This training methodology (Auer et al, 2009) was developed on the basis of the retrogenesis theory (Reisberg et al, 2002) using the

GDS staging as a framework. Developmental-stage, peer-training methodologies (as suggested in the theory of retrogenesis) (Reisberg et al, 2002) were adapted for each stage and tested for appropriateness. Stage-specific training is understood as a global stimulation training methodology consisting of cognitive and physical training elements. 'Global' means that not only memory functions are trained but also other cognitive and physical functions. People with dementia are encouraged to stay active for as long as possible. Training is based on the concept of 'stage specificity', since needs in the different stages are fundamentally different. The theory of retrogenesis perceives the person with dementia as an individual with competences despite diminished performance as judged from their highest achievement. The training tasks should be perceived by the person with dementia as meaningful and training time should be a joyful time. For later stages, important goals are the prevention of immobility and falls, and postponing frailty for as long as possible (Auer and Reisberg, 2006). The training is mainly organised as group training with additional opportunities for social interaction. In later stages or special hardship situations, single training (a trainer together with one person) is possible. People who present with subjectively perceived cognitive symptoms (GDS stage 2) are offered preventive group training.

Organisation and frequency of training groups

In very remote rural areas, the method of flexible group building is employed. Wherever there is a cluster of at least three to four people with dementia in an area, a local group opens, supervised by a trainer who lives in the area, using community rooms where available at no or low cost, thus saving on transport costs to supports further afield. Training groups meet once a week. Training duration is usually stage-specific, varying from one to three hours. For trainers, training material is available on the DSC website and accessible with a password.

Services for support providers

The DSC offers information, counselling and support groups for support providers. Specific training modules for support providers have been developed, based on the explanation of the disease symptoms following the GDS description. The GDS stages are translated into instructions for support providers, enabling them to improve their understanding of the situation of the person with dementia. Already during the pre-stages of dementia (subjective cognitive impairment [GDS 2] and mild cognitive impairment [GDS 3]), those affected by the condition are confronted with episodes of cognitive and functional loss. The person forgets names, misplaces objects and may develop problems at work. Reactions to these losses may include anxieties and depressive symptoms. Depressive symptoms substantially influence the person's relationship with a partner or other members of the family. In this phase, family members usually do not understand the origin of the symptoms and the support provider has not yet accepted their role as a caregiver. In stage 4, a medical dementia diagnosis is usually the main topic of discussion. Sometimes a diagnosis can come as a relief to the family. Professional guidance through this period is essential and can provide security and competence. For example, a person in this stage who has been responsible for financial affairs within the family will need assistance with this task. As dementia progresses, the person with dementia needs more intervention from the support provider. Without this help, survival is not possible (GDS stage 5). The protective function of the support provider in this stage needs to be clarified within the training groups and counselling sessions. At the same time, the person with dementia should be supported to live as autonomously as possible. This sometimes creates difficult situations and confusion. Anxieties and the feeling of helplessness on the part of the person experiencing the memory loss and their support provider are an important issue for discussion at this stage. Stage 6 involves the challenges of the caregiving function for the family. Without previous training in providing care, family members have to be able to support the person with dementia in dressing, bathing and toileting. For stages 6 and 7, support providers learn to change their communication style with the person with dementia. Understanding needs without explicit verbal communication is the challenge in this phase of the disease. Finally, physical care can be challenging for older support providers, and counsellors help with organising formal care within the home or if necessary in a nursing home.

Social events

The DSC provides regular social gatherings and events to which not only participants of the DSC but also other people from the community are invited. These events strengthen the community and foster friendship. Very importantly, these social events do not focus on dementia-related issues and connect affected people and their support providers to community life.

Table 6.2: Dementia Service Centre professionals and their responsibilities

Social worker	Clinical psychologist	Dementia trainer
Counselling (via telephone or face-to-face)	Psychological screening and referral for medical diagnosis, explaining medical reports to person with dementia and families	Creating an individualised training plan for a group/person
Coordination of appointments with families	Counselling (via telephone or face-to-face)	Organising/conducting group training or individual training (practical part)
Organising/developing educational modules for support providers	Supervising trainers (content and quality of the training)	First person to be approached by support provider in the training setting
Organising/conducting support groups for support providers	Conducting support providers' educational modules	Providing a training protocol for each training session
Organising/coordinating training groups for persons with dementia	Supervision of support groups	
Organising/coordinating available community services of other organisations		

Professionals working in a Dementia Service Centre

A DSC is run by a team consisting of a social worker (30 hours a week) and a psychologist (20 hours a week). These professionals coordinate and supervise a group of about ten dementia trainers per DSC. Dementia trainers are specialised in creating and delivering stage-specific training, and a specific certified curriculum (Schulz et al, 2012) has been developed. Across Austria, over 500 people have received the certificate thus far. Table 6.2 summarises the main tasks of all professionals employed in a DSC.

Is the Dementia Service Centre model fit for early detection?

As of 21 December 2017, the research database contained baseline data on 4,314 people in different stages of memory impairment and dementia, and their support providers (data were collected starting in 2001). Of these, 19 people were excluded because they did not sign the consent form, resulting in 4,295 records available for analysis. Of those who attended the DSC, 2,825 people (65.8 per cent) were female with a mean age of 79.3 years (SD=9.3), and 34.2 per cent were males (n=1,470) with a mean age of 77 years (SD=9.0). Overall ages ranged from 26 to 105 years. The median score of this population on the BEHAVE-AD (assessed in 76 per cent of the total population) was 13 points, and on the E-BEHAVE-AD (assessed in 99.9 per cent of the population) the median was one point, indicating that behavioural symptoms were not one of the main reasons for contacting a DSC.

Table 6.3 summarises the educational level of the population, their professions held before the illness or still being practised, and their living situation. About half of the analysed sample (52.1 per cent; n=2,090) completed nine years of Austrian compulsory education. Tertiary education was the least frequent level of education, attained by 248 people (6.2 per cent). The proportion of skilled workers was high (48.3 per cent) and interestingly nearly half of the people with unknown occupations did not complete compulsory schooling (n=311; 46.1 per cent). A substantial fraction (38.4 per cent) of the people approaching the DSC reported that they were living together with their partner or spouse and 22.1 per cent were living alone at baseline.

Information with respect to medical diagnosis was available for 4,178 of the 4,295 assessed individuals. On entering the services of the DSC, the majority of people (n=2,509; 58.4 per cent) had not received a medical dementia diagnosis. The most frequent dementia type diagnosed was Alzheimer's disease (n=737; 17.2 per cent), followed by the diagnosis of 'unspecified dementia', which was attested to 538 people (12.5 per cent). One-hundred-and-sixteen people (2.7 per cent) were diagnosed with mild cognitive impairment and three (0.1 per cent) with subjective cognitive impairment by a medical doctor (see also Table 6.4).

The GDS was scored in 4,081 (95 per cent) of people at baseline by the clinical psychologist. The results of the baseline assessment are presented in Figure 6.3. The cumulative number of people in stages 1 to 4 make up more than half of all assessed individuals (n=2,516; 61.7 per cent). Stage 4, the stage signifying the onset of a significant cognitive impairment, is the most frequent stage, with 1,263 people (30.9 per cent), followed by stage 5 with 1,071 people (26.2 per cent).

The MMSE was scored for 4,127 people (96.1 per cent of the population). The median score was 22 points.

In conclusion, 60 per cent of people entering the services of a DSC have no medical diagnosis of dementia. Only very few people

Table 6.3: Overview of the sociodemographic variables of the population at baseline

	n	%
Total population	4,295	100.0
Female	2,825	65.8[a]
Male	1,470	34.2[a]
Level of education	4,012	
Compulsory education (ISCED levels 1–2)*	2,090	52.1[b]
Secondary education (ISCED levels 3–4)	1,138	28.4[b]
No compulsory education	536	13.4[b]
Tertiary education (ISCED level 5–8)	248	6.2[b]
No information	283	6.6[a]
Occupations	3,621	
Skilled workers	1,768	48.8[c]
Unskilled labourers	594	16.4[c]
Homemakers	464	12.8[c]
Managers, technicians, professionals	459	12.7[c]
Other occupations	230	6.4[c]
Self-employed	106	2.9[c]
No information	674	15.7%[a]
Living situation	3,397	
With partner/spouse	1,305	38.4[d]
Living alone	749	22.0[d]
With children but in own household	424	12.5[d]
With children but in own household with partner/spouse	284	8.4[d]
In same household with children	265	7.8[d]
In same household with partner/spouse and children	145	4.3[d]
Assisted living	225	6.6[d]
No information	898	20.9[a]

Notes: [a] percentage of the total population; [b] percentage of participants for which the level of education is available; [c] percentage of participants for which information with respect to occupation is available; [d] percentage of participants for which living situation information is available.

* ISCED: International Standard Classification of Education 2011

accessing a centre have a medical diagnosis of dementia already in stage 4. Sixty-two per cent of people serviced in a DSC are in GDS stages 1 to 4. These stages correspond to no cognitive impairment (GDS stage 1), subjective cognitive impairment (GDS stage 2), mild

Table 6.4: Medical diagnoses on entering a Dementia Service Centre

Diagnostic category	n	%
Total population	4,295	100.0
No medical dementia diagnosis	2,509	58.4[a]
Dementia in Alzheimer's disease	737	17.2[a]
Unspecified dementia	538	12.5[a]
Dementia in other diseases classified elsewhere	125	2.9[a]
Vascular dementia	106	2.5[a]
Mild cognitive impairment	116	2.7[a]
Other dementia	44	1.0[a]
Subjective cognitive impairment	3	0.1[a]
No information	117	2.7[a]

Note: [a] percentage of the total population.

Figure 6.3: Distribution of Global Deterioration Scale for 4,081 persons at baseline

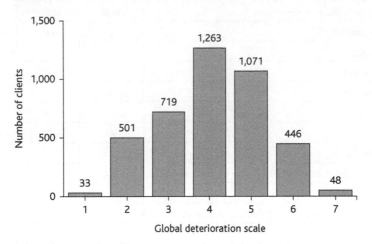

cognitive impairment (GDS stage 3) and mild dementia (GDS stage 4). These results suggest that more than half of the clients consult the DSCs for early detection of dementia, which is one of the main goals of the DSC model.

Longitudinal results of the 4,295 people analysed in our sample revealed that more than half of individuals (n=2,584; 60.2 per cent) participated at least once in a stage-specific training, 1,185 (27.6 per cent) were deceased and 825 (19.2 per cent) were institutionalised at the time of data extraction. The median time between the baseline screening and the institutionalisation date was 31 months. Institutionalisation rates after diagnosis without psychosocial support were lower than those reported in other studies. For example, Luppa and colleagues (2008) report an institutionalisation rate of 51 per cent after five years of follow-up. In their meta-review, a median time from study entry to institutionalisation of 30 to 40 months was estimated.

Additional evaluation studies during the developmental phase

To provide evidence for the stage-specific training and the services for the support provider, a three-and-a-half-year exploratory randomised controlled study was conducted. A total of 141 dyads of people with dementia and support providers visiting a DSC were recruited for the study. The 83 people with dementia who met the inclusion criteria were randomised to either treatment (stage-specific training and caregiver training) or the control condition (treatment as usual). The study showed a trend towards stabilisation of dementia progression for the treatment group on the GDS, MMSE and FAST measures (Auer et al, 2015). Other evaluation studies have focused on the acceptance of the DSC service and on carers' subjectively perceived burden (Mechtler, 2008). Among the support providers who participated in this evaluation, two thirds (66 per cent; n=144) reported a reduction of subjectively perceived burden. Furthermore, 85 per cent (n=157) of support providers were satisfied with the DSC service. On average (median), families used the service for 1.9 years (nine months to 3.6 years). These research results provided evidence for the effect of the stage-specific training that was suggested to people with dementia and their families and provided confidence for the DSC teams. The results of the research further influenced the decision of policy makers to promote the model for roll-out.

Current development and implementation status of the Dementia Service Centres

Since 2013, the DSC model has been piloted by the State Insurance Company and the county of Upper Austria. Interviews performed by project research staff reveal that support providers and support group leaders rate the service of the DSC positively and recommend the services to others. General practitioners report a reduction of work burden due to the existence of DSCs. Longitudinal data has demonstrated that people participating in stage-specific training remained longer in the early phases of the disease than those not participating in the training. The total duration of dementia was comparable, but the late stages were shortened in the training group. The training group also demonstrated fewer behavioural symptoms as measured by the BEHAVE-AD. Six DSCs were established during the model development, and an additional centre was opened during the Integrated Dementia Care project. Following the suggestion of the Austrian Dementia Strategy to organise easy-to-reach centres, other Austrian counties are currently adopting the DSC model. A manual has been developed for staff members and for other organisations setting up DSCs as well as a task list including legal guidelines for the different professional groups. The county of Upper Austria decided in September 2018 to roll out the DSC model and 11 centres will serve the communities starting in January 2020.

Challenges along the way

Organisational and financial issues are the biggest challenges for this rural care model. Since training should be stage-specific in order to meet the needs of people with dementia in a specific phase, training groups in rural areas are usually small (between two and ten people). Especially small groups (two to five people) are difficult to maintain and social workers and trainers need to be very flexible. Sometimes trainers have to travel long distances to reach the families and the group locations. Moreover, dementia trainers work under a 'freelance contract', which poses fiscal challenges.

Outlook on future developments

Currently, only 60 per cent of people attending a DSC accept stage-specific training. One of the future challenges will be to overcome even more hurdles in rural regions to optimise this percentage. To meet the needs of people affected early in their lives, special services for people with young onset dementia need to be developed. This is a special challenge for DSCs in rural areas since the number of affected people is small. Another issue faced is the development of services for people with dementia from different cultural backgrounds speaking different languages.

Organisations providing DSC services are set to work together within a common Upper Austrian Dementia Network. Common research projects, as well as international comparison studies, could be possible fields of research in the future. The DSC database is to be transferred to an openly accessible data repository, making further use of the data possible.

References

ADI (Alzheimer's Disease International) (2015) *World Alzheimer Report 2015. The global impact of dementia: An analysis of prevalence, incidence, cost and trends*, London: ADI. Available from: www.alz.co.uk/research/WorldAlzheimerReport2015.pdf [Accessed 26.09.2018].

Alzheimer Europe (2013) *Dementia in Europe Yearbook 2013*, Luxembourg City: Alzheimer Europe. Available from: www.alzheimer-europe.org/Publications/Dementia-in-Europe-Yearbooks [Accessed 26 September 2018].

Auer, S.R., Montciro, I.M. and Reisberg, B. (1996) 'The empirical behavioral pathology in Alzheimer's disease (E-BEHAVE-AD) Rating Scale', *International Psychogeriatrics*, 8: 247–66.

Auer, S.R. and Reisberg, B. (2006) 'Retrogenesis and communication with persons in the severe stages of dementia', *Les Cahiers de la Fondation Médéric Alzheimer*, 2: 126–35.

Auer, S.R., Gamsjäger, M., Donabauer, Y. and Span, E. (2009) 'Stadienspezifisches retrogenetisches Training für Personen mit Demenz: Wichtigkeit der psychologischen Merkmale der einzelnen Stadien' ['Stage-specific retrogenetic training for persons with dementia: importance of psychological features in the different disease stages'], in H. Schloffer, E. Prang and A. Frick (eds) *Gedächtnistraining: Theoretische und praktische Grundlagen*: Berlin and Heidelberg: Springer, pp 181–7.

Auer, S.R., Hofler, M., Linsmayer, E., Berankova, A., Prieschl, D., Ratajczak, P., Steffl, M. and Holmerova, I. (2018) 'Cross-sectional study of prevalence of dementia, behavioural symptoms, mobility, pain and other health parameters in nursing homes in Austria and the Czech Republic: results from the DEMDATA project', *BMC Geriatrics*, 18(1): 178.

Auer, S.R., Span, E. and Reisberg, B. (2015) 'Dementia service centres in Austria: a comprehensive support and early detection model for persons with dementia and their caregivers – theoretical foundations and model description', *Dementia*, 14(4): 513–27.

Barth, J., Nickel, F. and Kolominsky-Rabas, P.L. (2018) 'Diagnosis of cognitive decline and dementia in rural areas: a scoping review', *International Journal Geriatric Psychiatry*, 33(3): 459–74.

Bedard, M., Molloy, D.W., Squire, L., Dubois, S., Lever, J.A. and O'Donnell, M. (2001) 'The Zarit Burden Interview: a new short version and screening version', *Gerontologist*, 41(5): 652–7.

Cowan, R.A., O'Cearbhaill, R.E., Gardner, G.J., Levine, D.A., Roche, K.L., Sonoda, Y., Zivanovic, O., Tew, W.P., Sala, E., Lakhman, Y., Vargas Alvarez, H.A., Sarasohn, D.M., Mironov, S., Abu-Rustum, N.R. and Chi, D.S. (2016) 'Is it time to centralize ovarian cancer care in the United States?', *Annals of Surgical Oncology*, 23(3): 989–93.

Folstein, M.F., Folstein, S.E. and McHugh, P.R. (1975) '"Mini-mental state": a practical method for grading the cognitive state of patients for the clinician', *Journal of Psychiatric Research*, 12(3): 189–98.

Gleichweit, S. and Rossa, M. (2009) *Erster Österreichischer Demenzbericht Teil 1: Analyse zur Versorgungssituation durch das CC Integrierte Versorgung der österreichischen Sozialversicherung*, Vienna: Wiener Gebietskrankenkasse. Available from: www.cciv.at/cdscontent/loa d?contentid=10008.550842&version=1391172815 [Accessed 26 September 2018].

Koch, T. and Iliffe, S. (2010) 'Rapid appraisal of barriers to the diagnosis and management of patients with dementia in primary care: a systematic review', *BMC Family Practitioner*, 11: 52.

Lang, L., Clifford, A., Wei, L., Zhang, D., Leung, D., Augustine, G., Danat, I., Zhou, W., Copeland, J., Anstey, K. and Chen, R., (2017) 'Prevalence and determinants of undetected dementia in the community: a systematic literature review and a meta-analysis', *BMJ Open*, 7: e011146.

Logsdon, R.G., Gibbons, L.E., McCurry, S.M. and Teri, L. (1999) 'Quality of life in Alzheimer's disease: patient and caregiver reports', *Journal of Mental Health and Aging*, 5(1): 21–32.

Logsdon, R.G., McCurry, S.M. and Teri, L. (2007) 'Evidence-based interventions to improve quality of life for individuals with dementia', *Alzheimer's Care Today*, 8(4): 309–18.

Luppa, M., Luck, T., Brahler, E., Konig, H.H. and Riedel-Heller, S.G. (2008) 'Prediction of institutionalisation in dementia. A systematic review', *Dement Geriatr Cogn Disord*, 26(1): 65–78.

Mechtler, R. (2008) *Evaluierung der MAS Demenzservicestellen [Evaluation of the MAS Dementia Service Centres]*, Report of the IPG (Institut für Pflege- und Gesundheitsforschung), Linz: Johannes Kepler University.

Morgan, D., Kosteniuk, J., Stewart, N., O'Connell, M.E., Kirk, A., Crossley, M., Dal Bello-Haas, V., Forbes, D. and Innes, A. (2015) 'Availability and primary health care orientation of dementia-related services in rural Saskatchewan, Canada', *Home Health Care Services Quarterly*, 34(3–4): 137–58.

Morgan, D., Walls-Ingram, S., Cammer, A., O'Connell, M.E., Crossley, M., Dal Bello-Haas, V., Forbes, D., Innes, A., Kirk, A. and Stewart, N. (2014) "Informal caregivers' hopes and expectations of a referral to a memory clinic', *Social Science and Medicine*, 102: 111–18.

OECD (Organisation for Economic Co-operation and Development) (2018) *Care needed: Improving the lives of people with dementia*, Paris: OECD. Available from: www.oecd.org/health/care-needed-9789264085107-en.htm [Accessed 24.10.2018].

Olazaran, J., Reisberg, B., Clare, L., Cruz, I., Pena-Casanova, J., Del Ser, T., Woods, B., Beck, C., Auer, S., Lai, C., Spector, A., Fazio, S., Bond, J., Kivipelto, M., Brodaty, H., Rojo, J.M., Collins, H., Teri, L., Mittelman, M., Orrell, M., Feldman, H.H. and Muniz, R. (2010) 'Nonpharmacological therapies in Alzheimer's disease: a systematic review of efficacy', *Dementia and Geriatric Cognitive Disorders*, 30(2): 161–78.

Reisberg, B. (1988) 'Functional assessment staging (FAST)', *Psychopharmacolgy Bulletin*, 24(4): 653–9.

Reisberg, B. and Franssen, E. (2010) 'Alzheimer's disease', in H. Zaretsky, S.R. Flanagan and A. Moroz (eds) *Medical aspects of disability: A handbook for the rehabilitation professional* (4th edn), New York, NY: Springer, pp 25–64.

Reisberg, B., Borenstein, J., Salob, S.P., Ferris, S.H., Franssen, E. and Georgotas, A. (1987) 'Behavioral symptoms in Alzheimer's disease: phenomenology and treatment', *Journal of Clinical Psychiatry*, 48 Suppl: 9–15.

Reisberg, B. and Ferris, S.H. (1988) 'Brief Cognitive Rating Scale (BCRS)', *Psychopharmacol Bulletin*, 24: 629–36.

Reisberg, B., Ferris, S.H., de Leon, M.J. and Crook, T. (1982) 'The Global Deterioration Scale for assessment of primary degenerative dementia', *American Journal of Psychiatry*, 139(9): 1136–9.

Reisberg, B., Franssen, E.H., Souren, L.E., Auer, S.R., Akram, I. and Kenowsky, S. (2002) 'Evidence and mechanisms of retrogenesis in Alzheimer's and other dementias: management and treatment import', *American Journal of Alzheimer's Disease & Other Dementias*, 17(4): 202–12.

Schulz, H., Auer, S., Span, E., Adler, C., Donabauer, Y., Weber, S., Wimmer-Elias, J. and Meyer, M. (2012) 'A training program for dementia trainers: does this program have practical relevance?', *European Journal of Geriatrics*, 45(7): 637–41.

Statistik Austria (2017) 'Population since 2008 by provincial state', [online]. Available from: http://statistik.at/web_en/statistics/ PeopleSociety/population/population_censuses_register_based_ census_register_based_labour_market_statistics/totaL_population/ 078395.html [Accessed 24.10.2019].

Szymczynska, P., Innes, A., Mason, A. and Stark, C. (2011) 'A review of diagnostic process and postdiagnostic support for people with dementia in rural areas', *Journal of Primary Care & Community Health*, 2(4): 262–76.

Vernooij-Dassen, M.J., Moniz-Cook, E.D., Woods, R.T., De Lepeleire, J., Leuschner, A., Zanetti, O., de Rotrou, J., Kenny, G., Franco, M., Peters, V. and Iliffe, S. (2005) 'Factors affecting timely recognition and diagnosis of dementia across Europe: from awareness to stigma', *International Journal of Geriatric Psychiatry*, 20(4): 377–86.

Yesavage, J.A., Brink, T.L., Rose, T.L., Lum, O., Huang, V., Adey, M. and Leirer, V. O. (1982) 'Development and validation of a geriatric depression screening scale: a preliminary report', *Journal of Psychiatric Research*, 17(1): 37–49.

7

Key issues for people with dementia living in rural Ireland: social exclusion, models of care and policy change

Eamon O'Shea and Kieran Walsh

Introduction

The issue of rural ageing and dementia care has largely been neglected in Ireland. As populations age, the need to provide services to an increasing number of older people with dementia living in rural areas will become more acute, even if the share of older people living in rural areas is likely to decline in Ireland in the future. Concern for older people with dementia who continue to live in rural areas is based on a number of potential disadvantages arising from economic, social, geographical, environmental and demographic sources. There is a tendency for cumulative cycles of decline to occur in rural areas; poor employment opportunities tend to lead to out-migration which in turn leads to population decline, unbalanced age structures and falling economic activity, which reinforces unemployment issues and further out-migration (Milbourne and Doheny, 2012; Hanlon et al, 2015). This is quickly followed by a reduction in health and social care provision putting even more responsibility for care on people themselves and their shrinking networks and more dispersed families (Dwyer and Hardill, 2011; Skinner and Joseph, 2011; Warburton et al, 2014).

It is now routinely accepted in policy deliberations that social services in rural areas cannot always be provided to the same level as in urban areas for reasons of economies of scale. That leads to service objectives in rural communities (and sometimes even quality-of-life goals) being expressed in efficiency terms only, without reference to the distributional consequences of different policies in relation to infrastructure, connectivity and fairness. This is particularly true for older people with dementia. The potential for older people to experience multilevel and multifaceted forms of social exclusion across infrastructural, social and economic spheres (McDonald and Heath, 2008; Forbes et al, 2011; Peel and Harding, 2014) is very real – even before considering the ramifications of dementia symptoms, diagnosis and pathology. There are reasons, linked to relational, cultural and historical embeddedness of individuals, why older people want to remain in their rural communities, whether they have dementia or not (Herron and Rosenberg, 2017). Such reasons challenge us to think about orthodox service provision for people with dementia living in rural settings, in the context of the fullness of people's everyday experiences. How we think about people's lives at the intersection of dementia (Bond et al, 2004; Beard et al, 2009) and rurality (Herron et al, 2016), and how we should engage and recognise those lives (Grenier et al, 2017), is crucial to delivering more effective services and supports that can enable people to realise their full potential.

This chapter identifies some of the important distributional issues for older people with dementia living in rural areas in Ireland. It reframes these challenges in the context of social exclusion and its capacity to detract from full societal participation for people with dementia. Our purpose in this chapter is to harness the analytical frame of social exclusion, in contrast to the more policy-orientated construct of social inclusion, to help unpack complex and multiple challenges facing rural older people with dementia and illustrate the value in adopting a multifaceted approach to support full societal participation. The analysis draws on secondary data from a small number of recent studies carried out by the National University of Ireland Galway. The chapter opens with estimates of the prevalence of dementia in Ireland. This is followed by consideration of what is currently known about health and social care needs among people with dementia living in rural areas in Ireland. Social exclusion is explored using a framework developed by Walsh and colleagues (2019), with particular reference to people with dementia and the role of mediating factors in the exclusionary process. The subsequent analysis provides an argument for the recalibration of current dementia policy towards a broader social strategy for rural-dwelling people with dementia – one that focuses on supporting them to live well in rural communities through policies that act positively on mediating factors for social exclusion.

Dementia in Ireland

Ireland's population in 2016 stood at 4,757,976, of whom 637,567 people were aged 65 years and over (CSO, 2017). Estimating the number of people with dementia in the country is less straightforward, as the Census cannot directly provide us with such a figure. This is typically where epidemiological studies come into play. However, there are no Irish epidemiological studies to inform estimates of the prevalence of dementia in the country, a situation similar to many other European countries (Kiejna et al, 2010; Misiak et al, 2013). This is not surprising as epidemiological studies are costly, complex and time-consuming to undertake (Silman et al, 2018).

In the absence of Irish epidemiological studies, estimates of dementia prevalence for Ireland (O'Shea, 2007; Cahill et al, 2012; Pierce et al, 2013, 2019) use a methodology based on a meta-analysis of data (that is, combined data) from European epidemiological studies. Specifically, this involves the application of EuroCoDe dementia prevalence rates to Irish population data. The most recent estimates using this methodology suggests that there are 55,266 people with dementia in the country, two thirds of whom live at home in the community. While urban areas tend to have the highest absolute number of people with dementia, people with dementia as a proportion of the total population are much higher in the more rural western counties of Ireland, such as Mayo, Roscommon, Sligo, Leitrim, Donegal, Kerry and West Cork (Pierse et al, 2019). The majority of people with dementia have not been diagnosed, particularly those living at home, making it difficult to talk with certainty about their direct experiences, use of and barriers to formal service provision (Cahill et al, 2012; O'Shea et al, 2015). The distribution of memory clinics in Ireland is very urban-centred (O'Shea et al, 2017), making it more likely that diagnosis rates are higher in these locations compared with rural areas. People with dementia in rural communities face specific challenges in accessing services related to low population densities, diminished family support networks, distance and weak public transport (Innes et al, 2006; Dal Bello-Haas et al, 2014).

Social care for people with dementia: policy and practice

Social care provision for people with dementia living in rural areas in Ireland is a neglected area of research. Data on people with dementia living in rural areas are not routinely disaggregated in the official statistics covering community care provision for older people in Ireland. This is hardly surprising, given that most of those people have not been officially diagnosed with dementia and therefore have not come into contact with state services. All we know generally is that family carers are the main providers of home care, accounting for about 50 per cent of the overall cost of care (O'Shea et al, 2017). Formal home care is mainly funded by the state and is usually provided through direct Health Service Executive (HSE) service provision and by private or voluntary agencies paid for through state funding. An increasing, but so far undocumented, trend is for people to purchase home care directly out of pocket from private care agencies, sometimes in response to the cutbacks in public community-based care that have occurred in recent years. However, this is a trend that has been documented in other international contexts where, for one reason or another, there has been a narrowing of public responsibility for care (Dahlberg et al, 2018).

In common with other categories of dependent older people, the HSE provides a small number of formal supports for people with dementia focused mainly on public health nurse visits, home help services and, in more recent years, home care packages to support people living at home. While public health nurses are the cornerstone of community care provision for older people, the reality is that only a tiny proportion of people with dementia living at home actually receive any services from this source. People with a diagnosis of dementia must compete with many other categories of need emanating from a variety of patient groups, young and old, for the time and attention of the public health nurse (O'Shea et al, 2015; Donnelly et al, 2016).

The Home Support service now combines traditional home help provision and the home care package scheme, and provides support to older people to enable them to remain in their own homes for as long as possible. Home Support provides help to people with dementia with everyday tasks including getting in and out of bed, dressing and undressing, and personal care such as showering and shaving. The support provided depends on the individual needs of clients and care can be provided publicly or by external private providers, approved by the government. The most recent comprehensive data from the HSE (2017) shows that 17,094,000 million hours of Home Support are currently being provided to 50,500 older people, suggesting that the average weekly number of hours per client is 6.5 hours. There is no data on how many recipients of Home Support have a diagnosis of dementia. However, even when people with dementia receive Home Support, the amount of care provided is low relative to overall need (Donnelly et al, 2016).

Following the publication of Ireland's National Dementia Strategy (Department of Health, 2014), a small number of publicly funded intensive home care packages were made available to people with dementia to support additional personalised care services such as home care hours, physiotherapy and occupational therapy. These intensive packages are worth between €800 and €1,200 per week and were initially focused on people with dementia in eight acute hospitals to facilitate their return to their own homes following hospital treatment (Keogh et al, 2018). Since then the focus has been broadened to prevent admission of highly dependent people with dementia living at home to acute care and residential long-stay care. The latter initiative, while welcome, currently serves less than 300 people with dementia across the whole country and remains focused on urban settings, in keeping with its initial hospital focus (Keogh et al, 2018).

Other generic community-based services are also available to people with dementia, but an even smaller number of people with dementia are likely to be in a position to avail of these services, such is the general paucity of provision. For example, day care services and residential respite care are available in some areas, but dementia specific day care and respite care provision is very rare (O'Shea et al, 2015). Voluntary groups and other community organisations play a significant role in addressing other issues for people with dementia, such as poor nutrition and social isolation, through services such as Meals on Wheels and befriending groups. But provision is, once again, idiosyncratic and depends on local circumstances and organisation (O'Shea et al, 2017).

Economies of scale arguments, typically argued by statutory service and strategic planning agencies such as units within the HSE and Department of Health, are most frequently invoked to explain spatial differences in social services provision between rural and urban areas. Scale arguments are put forward as part of a wider efficiency rationale, which is commonly used to justify the rationalisation and curtailment of essential social services in rural areas. These arguments have generally not been contested in Ireland, because the debate has never moved beyond an economic efficiency narrative (O'Shea, 2009). The gap between need and provision for people with dementia is not unique to Ireland and there are many examples of underprovision and fragmented delivery systems in other countries, particularly in rural settings (Innes et al, 2006, 2011; Forbes et al, 2011; Herron et al, 2016). It is exacerbated in Ireland by the fact that people with dementia, as with the general older population, do not currently have any rights to home care supports, something that is due to change in the coming years as legislation is promised to give some level of statutory entitlement to home care services. Ageing and dementia have lagged behind the disability sector in relation to rights-based provision in Ireland. This is partly due to the dominance of the biomedical model within the health and social system of care, which is not well aligned with human rights thinking. It will take some time, therefore, even with new legislation, before people with dementia feel empowered to regain autonomy in their own space across different care settings (Cahill, 2018).

Rurality, ageing and social exclusion

There are more fundamental influences at play that incorporate and interact with health and social care provision for older people living in rural areas. They also implicate other areas of life that are intrinsic to experiences of living with dementia in rural environments. To unpack these elements, we now turn to a conceptual frame on age-related rural exclusion and the supporting international literature on rurality, ageing and social exclusion processes.

Figure 7.1 presents a conceptual framework on rural old-age social exclusion developed by Walsh and colleagues (2019), which is based on a qualitative study involving 106 older people across ten rural community sites in Ireland and Northern Ireland. The framework identifies a multilayered construction consisting of domains of social

Figure 7.1: Conceptual framework on old-age rural social exclusion

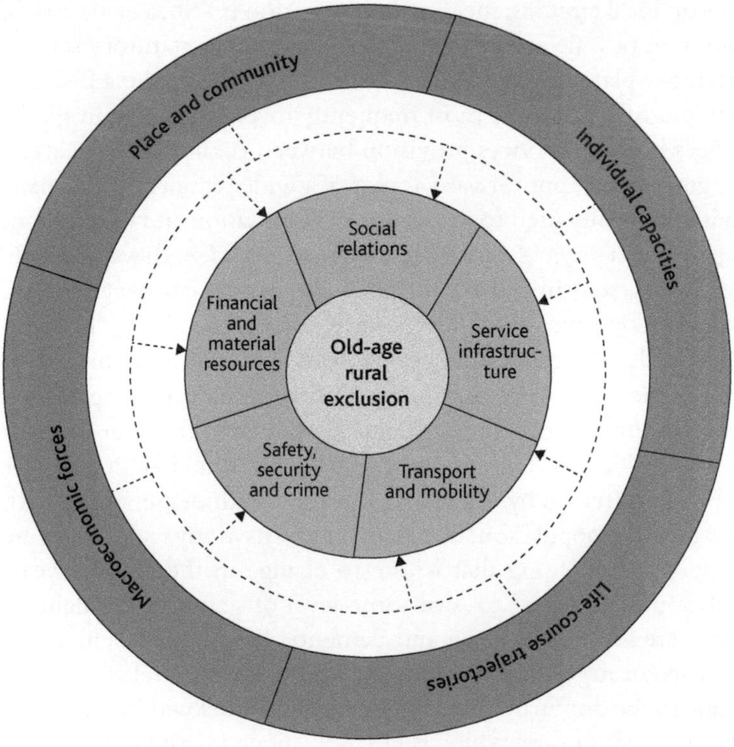

Source: Walsh et al (2019)

exclusion (that is, social relations; service infrastructure; transport and mobility; safety, security and crime; financial and material resources) and factors that serve to accentuate or diminish the potential of exclusion. Mediating factors operate singularly or in combination to intensify, or protect against, domain-specific experiences of disadvantage in the areas of social relations; service infrastructure; transport and mobility; safety, security and crime; and financial and material sources. The importance of agency and adaptive capacity for creating resilience reservoirs and later-life wellbeing outcomes has been explored by Wiles and colleagues (2012). Likewise, the significance of critical life transitions, such as dementia, in determining disadvantage trajectories has been well documented (Scharf et al, 2005; Elder and Shanahan, 2006). Place, its sociocultural context and its relationship to a sense of belonging, has been noted to have multifaceted impacts on older adults' experiences (Burholt et al, 2014; Walsh, 2015). And there is substantial research on the influence of macroeconomic forces on the rural economy, including population decline and demographic shifts (Giarchi, 2006; Phillipson, 2007).

This framework attempts to address how exclusionary processes intersect with diverse patterns of rural ageing and to contribute to gaps in our conceptual understanding around how rural places are involved in social exclusion in later life (Scharf and Bartlam, 2008; Walsh et al, 2017). The framework represents an initial effort to also explore how life-course experiences of older populations and the heterogeneity of their rural contexts (Glasgow, 1993; Keating, 2008) are involved in the inter-relationship between rurality, ageing and exclusion. As Walsh and colleagues (2019) note, residential tenure, status variables (such as socioeconomic position, gender and ethnicity), individual agency, and life-course shifts in personal circumstances (such as retirement, ill health and dementia) have the capacity to alter the potential for exclusion in later life (Scharf and Bartlam, 2008). The capacities of different rural settings, and the geographic and socioeconomic characteristics of such settings, have the potential to support and/or hinder people with dementia, particularly in their pursuit and protection of self-identity and personhood (Walsh et al, 2014; Scharf et al, 2016).

As highlighted earlier, there is compelling evidence as to why people with dementia might experience disadvantage in rural areas. Even for the general older population, lower population densities, migration outflows and changing social structure may undermine the connectedness and support networks of rural older individuals (Walker et al, 2013; Burholt and Scharf, 2014) and lead to the restructuring of public services (Dwyer and Hardill, 2011; Skinner and Joseph, 2011;

Warburton et al, 2014). However, rural communities can also be important sources of social opportunities and meaningful relationships (Wenger and Keating, 2008; Keating et al, 2013). Practices within place, whether social, cultural or even agrarian, can also represent important meanings that generate a sense of belonging (Eales et al, 2008; Wiles et al, 2012; Burholt et al, 2014) and affirmation of self-identity (Rowles, 1983; Walsh, 2015). Consequently, deep emotional attachments between people and places can emerge over time (Rubinstein and Parmalee, 1992; Gustafson, 2001). This can also apply to people with dementia and their family carers who can draw on positive aspects of rural environments (Blackstock et al, 2006; Egdell et al, 2010) and develop protective coping strategies that allow them to remain living at home (Branger et al, 2016).

Trying to locate people with dementia within rural social exclusion is not easy, given the absence of much information on rural dementia in Ireland, and indeed internationally. Therefore, the focus in the remainder this chapter is to highlight what we do know about the domains of rural social exclusion for people with dementia in Ireland, based on a very limited dataset. We have even less information on the impact of mediating factors, but it is important that they are acknowledged given their role in influencing policy to address older-age rural exclusion.

What is the evidence?

In this section we draw on material from a series of analyses completed by the authors on rural ageing in Ireland (Walsh et al, 2012, 2014, 2019) and two original datasets that explore stakeholder experiences of ageing in place in rural areas. While neither was designed for the purpose of exploring rural exclusion for people with dementia, they provide insights into how the dynamics of rurality, ageing and exclusion are considered in the context of living with the condition. Ethics for the collection of the original data was provided by the Research Ethics Committee at the National University of Ireland Galway. The data were generated through semi-structured interviews with a variety of stakeholders, including representatives from two dementia-specific, non-governmental, service providers (SPs), as well respondents from the National Dementia Office (NDO), which was established as part of the Irish National Dementia Strategy (Hennelly and O'Shea, 2017). Both service providers are directly involved in the care of people with dementia in rural areas. From the limited data, it is possible to identify three domains of exclusion – service infrastructure, transport and mobility, and social relations – and two mediating factors – place and community, and macroeconomic forces.

Service infrastructure

Enabling people with dementia to live in their own home for as long as possible and practicable is a key element of the government's strategy for the care of people with dementia in Ireland. However, poor service infrastructure remains a major impediment to keeping people living well with dementia in their own homes. In part, this implicates the wider general health and social care infrastructure in rural communities. Both in international contexts and in Ireland, such infrastructure has been noted to be increasingly under pressure through service retrenchment and a decoupling of public service infrastructure (Skinner and Hanlon, 2016; Warburton et al, 2017). In Ireland, heightened by public expenditure cuts due to the economic recessions, this has meant restrictions on public health nurse services, home help and home support allocations, and in some cases the closure of community hospitals in rural settings (Walsh et al, 2019). Evidence from stakeholder interviews confirms that community-based care specifically for people with dementia living in rural areas is weak and fragmented. Participants referenced the absence of appropriate supports in the community, citing economies of scale arguments for inadequate provision. The NDO talked about no services at all in some places, leading to isolation and exclusion for people with dementia living in rural areas.

> NDO: 'Responding to dementia in an urban setting and a rural setting and how it might be more difficult in a rural setting, because you don't have the services, the specific dementia specific services, because you don't have the numbers of people with dementia to make it pay.'

The implications of these circumstances were highlighted not just for the person with dementia but also for their families and carers, and it was also noted how these support networks can often be very much on their own in some of these contexts.

> SP2: 'In rural Galway there are some ... there are parts where there are no services whatsoever ... there's nothing for families, there's nothing for the person with dementia, in a lot of places in Galway, rural Galway.'

Transport and mobility

Transport is a particular challenge for rural older people who do not own a car (see Chapter 10 of this book for a full discussion of this issue). In Walsh and colleagues' (2012) study on rural ageing in Ireland, participants worried about reaching a stage when they might no longer be able to drive, or when they might have to depend on others to drive them to places should they fall ill. For people with dementia, the transition into cognitive decline and ill health means that this transition will be a reality for most of them. Public bus services in rural areas in Ireland have been rationalised, especially those serving unprofitable and remote rural communities (O'Shea, 2009). This has led to considerable hardship for people who continue to depend solely on public transport for getting around. Free travel for older people was introduced in Ireland because public transport has long been acknowledged as important in ensuring access to local services and facilities and in facilitating older people's engagement in social activities (Banister and Bowling, 2004). The irony is that while most people with dementia in Ireland have free travel, those living in rural areas have little opportunity to exercise that freedom. If the public transport system is weak or non-existent, it matters little that the entitlement is universal. Moreover, the lack of experimentation with social transport schemes in the country, such as community-based local interventions involving private citizen transport, and mobilising and pooling community buses from different organisations and sectors (such as the postal service), is hard to understand, given the potential for large gains to be made from more innovative use of existing social infrastructure. If we are to respond to rural care needs, it is important that transport is available to enable users to access the services (Innes et al, 2006). As this provider organisation points out, transport often serves as the core means to unlock not only the other service infrastructure in the local area and surrounding region, but also the therapeutic and quality of benefits that this infrastructure might be associated with:

> SP1: 'But if they're living out in rural Ireland and they have no car and they can't get to day centre and they can't get to a club, well then they don't have the stimulation and they don't have the ability to continue to live well.'

Social relations

Social relationships are key to maintaining inclusion pathways for older people and anything that undermines or weakens such relationships increases the risk of exclusion. So, for example, people with dementia without family and friends, living on their own, with little current attachment to community and without the opportunity or means for social contact are always likely to be at risk of exclusion (Herron and Rosenberg, 2017). As this stakeholder provider organisation highlights, this can simply limit daily social interactions:

> SP1: 'If you live alone in a rural community and you can't physically walk to your own shop, you might not talk to someone all day.'

If such a person is outside the sphere of influence of the community and not in receipt of basic services, that risk increases further. Older people living in rural areas keenly feel the absence of social connections and social relationships and are acutely aware of the debilitating impact of these absences on the quality of their lives (Walsh et al, 2014). Lower population densities, migration outflows and changing socialisation patterns can threaten elements of this social connectivity.

Research also testifies to how informal support networks are becoming more diverse in their composition (Knowles et al, 2016) and can involve family, friends and neighbours (Jacobs et al, 2016) and people with dementia themselves (Herron and Rosenberg, 2017). They can also be directly shaped by place characteristics, such as neighbourhood integration (Thomése et al, 2003). Recent studies demonstrate how hidden and stealth practices in rural places can draw in actors from multiple systems (private, public, community/voluntary) as primary (direct and regular support giving) and ancillary (sporadic monitoring and assistance) support givers (Hanlon et al, 2011; Walsh et al, 2014). Added to this are rural characteristics that influence the effectiveness of social and support networks. Remoteness, poor weather, difficult terrain and lack of accessibility compound issues for people with dementia around accessing support to help negotiate their environment, as places become less familiar (Herron et al, 2016).

Family support is also integral to allowing older people with dementia to remain active and connected in their rural communities, which makes the absence of that support an important risk factor, particularly if other mediating factors are at play, such as stigma, burnout or the absence of connectivity platforms, such as rural broadband.

> SP1: 'So you can imagine why people, it's easier sometimes to isolate themselves and become socially isolated ... so there would be a lot of times that people with dementia

become socially isolated very, very quickly … if you go back to the internet and the broadband spread in Ireland, there's a lot of places are still quite rural and quite isolated so … there is a difference between rural and urban, yeah.'

Mediating factors

As found by Walsh and colleagues (2019), place, as an embodiment of a geographic location and a community of people, is a pervasive dimension of the lived experiences of people with dementia. Place and community do not function simply as a location, but are constructed from both real, imagined and perceived experience. These elements have a multifaceted impact on the lives of people with dementia and serve to determine the quality of the accord between themselves and their rural places, and ultimately their sense of identity, belonging and attachment to these places (Kelly and Yarwood, 2018; Walsh et al, 2019). Continuing to age in place can help preserve life-course connection with place, relational connectedness, and, even for those with memory loss, a set of meanings around identity manifest in routines and environmental cues (Clarke and Bailey, 2016; Walsh, 2018).

> SP1: 'Place … is hugely important and hugely important to somebody with Alzheimer's as well because they will lose their short-term memory. So they will remember, you know, where they were born, they will remember where they were, they will remember neighbours, they will remember where they went for walks, they will have all that … so all of that long term memory becomes very, very different for them.'

As Walsh and colleagues (2019) assert, place attachment may, therefore, help compensate for some of the impacts and processes of age-related rural exclusion. This includes those that are fundamentally place-based, such as depleted services and shifts in local collective socialisation patterns.

> NDO: 'The physical environment is really important as well. I'm talking about the community and then, you know, you talk about your home, where you live and having your things around you and the familiarity of that is so important, particularly for people with dementia.'

> SP1: 'And then people don't want to move from their own community, they want to generally stay where they are if they've been living in an area and their family are there, their neighbours are there, their friends are there and that's where they're known and that's where people can actually look out for them. So many people now with dementia who I know, they will actually tell their friends and neighbours if you find me wandering, please bring me back. And then people look out for them, if they see them in an unusual place they will then go over to them and talk to them and make sure that they know and how they're getting back etc.'

Family circumstances in rural areas are affected by macroeconomic influences; local economic decline tends to lead to increased emigration, resulting in the vibrancy of the local community being diminished or permanently damaged. Having good neighbours never fully compensates for the absence or loss of immediate family, who may have to leave the local community for education and work. That loss is particularly felt later in life should people require high levels of care resulting from a diagnosis of dementia.

> SP2: 'There's a lot of social exclusion, particularly in rural areas. I'm sure it happens in built-up areas as well, but mostly it's in the far-flung places where maybe all their family have left (for work), maybe not the country but they might be living in Dublin or whatever, and their friends may have died.'

> SP2: 'And a lot of these areas, there's been a lot of emigration; so there aren't the pool of people to draw on.'

But aside from the impact on relational communities and the social sustainability of these sites, studies in Ireland have highlighted that macro-forces were perhaps most acute and significant in terms of the impact of the global economic crisis and to subsequent programmes of austerity (Walsh et al, 2019).

Policy implications

This section explores the policy and practice issues for people with dementia living in rural communities, beginning with the need to set explicit social objectives alongside conventional economic goals in relation to rural development in Ireland. There is significant unmet personal and social need in rural communities, across a range of vulnerable groups, especially people with dementia. Economies of scale arguments are most frequently invoked to explain spatial differences in social services provision between urban and rural areas. These arguments have not been contested in Ireland, because the debate has never moved beyond an economic efficiency framework.

But clearly social objectives are also important, and for lasting changes to occur there will have to be a radical reassessment of the relative weighting given to efficiency and equity in public policy making. The Irish National Dementia Strategy is predicated on two overarching principles, personhood and citizenship, neither of which are clearly defined in the strategy document. They do imply, however, that people with dementia are enabled and supported, even if sometimes only in a partial way, to maintain their resilience and dignity in the face of the disease; and that they remain valued, independent citizens who have the right to be fully included as active citizens in society. But if these sentiments are to have any meaning, the social and distributional consequences of public policy for dementia will have to be given much higher priority than is currently the case. Poor social infrastructure is undermining both personhood and citizenship for people with dementia living in rural areas.

The model developed earlier in this chapter can facilitate new ways of looking at dementia policy in the country, emphasising the need to unpack complex and multiple challenges facing older people with dementia in rural settings and to adopt a multifaceted approach to supporting the participation of rural people with dementia as full citizens. This encompasses a now much-advocated call for a shift away from the medical lens (Cahill et al, 2012; Cahill, 2018) to viewing people with dementia as holistic, rights-based citizens embedded and invested in our communities. New social indicators can help shift the focus towards citizenship and participation for people with dementia living in rural areas. Benchmarks need to be established and progress measured with respect to social care provision, social networks, transport solutions, technology, housing and general quality-of-life issues for people with dementia living in rural communities. Benchmarking and measurement has contributed to the alleviation of poverty in Ireland through focusing attention on policy instruments, programmes and outcomes (O'Shea, 2009). The same strategy could serve an equally important function in addressing deficits in social care provision for people with dementia living in rural areas, including deficits that serve to undermine, and in some circumstances dismantle, the personhood of those affected by the disease. The challenge is to secure more tangible pathways to reducing social exclusion and marginalisation for rural-dwelling people with dementia. Strategies to offset social exclusion and support greater engagement in society are beginning to emerge in primary and public health internationally (O'Donnell et al, 2018). Similar design goals will be necessary when developing practical interventions in community and social care spaces to offset exclusion for people with dementia.

One of the main issues for people with dementia living in rural areas is the gap between need and provision. Responsibility for provision for people with dementia is largely the domain of the HSE funded through the health budget. The reality is that many of the problems facing people with dementia living in rural communities go beyond individual health and are firmly rooted within the broad psychosocial space. Unfortunately, very little attention has focused on alternative ways of addressing unmet social need in rural areas among people with dementia. One possible solution is to make better use of latent social entrepreneurship within local communities to address some of the exclusion domains identified by stakeholders (O'Shea, 2009). The development of social entrepreneurship, to address gaps in service provision, transport and social relations, does not have to start from scratch, as there already exists a pool of potential entrepreneurs in many parts of Ireland, many currently operating as volunteers, who wish to make a contribution to social provision. However, more will have to be done by government to encourage and support social entrepreneurship within rural communities to address social exclusion issues for people with dementia. This means the introduction of seed capital and start-up grants for social production, using similar schemes to those currently available to economic entrepreneurs. Entrepreneurs should be given support in identifying commercial social opportunities and generating realistic business plans that match economic imperatives with the realities of current social provision for people with dementia. Some failures will undoubtedly occur, but that is only to be expected given the nature of the production and the risks associated with new initiatives in this field. Training schemes will also have to be introduced for workers in any newly emerging social economy for people with dementia in order to maintain acceptable standards of care. But above all a mind-set change is necessary to move dementia care out of health and into social production. Only by doing this can we respect and address the principles of personhood and citizenship that underpin the National Dementia Strategy.

The maintenance of rural communities and the protection of both culture and way of life across the life course should be a fundamental goal for the Irish government. Up to now, the only approach to maintaining rural communities has been the strategy of promoting various types of rural economic development. This is a necessary but not a sufficient condition for the maintenance of a sustainable rural tradition in the country. Economic development means little if the quality of life of rural people, and particularly those with dementia, is poor because social models of care are so weak. There must be a dual approach to development that recognises the importance of the economic and the social in the lives of the people, including those with dementia. Specifically, progress is required in the following areas:

- measurement of social progress and social gain in rural communities through an annual social audit of quality of life;
- development of citizenship indicators for people with dementia in rural areas;
- establishment of personhood criteria for the development of social care provision for people with dementia in rural areas;
- identification and nurturing of social entrepreneurs for dementia within rural communities, building on the existing network of volunteer providers;
- provision of basic seed and start–up capital grants for rural projects meeting specific social inclusion criteria within the dementia field.

Some people might argue that many of these activities already fall under the control of existing statutory agencies, like the HSE or the local authorities, but the reality is that these agencies, by definition, are not geared to social production. The HSE is too focused on the medical model of health production, while local authorities are mainly concerned with economic activity. The key element in the sustainability of rural communities is a broader vision of the potential and regenerative nature of rural society. Development has been too narrowly defined to encompass only economic effects and the social needs of people are being neglected. This is potentially catastrophic for people with dementia. People living in rural communities experience life in economic terms certainly, but also in social and cultural terms. A vibrant social economy dedicated to meeting the social needs of the community would allow people with dementia living in rural areas continue to realise their human potential, even when cognitive decline has taken hold. Making use of the conceptual framework on rural exclusion outlined in this chapter to inform public policy for people with dementia can play an important role in making this happen.

References

Banister, D. and Bowling, A. (2004) 'Quality of life for the elderly: the transport dimension', *Transport Policy*, 11(2): 105–15.

Beard, R.L., Knauss, J. and Moyer, D. (2009) '"Managing disability and enjoying life": how we reframe dementia through personal narratives', *Journal of Aging Studies*, 23: 227–35.

Blackstock, K., Innes, A., Cox, S., Smith, A. and Mason, A. (2006) 'Living with dementia in rural and remote Scotland: diverse experiences of people with dementia and their carers', *Journal of Rural Studies*, 22: 161–76.

Bond, J., Corner, L. and Graham, R. (2004) 'Social science theory on dementia research: normal ageing, cultural representation and social exclusion', in A. Innes, C. Archibald and C. Murphy (eds) *Dementia and social inclusion: Marginalised groups and marginalised areas of dementia research, care and practice*, London: Jessica Kingsley, pp 220–36.

Branger, C., Burton, R., O'Connell, M., Stewart, N. and Morgan, D. (2016) 'Coping with cognitive impairment and dementia: rural caregivers' perspectives', *Dementia: The International Journal of Social Research and Practice*, 15(4): 814–31.

Burholt, V. and Scharf, T. (2014) 'Poor health and loneliness in later life: the role of depressive symptoms, social resources, and rural environments', *The Journals of Gerontology Series B*, 69: 311–24.

Burholt, V., Curry, N., Keating, N. and Eales, J. (2014) 'Connecting with community: the nature of belonging among rural elders', *Countryside connections: Older people, community and place in rural Britain*, 95–124.

Cahill, S. (2018) *Dementia and human rights*, Bristol: Policy Press.

Cahill, S., O'Shea, E. and Pierce, M. (2012) *Creating excellence in dementia care: A research review for Ireland's National Dementia Strategy*, Dublin and Galway: Trinity College Dublin and National University of Ireland Galway.

Clarke, C.L. and Bailey, C. (2016) 'Narrative citizenship, resilience and inclusion with dementia: on the inside or on the outside of physical and social places', *Dementia*, 15(3): 434–52.

CSO (Central Statistics Office) (2017) *Census of Population 2016*, Cork: Central Statistics Office.

Dahlberg, L., Berndt, H., Lennartsson, C. and Schön, P. (2018) 'Receipt of formal and informal help with specific care tasks among older people living in their own home. National trends over two decades', *Social Policy & Administration*, 52: 91–110.

Dal Bello-Haas, V., Cammer, A., Morgan, D., Stewart, N. and Kosteniuk, J. (2014) 'Rural and remote dementia care challenges and needs: perspectives of formal and informal care providers residing in Saskatchewan', *Rural and Remote Health*, 14: 2747.

Department of Health (2014) *The Irish National Dementia Strategy*, Dublin: Department of Health.

Donnelly, S., O'Brien, M., Begley, E. and Brennan, J. (2016) *"I'd prefer to stay at home but I don't have a choice." Meeting older people's preference for care: Policy, but what about practice?*, Dublin: University College Dublin.

Dwyer, P. and Hardill, I. (2011) 'Promoting social inclusion? The impact of village services on the lives of older people living in rural England', *Ageing & Society*, 31: 243–64.

Eales, J., Keefe, J. and Keating, N. (2008) 'Age-friendly rural communities', in N. Keating (ed) *Rural ageing: A good place to grow old?*, Bristol: Policy Press, pp 109–20.

Egdell, V., Bond, J., Brittain, K. and Jarvis, H. (2010) 'Disparate routes through support: negotiating the sites, stages and support of informal dementia care', *Health & Place*, 16(1): 101–7.

Elder, G.H. Jr and Shanahan, M.J. (2006) 'The life course and human development', in W. Damon and R.M. Lerner (eds) *Handbook of child psychology. Volume 1: Theoretical models of human development* (6th edn), Hoboken, NJ: John Wiley & Sons, pp 665–715.

Forbes, D., Ward-Griffin, C., Kloseck, M., Mendelsohn, M., St-Amant, O., DeForge, R. and Clark, K. (2011) '"Her world gets smaller and smaller with nothing to look forward to": dimensions of social inclusion and exclusion among rural dementia care networks', *Online Journal of Rural Nursing and Health Care*, 11(2): 27–42.

Giarchi, G.G. (2006) 'Older people "on the edge" in the countrysides of Europe', *Social Policy and Administration*, 40(6): 705–21.

Glasgow, N. (1993) 'Poverty among rural elders: trends, context, and directions for policy', *Journal of Applied Gerontology*, 12(3): 302–19.

Grenier, A., Lloyd, L. and Phillipson, C. (2017) 'Precarity in late life: rethinking dementia as a "frailed" old age', *Sociology of Health & Illness*, 39: 318–30.

Gustafson, P. (2001) 'Meanings of place: everyday experience and theoretical conceptualisations', *Journal of Environmental Psychology*, 21(1): 5–16.

Hanlon, N., Halseth, G. and Ostry, A. (2011) 'Stealth voluntarism: an expectation of health professional work in underserviced areas?', *Health & Place*, 17: 42–9.

Hanlon, N., Skinner, M., Joseph, A., Ryser, L. and Halseth, G. (2015) 'New frontiers of rural ageing: resource hinterlands', in M. Skinner and N. Hanlon (eds) *Ageing resource communities: New frontiers of rural population change, community development and voluntarism*, Abingdon and New York, NY: Routledge.

Health Service Executive (HSE) (2017) *HSE National Service Plan 2018: Increased supports for older people and streamlining of home support services*, Dublin: HSE.

Hennelly, N., and O'Shea, E. (2017) 'Personhood, dementia policy and the Irish National Dementia Strategy', *Dementia*, 18(5): 1810–25.

Herron, R.V. and Rosenberg, M.W. (2017) '"Not there yet": examining community support from the perspective of people with dementia and their partners in care', *Social Science & Medicine*, 173: 81–7.

Herron, R.V., Rosenberg, M.W. and Skinner, M.W. (2016) 'The dynamics of voluntarism in rural dementia care', *Health & Place*, 41: 34–41.

Innes, A., Cox, S., Smith, A. and Mason, A. (2006) 'Service provision for people with dementia in rural Scotland: difficulties and innovations', *Dementia*, 5:249–70.

Innes, A., Morgan, D. and Kostenuik, J. (2011) 'Dementia care in rural and remote settings: a systematic review of informal/family caregiving', *Maturitas*, 68(1): 34–46.

Jacobs, M., Van Tilburg, T., Groenewegen, P. and Van Groenou, M. (2016) 'Linkages between informal and formal care-givers in home-care networks of frail older adults', *Ageing & Society*, 36: 1604–24.

Keating, N. (2008) *Rural ageing: A good place to grow old?*, Bristol: Policy Press.

Keating, N., Eales, J. and Phillips, J.E. (2013) 'Age-friendly rural communities: conceptualizing "Best-Fit"', *Canadian Journal on Aging*, 32(4): 319–32.

Kelly, C. and Yarwood, R. (2018) 'From rural citizenship to the rural citizen: farming, dementia and networks of care', *Journal of Rural Studies*, 63: 96–104.

Keogh, F., Pierce, M., Neylon, K., Fleming, P., O'Neill, S., Carter, L. and O'Shea, E. (2018) *Supporting people with complex needs at home: Evaluation of the HSE Intensive Home Care Package initiative*, Dublin: Genio.

Kiejna, A., Frydecka, D., Asdanowski, T., Bickel, H., Reynish, E., Prince, M., Caracciolo, B., FratiglioniI, L. and Georges, J. (2010) 'Epidemiological studies of dementia in Eastern and Middle European countries', *International Psychogeriatrics*, 26: 111–17.

Knowles, S., Combs, R., Kirk, S., Griffiths, M., Patel, N. and Sanders, C. (2016) 'Hidden caring, hidden carers? Exploring the experience of carers for people with long-term conditions', *Health and Social Care in the Community*, 24(2): 203–13.

McDonald, A. and Heath, B. (2008) 'Developing services for people with dementia: findings from research in a rural area', *Quality in Ageing: Policy, Practice and Research*, 9: 9–18.

Milbourne, P. and Doheny, S. (2012) 'Older people and poverty in rural Britain: material hardships, cultural denials and social inclusions', *Journal of Rural Studies*, 28(4): 389–97.

Misiak, B., Cialkowska-Kuzminska, M., Frydecka, D., Chladzinka-Kiejna, S. and Kiejna, A. (2013) 'European studies on the prevalence of dementia in the elderly: time for a step towards a methodological consensus', *International Journal of Geriatric Psychiatry*, 28: 1211–21.

O'Donnell, P., O'Donovan, D. and Elmusharaf, K. (2018) 'Measuring social exclusion in healthcare settings: a scoping review', *International Journal for Equity in Health*, 17: 15.

O'Shea, E. (2007) *Implementing policy for dementia in Ireland: The time for action is now*, Dublin: Alzheimer Society of Ireland.

O' Shea, E. (2009) 'Rural ageing and public policy in Ireland', in J. McDonagh, T. Varley and S. Shortall (eds) *A living countryside? The politics of sustainable development in rural Ireland*, Farnham: Ashgate, pp 269–86.

O'Shea, E., Cahill, S. and Pierce, M. (2015) 'Reframing policy for dementia', in K. Walsh, G. Carney and Á. Ní Léime (eds) *Ageing through austerity: Critical perspectives from Ireland*, Bristol: Policy Press, pp 97–112.

O'Shea, E., Cahill, S. and Pierce, M. (2017) *Developing and implementing policy in Ireland*, Galway: National University of Ireland Galway.

Peel, E. and Harding, R. (2014) ' "It's a huge maze, the system, it's a terrible maze": dementia carers' constructions of navigating health and social care services', *Dementia*, 13(5): 642–61.

Phillipson, C. (2007) 'The "elected" and the "excluded": sociological perspectives on the experience of place and community in old age', *Ageing & Society*, 27(3): 321–42.

Pierce, M., Cahill, S. and O'Shea, E. (2013) 'Planning dementia services: new estimates of current and future prevalence rates of dementia for Ireland', *Irish Journal of Psychological Medicine*, 30: 13–20.

Pierse, T., O'Shea, E. and Carney, P. (2019) 'Estimates of the prevalence, incidence and severity of dementia in Ireland', *Irish Journal of Psychological Medicine*, 36(2): 129–37.

Rowles, G.D. (1983) 'Place and personal identity in old age: observations from Appalachia', *Journal of Environmental Psychology*, 3(4): 299–313.

Rubinstein, R.L. and Parmalee, P.A. (1992) 'Attachment to place and the representation of life-course by the elderly', in I. Altman and S.M. Low (eds) *Place attachment*, New York, NY: Plenum Press, pp 139–63.

Scharf, T. and Bartlam, B. (2008) 'Ageing and social exclusion in rural communities', in N. Keating (ed) *Rural ageing: A good place to grow old?*, Bristol: Policy Press, pp 97–108.

Scharf, T., Phillipson, C. and Smith, A.E. (2005) 'Social exclusion of older people in deprived urban communities of England', *European Journal of Ageing*, 2: 76–87.

Scharf, T., Walsh, K. and O'Shea, E. (2016) 'Ageing in rural places', in M. Shucksmith and D. Brown (eds) *International handbook of rural studies*, Abingdon and New York, NY: Routledge, pp 80–91.

Silman, A.J., Macfarlane, G.J. and Macfarlane, T. (2018) *Epidemiological studies: A practical guide*, Oxford: Oxford University Press.

Skinner, M. and Hanlon, N. (2016) 'Introduction to ageing resource communities', in M. Skinner and N. Hanlon (eds) *Ageing resource communities: New frontiers of rural population change, community development and voluntarism*, Abingdon and New York, NY: Routledge, pp 106–18.

Skinner, M.W. and Joseph, A.E. (2011) 'Placing voluntarism within evolving spaces of care in ageing rural communities', *GeoJournal*, 76(2): 151–62.

Thomése, F., Tilburg, T.V. and Knipscheer, K.C. (2003) 'Continuation of exchange with neighbors in later life: the importance of the neighborhood context', *Personal Relationships*, 10: 535–50.

Walker, J., Orpin, P., Baynes, H. and Stratford, E. (2013) 'Insights and principles for supporting social engagement in rural older people', *Ageing & Society*, 33: 938–63.

Walsh, K. (2015) 'Interrogating the "age-friendly community" in austerity: myths, realties and the influence of place context', in K. Walsh, G. Carney and Á. Ní Léime (eds) *Ageing through austerity: Critical perspectives from Ireland*, Bristol: Policy Press, pp 9–95.

Walsh, K. (2018) 'Constructions of old-age social exclusion: in place and shaped by place', in M. Skinner, G. Andrews and M. Cutchin (eds) *Geographical gerontology: Concepts and approaches*, Abingdon and New York, NY: Routledge, pp 252–6.

Walsh, K., O'Shea, E. and Scharf, T. (2012) *Social exclusion and ageing in diverse rural communities: Findings of a cross-border study in Ireland and Northern Ireland*, Galway: National University of Ireland Galway.

Walsh, K., O'Shea, E. and Scharf, T. (2019) 'Rural old-age social exclusion: a conceptual framework on mediators of exclusion across the life course', *Ageing & Society*, 1–27, doi: 10.1017/S0144686X19000606.

Walsh, K., O'Shea, E., Scharf, T. and Shucksmith, M. (2014) 'Exploring the impact of informal practices on social exclusion and age-friendliness for older people in rural communities', *Journal of Community & Applied Social Psychology*, 24(1): 37–49.

Walsh, K., Scharf, T. and Keating, N. (2017) 'Social exclusion of older persons: a scoping review and conceptual framework', *European Journal of Ageing*, 14(1): 81–98.

Warburton, J., Cowan, S., Winterton, R. and Hodgkins, S. (2014) 'Building social inclusion for rural older people using information and communication technologies: perspectives of rural practitioners', *Australian Social Work*, 67(4): 479–94.

Warburton, J., Scharf, T. and Walsh, K. (2017) 'Flying under the radar? Risks of social exclusion for older people in rural communities in Australia, Ireland and Northern Ireland', *Sociologia Ruralis*, 57: 459–80.

Wenger, G.C. and Keating, N. (2008) 'The evolution of networks of rural older adults', in N. Keating (ed) *Rural ageing: A good place to grow old?*, Bristol: Policy Press, pp 33–42.

Wiles, J.L., Leibing, A., Guberman, N., Reeve, J. and Allen, R. (2012) 'The meaning of "aging in place" to older people', *The Gerontologist*, 52: 357–66.

PART III

Practice challenges

8

Developing collaborative relationships with rural-dwelling older men with dementia in the UK: lessons learned from a community technological initiative

Ben Hicks and Anthea Innes

Introduction

This chapter discusses the process of developing collaborative working relationships with rural-dwelling older men with dementia in the UK. This population warrants further exploration in its own right, as often facilitators do not acknowledge and address the issues that can be specific to it, resulting in increased risks of social isolation and poorer health outcomes. The chapter outlines the potential challenges that can be encountered when seeking to engage this hard-to-reach group as well as solutions to address them. The lessons considered throughout the chapter are underpinned by theoretical knowledge and have been informed by reflexive practice through research that has sought to enhance social inclusion in rural-dwelling older men with dementia using a technological initiative. This will be discussed in more detail later in the chapter. While there were many challenges throughout this applied research, some of which will be examined later, the initiatives were warmly received by the men and successfully adopted within all three rural communities. They continue to this day, four years after the completion of the study, with funding obtained from local organisations, thereby highlighting their success.

Prior to discussing the lessons learned for successful collaboration with rural-dwelling older men with dementia, it is necessary to situate them within the wider context of the dementia-care field as well as provide an overview of the technological initiative that helped to inform them.

Context: why is there a need to better understand how to support community-dwelling older men with dementia?

Some current political and academic discourses highlight the importance of community initiatives for ensuring a cost-effective means to support the wellbeing (Kenigsberg et al, 2016; ADI, 2017, 2018) and psychological needs (Nyman and Szymczynska, 2016) of people living with dementia. For these initiatives to be successful, it is important that people with dementia are engaged as collaborators throughout their design, implementation and delivery, thereby ensuring that the outcomes are meaningful to them (Øksnebjerg et al, 2018). Despite this, research has consistently demonstrated the reluctance of older men (65 years and over) more generally, as well as those with dementia, to engage with traditional health and social care initiatives, thereby increasing their risk of isolation, social exclusion and poorer health outcomes (White, 2011; White et al, 2011; Milligan et al, 2015). This has resulted in some countries adopting specific male-health policies to focus on and address these challenges such as Australia (Australian Government, 2010), Ireland (Baker, 2015) and Brazil (Spindler, 2015).

The difficulties when engaging older men with dementia in community initiatives can be partly attributed to men's health-seeking behaviours, which, in turn, can be linked to their perceptions of masculinities. These are the cultural attitudes and beliefs they hold, and the actions they undertake, to establish themselves as 'male' in the eyes of others (Courtenay, 2000; Connell and Pearse, 2015). These masculinities have been developed and reinforced throughout an individual's lifetime in accordance with the culture of their society for that particular time and place (Connell, 2005; Thompson and Bennett, 2015). Consequently, by adulthood, the majority of men will be aware of the standards and expectations that are associated with masculinity (Connell and Messerschmidt, 2005; Connell and Pearse, 2015) and these will continue to influence their experiences and actions as they age, with or without dementia (Thompson and Langendoerfer, 2016; Sandberg, 2018; Twigg, 2018). For some men as they age, and in response to life changes, their masculinities evolve and are reinterpreted to favour family life over work (Wentzell, 2013) and acknowledge their own vulnerability and health issues (Courtenay, 2000; Clarke and Lefkowich, 2018). Others, however, remain rigid and closely aligned with the traditional Western or 'hegemonic ideals' (Connell, 2005) they demonstrated during their younger years (Thompson and Langendoerfer, 2016). It is likely that these latter individuals, who may prefer stoicism and the 'stiff upper lip' mentality as well as the display of attributes such as physical strength, competitiveness, capability and control (Coston and Kimmel, 2013; Thompson and Langendoerfer, 2016), will have difficult late-life experiences (Coston and Kimmel, 2013) as they downplay health concerns (Clarke and Bennett, 2013), avoid seeking help (Sloan et al, 2015; Yousaf et al, 2015) and resist community-based health services and preventative health activities (White, 2011; White et al, 2011; Milligan et al, 2015) for fear of the detrimental impact such concerns may have on their sense of masculinities. This may be particularly pertinent in rural-dwelling men who can align more closely with these masculine ideals than their urban counterparts (Levant and Habben, 2003; Hammer et al, 2013).

Consequently, if these challenges are to be addressed it is imperative that researchers and practitioners acknowledge the impact of masculinities on older men's experiences of dementia and their willingness to engage with community initiatives and seek support (Hicks et al, 2019). Unfortunately, at present, there is a tendency to view those with dementia as a homogenous and androgynous population (Hulko, 2009; Milligan et al, 2015; Bartlett et al, 2016), thereby assuming that a 'one-size-fits-all' approach to dementia care will be successful. Continuing in this vein is likely to yield limited positive results for older men with dementia and so a change is urgently required that draws on academic theory and the reflexive lessons learned through practice. Addressing this challenge is even more pertinent within rural communities, where financial resources and formal dementia support services can be limited or redistributed to urban areas (Clarke and Bailey, 2016; Bowes et al, 2018), meaning those community initiatives that do exist must be fit for purpose and appeal to and benefit the older men with dementia residing there.

What is a technological initiative?

The lessons discussed in this chapter have been informed through the authors' delivery of technological initiatives to people living with dementia (Cutler et al, 2016; Hicks et al, 2019) and in particular the reflexive practice of the lead author who was responsible for delivering a technological initiative as part of a three-year Doctoral Study. Although more details of the initiative can be found elsewhere (Hicks, 2016), this section provides a brief overview of this applied research study.

During the summer of 2014, the initiative was delivered across three rural locations of England, to enhance the generalisability of the research, and targeted at community-dwelling older men (65 years and over) with dementia, a population the funding charity was finding difficult to engage. One of the locations (L1) was typical of a 'bypassed' community (Keating et al, 2013), with poor services and transport links and the majority of funding being directed towards a nearby urban conurbation, whereas the other two locations (L2 and L3) were more consistent with 'bucolic' rural communities (Keating et al, 2013), with good resources and assets that were attracting wealthy retirees and second-home owners. Within each location the initiative continued for a total of nine weeks, with one session per week lasting for two hours including breaks for refreshments and informal discussions.

Off-the-shelf digital gaming technology, including iPads, Nintendo Wii, Nintendo Balance Board and Microsoft Kinect, was selected as the medium to engage the older men. This technology was selected as it is widely available within society, making it easier for dementia practitioners to purchase and use than more dementia-specific devices, and it may not be associated with the same stigma that can accompany these other technologies (Meiland et al, 2017). This made it an interesting medium to explore with the men, particularly as the rural–urban digital divide (Baker et al, 2017) meant that many of them were not already accustomed with such devices.

In accordance with other research (Joddrell and Astell, 2016; Dove and Astell, 2017; Kenigsberg et al, 2017; Cutler, 2018), the initiative aimed to provide leisure activities that enhanced the social inclusion of people with dementia, rather than ameliorate the deterioration of their condition. Specifically, it sought to provide people with 'in-the-moment' benefits for their wellbeing, including opportunities for mental, physical and social stimulation as well as lifelong learning. The technological activities were delivered predominantly within a group environment, to encourage social interaction, and the games and applications varied across the three rural locations so as to cater for the interests and capabilities of the men, as advocated by a person-centred approach (Cohen-Mansfield et al, 2010; Kolanowski et al, 2011). On the first session of each technological initiative, the men were asked to name their groups and these names were used throughout the study (L1 – Old Boys, L2 – Done Roaming, L3 – Marching On). A breakdown of the activities undertaken within the initiative, as well as their purpose, benefits and challenges, can be seen in Table 8.1.

Tips to successfully engage rural-dwelling older men with dementia in community initiatives

Although the lessons outlined in this chapter have been informed by the successful delivery of a technological initiative to rural-dwelling older

Table E.1: Theme of activities

Theme of activities	Purpose of the activities	Name and details of games	Platform(s)	Benefits	Potential challenges
Getting to know the participant games	Great ice-breaker activities, appropriate during the first few sessions. The activities should aim to promote conversations between the participants and alleviate any fear of the devices. These activities will help practitioners and other group members develop a better understanding of one another. This will enable future activities to be tailored to participants' interests. During these discussions, practitioners could share information about themselves, their hobbies and interests, and places they have visited. It is important that they are seen as a member of the Technology Club and not just a practitioner.	**Photography** Using the camera application, players take a photograph of another member of the group (with their consent). Once their photograph has been taken, the player can introduce themselves and says a little about their interests and hobbies.	iPad	Players become accustomed to using the camera function and holding the iPad. It also enables them to develop an understanding of the touchscreen. Applications can also be download that allow users to distort pictures. This can add an element of humour to the discussions.	Some participants may struggle to hold the iPad and use the camera application. The practitioner can support this by holding the iPad while the participant lines up the camera shot and pushes the button.
		Popular songs, films, videos or pictures Participants are invited to think of a song, film or television programme they enjoy. Practitioners can then work with participants to find the chosen item on an application such as YouTube, and discuss its meaning for each participant as it plays. If everyone enjoys, for example, a particular	iPad	This type of media can enable the conversations to flow and may encourage other group members to join in. This is a particularly useful activity during one-to-one conversations with participants.	Some participants may struggle to remember or talk about aspects of their life, or not feel confident in doing so.

Table 8.1: (continued)

Theme of activities	Purpose of the activities	Name and details of games	Platform(s)	Benefits	Potential challenges
	Also, when discussing participants' lives, practitioners should ensure they draw comparisons between other members of the group (if applicable). This will highlight commonalities between participants and may facilitate future conversations during or after the activities.	song, it could even become the Technology Club theme tune, which can be played at the start and end of each session. Practitioners can also encourage participants to find videos or pictures to provide illustrations for their discussions, for example, photographs of the school they attended.			
		The Game of Life This board game is used in conjunction with the iPad. Players navigate the board, making certain life choices while interacting with mini-games on the iPad and collecting fake money.	iPad	This is a great game for learning more about the participants' lives, as practitioners can ask them why they chose certain paths on the game, and whether they correlate with choices they made in their own life. The 'banker' role can be offered to interested players, thereby providing them with a role of responsibility within the game. A sense of achievement and pride can be developed when participants emerge winner of the game.	Some of the mini-games on the iPad may be challenging for participants. Numbers permitting, people can be paired up to play in teams and support each other with the mini-games. The banker role should be given to someone who is confident about adding up and distributing money.

Google Earth This is a free application that provides satellite images of the world, which can be used to support conversations about participants' lives.	iPad	Players can be encouraged to talk more about their lives or revisit areas that they were once interested in, such as places where they grew up or went on holiday, or famous landmarks. This is important for participants' sense of identity.	Some participants may find it difficult to navigate the virtual earth and may struggle with orientation. In these instances, it is useful for practitioners to support participants with the navigation and encourage them to lead the discussions.
Creating a Mii character Participants are invited to create their own Mii character to represent their Technology Club. If playing within a group, each participant can take turns in selecting a feature for the virtual character, including their gender, height, weight, eye colour and hairstyle. This newly created character can be used to play a range of other games on the Nintendo Wii, thereby creating an element of consistency throughout future activities.	Nintendo Wii	This is a great introductory game to the Nintendo Wii controls. The activity can generate a lot of discussion and laughter, and so is ideal for social bonding. It can also establish a virtual identity for each player.	Participants may initially struggle to use the controller. If used as part of a group activity, participants can support one another with the game mechanics.

Table 8.1: (continued)

Theme of activities	Purpose of the activities	Name and details of games	Platform(s)	Benefits	Potential challenges
Sporty games	These games run on sensor technologies and require participants to simulate physical actions such as golf swings, bowling and dart throwing. They are a great way to promote mild physical exercise as well as mental stimulation and social interaction. It is important that practitioners consider tailoring the games to the abilities of the participants (based on the participants' evidenced abilities and/or preferences). Practitioners are advised to introduce the simpler, slower games first to enable participants to become comfortable with the technology before moving on to more complicated games.	**Bowling (Wii Sports and Brunswick Bowling)** Similar to ten-pin bowling, participants position themselves on the screen before bowling the ball. The objective is to knock down as many skittles as possible over the course of a match (ten rounds).	Nintendo Wii and Microsoft Kinect	This is a slow-paced and relatively straightforward activity, making it a great introductory game for either technological device. If it is played in a group, practitioners can consider arranging players into teams (two per team with players alternating their turns) to promote friendly competition and teamwork.	On Wii Sports, players perform bowling actions while simultaneously releasing a button at the appropriate time. This adds a level of complexity to the game compared with Brunswick Bowling where no buttons are required. Practitioners should not be put off using Wii Sports, however, as players are likely to develop quickly the skills required to play successfully.
		Boxing (Wii Sports) This game requires both the Wii controller and the Nunchuck (additional part of the controller). Holding both devices (one in each hand), players swing either hand to simulate hitting their opponent. Similar to boxing, the objective of the game is to knock your opponent to the floor for a count of ten.	Nintendo Wii	This is a relatively straightforward game with a simple objective, which makes it a good choice for preliminary Technology Club sessions. Players can virtually fight against other members of the Technology Club (if applicable), to promote friendly competition, or against a computer opponent.	The mildly aggressive nature of the game may not appeal to everyone, so it is important that practitioners consult participants before introducing it. Practitioners should not be put off by games that use a combination of the hand-held controller and Nunchuck (sometimes simultaneously), as players are likely to develop quickly the skills required to play successfully.

Darts (Kinect Sports) Players simulate the action of throwing a dart on to a virtual dartboard to score points. Similar to darts, the aim is to knock their score down from 360 to 0.	Microsoft Kinect	The objective is relatively straightforward and the game is slow-paced, making it a good choice for preliminary sessions. Players can play together in teams (taking one round of darts each) to promote teamwork.	Some players may find the required hand-eye coordination challenging, and may also have difficulty with keeping their hand steady when lining up the darts with the board.
Golf (Wii Sports and Kinect Sports) Players move their arms to simulate the swing of a golf club. The objective is to hit the ball into the hole in as few shots as possible.	Nintendo Wii and Microsoft Kinect	This is a slow-paced and relatively straightforward activity, making it a great introductory game for either technological device. Practitioners can promote friendly competition by having players compete against one another over the course of a match. Alternatively, participants can play a round of nine holes (one hole each) against the computer opponent to encourage teamwork and camaraderie.	Those who have played golf in the past are likely to adopt the appropriate stance quickly, but those who have no experience of golf may take more time and require more support.

Table 8.1: (continued)

Theme of activities	Purpose of the activities	Name and details of games	Platform(s)	Benefits	Potential challenges
		Tennis (Wii Sports and Kinect Sports) Players move their arms to simulate the swing of a tennis racket to connect with the ball at the appropriate time. The movements required are either up and down, when serving the ball, or forwards and backwards, when returning shots. Similar to tennis, the aim is to outscore your opponent over the course of the match.	Nintendo Wii and Microsoft Kinect	Practitioners can encourage participants to play against other members of the Technology Club (if applicable) to promote friendly competition.	Although the games are straightforward, they can be fast-paced, meaning some players may struggle to time their shots. However, practitioners should not be put off using them; with practice, participants can improve. Those with previous tennis experience may find these games easier to play.
Driving games	Following a diagnosis of dementia, affected people often have their driving licence revoked, and for some this can be a huge loss. These games may be a good way to enable them to reconnect with this experience as well as provide a lot of humour and entertainment.	**Mario Kart** Holding the Wii controller in both hands to simulate a steering wheel, players navigate a series of racing tracks that increase in difficulty the further they progress through the game.	Nintendo Wii Microsoft Kinect	Participants can compete against other members of the Technology Club (if applicable) to promote friendly competition, or against computer opponents. Practitioners can also set up time trial laps to encourage players to beat their own scores.	Some of the tracks can be difficult to navigate, so it is best to begin on the easier levels when introducing the game. The steering wheel accessory may facilitate players' interactions with the game as well as enhance their whole driving experience.

The objective of the game is to finish ahead of the other racers. While racing, players can collect objects that give them advantages over their opponents, as well as add humour to the overall gaming experience. These advantages include being able to shrink your opponents, leaving banana skins for your opponents to slip on, or turning yourself into a bullet to fly past everyone.

Joy Ride Turbo

Using either a steering wheel accessory or hand movement alone, players navigate a series of racing tracks that increase in difficulty the further they progress through the game. The objective of the game is to finish ahead of the other racers.

The driving game relies on hand movements alone. This can become confusing to some participants as there is no physical object connecting their movements to the screen. Practitioners may wish to consider using a steering wheel accessory to ameliorate these issues.

Table 8.1: (continued)

Theme of activities	Purpose of the activities	Name and details of games	Platform(s)	Benefits	Potential challenges
Music and dance games	Musical games are likely to be popular within Technology Clubs. They can be a useful way for people with dementia to express themselves, particularly if they have difficulties with verbal communication. All of the technological devices provide opportunities for accessing musical games.	**Keyboard bongos** These are free applications. In essence, the device becomes the musical instrument (either a keyboard or a bongo drum) and responds to a player's touch, enabling them to play along with songs or freestyle. **Just Dance** These are dance-based games that allow players to hold on to a controller or have their movements tracked via a sensor as they copy dance sequences on the screen with the accompaniment of well-known musical tracks.	iPad Microsoft Kinect and Nintendo Wii	These are useful applications for introducing iPad touchscreen technology and discussing participants' musical interests. With groups, practitioners may consider setting up a range of musical instruments on different iPads to form a Technology Club band. These are good games for encouraging physical and mental stimulation and promote an enjoyable, humorous and supportive environment.	With free applications, advertisements sometimes appear on the screen, interrupting the game play. To prevent this, practitioners could consider purchasing the application (for a minimal amount). Not all participants will want to take part in a dance-based game for reasons of preference, ability, or health/mobility. Practitioners may wish to consider alternative activities for those who do not want to play this game.

Balance and movement games	**Wii Motion Play** This comprises various mini-games that challenge participants to perform intricate movements with their wrists, as they hold the Wii controller. The games are fairly slow-paced and enable players to engage in a number of humorous tasks, such as catching ice creams on a cone as they fall from the sky or whacking moles around the head as they steal your vegetables.	Nintendo Wii Motion	Practitioners can encourage other members of the Technology Club (if applicable) to compete against one another for the best score. This will provide elements of friendly competition and encourage participants to keep playing.	Some participants may find it challenging to undertake the intricate movements required for the games. However, players are likely to become more confident and competent with the games the more they practise.
These games are a great way for participants to practise their balance and fine motor control skills. Some of these games may be complicated for participants, so practitioners should be steered by the participants and recognise when to increase or lower the challenge level.	**Wii Fit Balance** This comprises various mini-games that challenge participants to perform a range of lower body movements while standing on the balance board. These include shifting their weight between their feet to maintain their balance on a tightrope or bending and straightening their knees to tackle the ski slalom. These games are fun but can require a lot of practice, particularly those that are fast-paced.	Nintendo Balance Board	These mini-games are good at promoting some mild physical exercise as well as balance. Mental stimulation is also promoted through these games as often coordination is challenged and so participants need to consider their movements carefully.	Some of the games can be fast-paced and so may require a lot of practice from participants. Some players may struggle to bend their knees. In such cases, practitioners may wish to avoid using these games or encourage participants to practise movements on the floor prior to using the balance board.

Table 8.1: (continued)

Theme of activities	Purpose of the activities	Name and details of games	Platform(s)	Benefits	Potential challenges
Virtual board games	Traditional board games that participants may enjoy are also available on technological devices. This is beneficial as players can challenge a computer opponent (as well as any other Technology Club members) and the games often provide hints and tips if players are struggling with their next move, enabling them to engage with the game independently.	**Backgammon, cards, dominoes, chess and jigsaws** All of these classic, traditional games are available to download free. The objective of each game is similar to its traditional board-game counterpart and participants can play them alongside or against other Technology Club members (if applicable) or on their own against a computer opponent. The difficulty level of the games can be adjusted, and it is important that they are set appropriately for the player's ability.	iPad	These games are particularly good for one-to-one interactions, where the practitioner can work with the participant to encourage and support them to learn a new game or re-engage with one they used to play. Certain versions of the games are more interactive than others, thereby potentially enhancing their appeal. These might include Battle Chess (where chess pieces fight on the screen) or jigsaw puzzles made from participants' own selfies that have been downloaded on to the iPad.	With free applications, advertisements sometimes appear on the screen, interrupting the game play. To prevent this, practitioners could consider purchasing the application (for a minimal amount).

men with dementia, they are discussed within the context of the wider academic literature. This demonstrates how they can be applied more generally by facilitators wishing to establish rural community initiatives that will appeal to and benefit this difficult to reach population.

Establishing a collaborative working partnership

As a facilitator, it is imperative to adopt a collaborative approach from the outset that includes listening to the voices of other health and social care professionals, key community organisations and personnel, and men with dementia and their care partners. This is widely advocated by scholars who stress the need for incorporating and valuing diverse perspectives during any decision-making process (Dupuis et al, 2012, 2016; Wiersma et al, 2016; Bartlett and Brannelly, 2018).

Setting up consultation sessions with key informants to discuss the planned initiative can ensure that it is fit for purpose and has the best possible chance of succeeding. These sessions can be used by facilitators to promote their idea and outline the potential benefits for people with dementia, their care partners and the wider rural community, as well as glean information on the rural community as a whole and those areas that may be most receptive to and benefit the most from the initiative, thereby ensuring resources are used effectively. These discussions will also be vital for obtaining the buy-in of influential gatekeepers who can act as ongoing advisers for the initiative as well as promoting it among the rural communities. This is likely to mean it will be perceived with a greater sense of credibility by the target population. This is particularly important for 'outsider' facilitators who are unknown to the rural community and may initially be treated with scepticism and mistrust (Szymczynska et al, 2011). Older men with dementia, and particularly those who align with traditional masculinities, may feel more confident discussing their vulnerabilities and concerns about the initiative with a trusted member of the community rather than an unknown facilitator. In turn, these trusted community members can reassure them and relay any important information back to the facilitator, so that any foreseeable barriers to older men's engagement can be resolved at an early stage. For instance, during the planning phase of the technological initiative, some older men in L1 raised concerns with local memory support workers about travelling to and from the location. When this information was passed to the lead researcher, he was able to work with a local charity in the area that agreed to provide a shuttle bus service for a minimal fee. Furthermore, at another location, health professionals promoting the initiative to older men with dementia reported that the stigmatised label of 'dementia' was preventing some potential participants from registering their interest. Consequently, the initiative was promoted as something targeting 'men with memory problems', as this term was considered more acceptable within this rural community. It should be noted, however, that in this instance, while it was necessary at the beginning to aid recruitment, once people began attending the group the word 'dementia' was no longer avoided (if these discussions were initiated by the men, as discussed later) so as not to further stigmatise the condition.

Working within collaborative partnerships with people with dementia also requires positioning them as 'experts by experience' and seeking to ascertain and act on their opinions and advice. Researchers have demonstrated that including these often marginalised and silenced voices can improve the decision-making process and ensure any initiatives are suitable for their intended target population, as well as empower people with dementia by enabling them to enact their rights for social citizenship and inclusion (Wiersma et al, 2016; Øksnebjerg et al, 2018). Western older men with dementia are likely to be receptive to this approach, particularly if they have been accustomed throughout their lifetime to a role as head of the family and have been responsible for making important decisions. Consequently, facilitators seeking to implement and deliver community initiatives for this population would be advised to democratise the process by situating the men as collaborators and working with them in an equal power relationship. This will ensure they do not unintentionally impose any undue threats to men's masculinities that may result in them suppressing thoughts and feelings during interactions and disengaging with the initiatives as a means of preserving these masculinities. Within the work drawn on here, the democratisation of the research process began from the very start, with older men with dementia being consulted during the development and implementation of the technological initiative as well as throughout its subsequent delivery and evaluation within the three rural locations. Four one-off 'taster' sessions were held with older men with dementia and their care partners to consult them on the proposed idea and the planned structure of the groups, as well as provide them with an opportunity to engage with the technology. During these sessions, the men provided invaluable information on the technology to include within the main initiative as well as the terminology to use when promoting it. For instance, they suggested that the Nintendo DS be excluded as the screen was small and difficult to navigate with the stylus, and that the word 'technology' be removed from advertisement flyers, as it may have evoked fear in some potential participants, and replaced with words such as 'gadgets' and 'gismos'. Furthermore, during the subsequent delivery and evaluation of the technological initiatives, the men were also engaged as part of the collaborative working relationship. This included providing feedback at the end of every session on the success of the activities and the layout of the room, as well as making suggestions on future games and applications they would like to play on the various devices. This ensured that the groups sustained their appeal throughout the research. In addition to this, the men contributed to the successful funding applications that were used to obtain money to maintain the initiatives, including taking photographs depicting their experiences of participating in the initiatives and providing quotes that highlighted their achievements. This collaborative approach empowered the men and was an important contributing factor for the success of the technological initiative.

Having a flexible and adaptable approach

The aim of all facilitators collaborating with people living with dementia, and particularly facilitators who are unknown to the rural community, is to become accepted and trusted by the group, moving from a position of 'outsider' to 'insider' (Bryce, 2013). This will ensure that richer and more honest feedback can be collected throughout the delivery of the initiative, thereby guaranteeing it remains appealing to those attending. When forming working partnerships with older men with dementia, it is likely that facilitators will need to be flexible and adaptable in their approach, and perhaps move outside of their comfort zone, to successfully engage with the multiple masculinities that will inevitably be at play. For instance, in the work drawn on here, it was notable that some men aligned with more performative masculinities that demonstrated physical strength and capability as well as competitiveness. In these cases, it was necessary for the facilitator to adopt a more outgoing persona and engage in activities such as ten-pin bowling, boxing, darts or golf, either competing against the men or teaming up with them against a computer avatar, as a means to develop rapport. Other men preferred to demonstrate their masculinities and garner respect from others through discussing their achievements and highlighting their intellectual capabilities or sense of worldliness. These interactions and activities were often more sedentary and relaxed, using the iPad and applications such as Google Earth, to give the men and the facilitator the space and time to share aspects of their life and so develop mutual respect. This highlights the importance of workers not only joining in with the initiative and sharing aspects of their life, to be perceived as part of the group rather than solely its facilitator, but also tailoring their approach accordingly so that they can develop rapport with the men in a way that is likely to be preferred by them.

Furthermore, it is essential that facilitators are flexible in their approach when seeking feedback from older men with dementia regarding the initiative. While some men may be more willing to speak in groups and discuss difficulties encountered when engaging with activities, others may perceive these vulnerabilities as a threat to their masculinities and so withhold this information from other members. In these instances, and certainly during the early stages of the initiative, it may be prudent for facilitators to follow up any group feedback discussions with quick, informal, one-to-one conversations with the men to elicit potentially more insightful information.

Finally, linked to this point, it is necessary for facilitators to be mindful of how their gender may influence relationship dynamics when they seek to develop working collaborations with older men with dementia. Some men, particularly those who value more traditional masculine ideals, may not feel comfortable expressing themselves or admitting their vulnerabilities to women, and so this can prevent them from fully engaging with female facilitators, certainly in the short term. Consequently, it is even more important for female facilitators targeting older men with dementia to be mindful of this and adapt their approach and communication techniques in a flexible way that will enable them to connect and develop rapport with their participants. This is likely to involve participating in the activities, so that they are seen as 'one of the lads', and also focusing any conversations on the men's interests and capabilities rather than their vulnerabilities.

Seeking to create physically and conceptually safe environments for expression

Researchers have acknowledged the importance of creating community initiatives for people with dementia that are both physically safe and encourage them to freely express themselves without fear of reprimand (Phinney et al, 2016). The former aspect can be easily achieved by facilitators through undertaking a risk assessment prior to the delivery of any initiative and identifying and addressing potential hazards for the men's participation in the planned activities. During the technological initiative, venues were selected with the support of an advisory group (established during the consultation period) that were well connected in the rural community (on bus routes or with parking facilities), spacious, accessible for wheelchair users and allowed a lot of natural light in. This ensured safe communal spaces that enabled people to move around freely when engaging with motion sensor technology, such as the Nintendo Wii or Microsoft Kinect, without tripping over wires or hitting others who were watching. The spaciousness of the rooms also meant that more intimate spaces for discussions and smaller group activities on the iPads could be set up away from the group activities. These more intimate spaces were also particularly useful for men to retreat to, if at times they needed some respite from the group.

As well as creating physically safe environments, it is important for facilitators to develop spaces that are psychologically safe and comforting for people with dementia. To achieve this, they must be mindful of the factors that may inhibit or encourage free expression. When working with older men, this requires facilitators to acknowledge the gendered experiences of living with dementia. Consistent with other research within this field (Milligan et al, 2015; Carone et al, 2016), the work we draw on here determined two mechanisms that worked in tandem and contributed to the creation of a psychologically safe space for rural-dwelling older men with dementia. These were a male-only environment consisting solely of older men with dementia, as well as a 'dementia-free' zone where the topics of conversations focused on the men's interests and capabilities rather than their condition and any difficulties they faced (although these were not ignored if the conversations were initiated by the men). Adopting a 'dementia-free' zone is beneficial for those men who are eager to retain a stoic resolve and suppress emotional concerns that might be viewed as feminine, thereby threatening their sense of masculinity. Although the emotional and physical difficulties that men with dementia face are 'unspoken' in this environment, research has shown that they are still acknowledged (Hicks et al, 2019), and this helps to create a sense of community and solidarity that is important for the success of any initiatives targeted at people with dementia (Keyes et al, 2016).

A male-only environment tends to be a novel concept in the lives of rural-dwelling older men with dementia, who often lead a fairly feminised and closed world, speaking and engaging predominantly with their informal care partners and/or dementia support workers, many of whom are women. However, it is an environment that many older men would have been accustomed to during their younger masculine years and as such would feel confident expressing themselves in, without fear of having to curb their language to 'protect' any women present (Milligan et al, 2015). Ensuring the initiative is only attended by men with dementia is likely to enhance its inclusivity by reducing the threat posed to these men of being 'othered' and silenced by some older men without dementia who may seek to exert their perceived superior masculinities and separate themselves from those they view as representing the maligned 'Fourth Age' (McParland et al, 2017), commonly associated with dependency, inferior masculinity and death. When running groups we have noted that within initiatives where care partners wish to stay and watch the activities, this beneficial male-only group atmosphere can be created by ensuring that care partners are seated out of earshot of the activities but still able to view them. In these instances, care partners often use the initiatives as informal support groups for themselves, and some men appreciate the arrangement as it provides them with comfort knowing their care partner is close by.

Adopting a male-only environment is also likely to mean that facilitators will need to recruit male volunteers to support the delivery of any activities. Our work suggests that volunteers did not require previous knowledge of the technology or dementia (and indeed engaging in the groups enhanced their understanding in each of these areas), but that it was essential that they remained open-minded and willing to participate in the group. For instance, during the preliminary stages of the technological initiative, some volunteers were reluctant to engage with the activities and keen to disassociate themselves from the other men in the group who had dementia, thereby hindering the development of a socially cohesive group. Facilitators can overcome this by meeting with the volunteers prior to the commencement of any initiative and outlining their aims for the group and what is expected from them.

Providing meaningful activities that enable the expression of masculinities

Research has stressed the importance of selecting activities that are meaningful to people living with dementia, enabling them to participate in an enjoyable activity that maintains their interests and physical abilities, promotes a sense of purpose and lifelong learning and addresses any psychological needs (Roland and Chappell, 2015; Nyman and Szymczynska, 2016). As such, it is important that facilitators consider their target population beforehand and select activities that fulfil these important criteria. Currently, initiatives that have sought to specifically engage men with dementia have used either football (Solari and Solomons, 2012; Tolson and Schofield, 2012; Carone et al, 2016) or 'shed' activities, including wood work (Milligan et al, 2015). These initiatives have been successful, although, given that older men seek to maintain activities they have undertaken throughout their lives (Genoe and Singleton, 2006; Phinney et al, 2013), they may be limited in scope and only appeal to those with prior interests in football or 'shed' activities during their younger masculine years. As such, facilitators wishing to successfully engage older men with dementia would be advised to consider community initiatives that provide opportunities for participants to engage with a wide range of activities that can be tailored towards their multiple interests and masculinities. An initiative using a range of technological devices that enable access to a vast array of applications and games is likely to offer an important means for facilitators to appeal to and sustain the social inclusion of this hard-to-reach population. This is even more the case given the gendered nature of technology (Ravneberg, 2012), commonly seen as something that is more attractive to men than women.

When selecting activities to run for older men with dementia, facilitators would also be advised to think a little 'outside of the box'. As scholars have posited, some activities can quickly become perceived as typical, or most appropriate for people with dementia (Genoe, 2010). This can result in them becoming the 'go-to' option when dementia practitioners are considering setting up an initiative within a rural community. This is dangerous, as it can perpetuate the myth that people with dementia are a homogenous population, who are only capable of engaging with a few limited activities. Consequently, these initiatives provide few opportunities for participants to challenge public misconceptions of their competencies or to learn new skills that will enable them to continue their lifelong learning, facets that are vital for their sense of social inclusion and wellbeing (Bartlett and O'Connor, 2010; Cutler et al, 2016). If the 'dementia-friendly communities' agenda is to be realised (ADI, 2017), people with dementia must feel socially included within society and be provided with the opportunities to challenge the stigma and public misunderstandings of the condition that can be detrimental to their wellbeing. Our work suggests that a technological initiative may be one means for facilitators to achieve this. First, it provides people with dementia the means to engage with commercially available technology that is ubiquitous within society, rather than the potentially stigmatised dementia-specific devices, and so challenge their own perceptions of their capabilities. This is important for enhancing participants' sense of self-esteem and confidence in their abilities. Second, it provides them with the space to contest public perceptions of their abilities, and particularly for older men, the negative social constructions associated with an 'old man' that can detrimentally affect their willingness to participate in activities (Wiersma and Chesser, 2011). Again, this is important for participants' wellbeing and is unlikely to be achieved through 'shed' activities that are typically associated with the 'old man'. Finally, it gives people an opportunity to reconnect and feel socially included within contemporary culture. This can be particularly appealing for older men with dementia, who during their younger masculine years may have perceived themselves as being at the forefront of society.

When delivering the community initiative, facilitators would be advised to use activities that give older men with dementia the opportunity to connect with others in the group as well as express themselves verbally and physically, thereby catering for the multiple masculinities that are likely to be at play within the group. Physical activities may appeal to those men who favour performative masculinities as they will enable them to demonstrate facets of strength, success, capability and competitiveness, and so garner respect from others present within the group. A particularly important trait that is appealing to some older men with dementia, but often overlooked in community initiatives, is the need for competition. This can be achieved during a technological initiative through the introduction of motion sensor technology such as the Nintendo Wii and Microsoft Kinect that requires people to perform certain actions such as bowling or golf to be successful at the game. Workers can encourage competition during these games by having people compete against others in the group or team up to challenge a computer opponent, such as playing a hole each on a nine-hole golf game against a computer avatar. Furthermore, research has demonstrated that having care partners present to watch such activities (but not participate) can be a useful mechanism to enhance the competitiveness, and positive feelings associated with this, during community initiatives for older men with dementia (Hicks et al, 2019). As posited by other research, this may be due to men using this environment and activity to compete for the respect of their care partner, and so increase their ranking and sense of masculinity compared with the other men present within the group (Genoe and Singleton, 2006). Again, as discussed earlier, it is therefore important for facilitators to consider whether they wish to have care partners present at the initiative and how this will be managed. Encouraging partners to stay within eyeshot but out of earshot may be one way to achieve this without restricting the autonomy of older men with dementia.

Facilitators are also encouraged to provide activities within their initiative that encourage older men with dementia to provide a narrative account of their life and achievements, which is a secondary means for them to garner respect from others present. This may be favoured particularly by those men who do not subscribe to performative masculinities. Research has demonstrated that older men often prefer 'shoulder-to-shoulder' communication when discussing aspects of their life (Milligan et al, 2015). This refers to the concept of talking while engaged in other hands-on tasks as opposed to solely sitting and discussing topics of conversation. Again, our work suggests that technological initiatives provide a useful medium for achieving this appealing 'shoulder-to-shoulder' communication; in our initiatives, the men were more likely to discuss their lives while navigating a technological device such as the iPad and using applications such as Google Earth, YouTube and Game of Life. It was particularly beneficial to introduce these activities early on in the group formation, as the conversations they promoted highlighted the similar interests that the men shared, and so encouraged them to develop friendships. Furthermore, as suggested by other research (Joddrell and Astell, 2016), the iPad was able to stimulate and 'scaffold' conversations through various relevant media (such as video clips or pictures) that could be obtained in that moment and so support more sustained and in-depth discussions as well as ameliorate any memory difficulties the men may have been experiencing. Consequently, this provided them with greater opportunities to talk more confidently and competently about their life experiences and achievements associated with their masculinities.

When delivering activities for older men with dementia, it is important for facilitators to reduce the amount of pressure placed on the men to perform to a certain standard. This can be achieved through creating a psychologically safe environment, as discussed previously, but also through using activities that are fun and are tailored towards their capabilities rather than emphasising their difficulties. When delivering technological initiatives, it is imperative that facilitators trial the devices and applications prior to introducing them to the group and consider the difficulties that some attendees may experience as well as potential solutions. For instance, our work suggests that some people with dementia may find it difficult to use their fingers to engage with the iPad and so a stylus may be more intuitive for them. A list of potential difficulties as well as solutions for each device can be seen in Table 8.2. To further reduce any pressure or fear that people with dementia may experience when engaging with off-the-shelf gaming technology, facilitators would be advised to take the following steps:

- Introduce games that are slow-paced and have simple objectives within the preliminary sessions of the initiative. This will ensure that people have adequate time to engage with them and develop their confidence with the technology.

- Ensure that the volume on the games is turned up, as the music is often entertaining and will create a playful and relaxed atmosphere that will encourage participation.
- Do not set people up to fail. Ensure that the games are initially set at the easiest level; it can always be increased as the players improve.
- Invite those who are more confident about engaging with the technology to go first. This is likely to encourage others to participate. Alternatively encourage the more apprehensive participants to pair up with other members of the group or with others known to them. This may give them more confidence to explore the technology together.

As the technological initiative progresses, it is likely that men's confidence with the technology will increase. At this point, it may be feasible to introduce more complicated games and/or increase the difficulty levels. However, it is important that before doing this, facilitators have developed a socially cohesive and friendly group atmosphere. This can serve to relieve any tension or disappointment that men may feel if struggling to engage with the games. The time to achieve this is likely to vary from group to group and within different settings. For instance, our own experiences are consistent with wider research that has posited that people living in 'bypassed' rural communities may develop a stronger sense of solidarity than those living in 'bucolic' rural communities (Keating et al, 2013). Consequently, the time to introduce these more complicated technologies and games should be left to the discretion of the facilitator.

Furthermore, our work highlighted the need for facilitators to be mindful when introducing games to older men with dementia that are associated with their previous leisure interests. This can inadvertently evoke a sense of pressure for participants to perform to a high standard, particularly if they were once adept at the activity. This can be detrimental to their wellbeing if the expected standard is not achieved, emphasising participants' current shortcomings compared with the younger masculinities they once aligned with. Facilitators can seek to ameliorate such situations by situating the blame for the men's performance on the technology and so diffusing any potential threat to their masculinities. In these situations, it is also advantageous for the men to be surrounded by a supportive group.

Managing masculinities and creating a cohesive group

The aim for any community initiative is to create a cohesive group. This can be particularly challenging for workers within 'bucolic' rural communities that may not have the sense of camaraderie and 'underdog' spirit that is common with 'bypassed' communities (Keating et al, 2013), and when seeking to create an environment that does not temper the masculinities of older participants with dementia. Our research demonstrated that open environments could sometimes encourage sexist, racist and homophobic conversations, with some men using deriding language as a means to express and exert their masculinities over those populations they perceived to be inferior to them. While such views can be difficult to listen to as a facilitator, it is important to continue to encourage the men to express their opinions, but, of course, to challenge them where appropriate. On occasion it may be beneficial for facilitators to establish a set of ground rules at the beginning of the initiative that outline the topics of conversation that the group agrees are suitable.

Furthermore, encouraging men to express themselves may highlight the juxtaposition of their perceived social positioning, interests and masculinities within the group, thereby leading to tensions and the formation of an 'us' and 'them' mentality. Facilitators should carefully manage such situations so as to create a cohesive group that is supportive when activities are introduced. Where differences and tensions result from participants' initial unwillingness to engage with other men with dementia, whom they associate with lesser forms of masculinity, facilitators can manage the situation by removing the 'dementia' focus from the group and encouraging discussions that centre on people's lives and interests, particularly within the early stages of group formation. Highlighting the commonalities between participants, over and above their dementia, can enable them to become a more cohesive unit over time. However, it is also important to be mindful that on occasion, such masculinities may clash so violently that any attempts to highlight commonalities are futile and harmony may only occur within the group following the departure of any disruptive participants. It is important not to take this to heart. Remember, people with dementia are a heterogeneous group and so it is always likely that some personalities will never get on, just as you would expect in all walks of life.

This section has drawn on our own experiences of running a technological initiative within rural communities and situated these within the wider academic literature to provide lessons for facilitators wishing to successfully engage older men with dementia. It has emphasised the importance of developing these collaborative working relationships with older men with dementia from the design phase of the initiative and sustaining them throughout the subsequent implementation, delivery and evaluation phases. To achieve this, it is important that facilitators acknowledge the influence of masculinities on the lived experience of dementia and seek to engage older men in ways that enable them to express and reaffirm these experiences. This will require facilitators to be flexible in their approach and to provide activities that are tailored towards the interests, capabilities and masculinities of the men within a physically and psychological safe space. Drawing on the lessons highlighted here, we now provide a list of recommendations for people interested in developing and delivering community activities for older men with dementia in rural areas.

Recommendations

To develop successful collaborative working relationships with rural-dwelling older men with dementia, facilitators are advised to take the following steps:

- Democratise all phases of the planning, implementation, delivery and evaluation of community initiatives, and position rural–dwelling older men with dementia as the 'experts by experience' throughout. This is likely to appeal to participants' masculinities and provide them with a sense of empowerment that will ensure their sustained engagement and so contribute to the continued success of the initiative.
- Be flexible when engaging with older men with dementia and be mindful that a facilitator's approach as well as their gender may promote or threaten men's sense of masculinities, thereby influencing their willingness to contribute. Tailoring the approach according to the individual and focusing conversations around the strengths, achievements and capabilities of the older men is likely to reap the most rewards.
- Provide multiple activities that can be tailored towards the interests, capabilities and masculinities of the older men. This will ensure that the activities are meaningful to them, providing them with a sense of purpose as well as the opportunity to express their masculinities

and so garner respect from others present. However, it is important to be mindful that some activities may evoke a sense of pressure on participants to perform to certain standards. The perceived failure to achieve such standards may be detrimental to the men's wellbeing. In these instances it is important that facilitators provide reassurance and potentially look to situate the blame on other external factors, such as the technology, so as not to pose a threat to participants' masculinities.

- Think 'outside of the box' and offer activities that are not typically associated with people with dementia. These activities are likely to appeal to older men and will help them to challenge their assumptions of their capabilities as well as provide them with a platform to resist the negative social constructions associated with dementia and the 'old man', Promoting the benefits of such non-typical dementia activities will help to raise dementia awareness and positively contribute to the wider social inclusion agenda.

- Create physically and psychologically safe spaces where older men are enabled to express and reaffirm their masculinities. To this end, facilitators may find it useful to promote male-only environments that consist solely of older men with dementia as well as introduce 'dementia-free' zones.

- Be positive! Remember that people with dementia are a heterogeneous population. Supporting older men with dementia to express and enact their masculinities is likely to emphasise their differences and so lead to personality clashes. While it may be possible to manage differences in some situations, in others it is likely that any such efforts will prove futile. In these instances, it may be that a socially cohesive unit can only be formed after certain participants have left the group.

This chapter has outlined the urgent need for facilitators of services and community initiatives to improve their approaches to dementia care so that they can better appeal to and engage rural-dwelling older men with dementia with community initiatives that are likely to enhance their wellbeing and sense of social inclusion. Although this can often be challenging, due in part to the health-seeking behaviours of some older men with dementia, it is important that facilitators learn from our experiences and adopt a more refined approach when working with this population that acknowledges their gendered identities and provides safe spaces where older men can enact and maximise their masculine capital.

Table 8.2: The benefits, challenges and potential solutions to using off-the-shelf gaming technology

Technology	Description	Benefits	Challenges	Potential solutions
Apple iPad	Touchscreen tablet	Portable, allowing freedom of movement and use in any room Range of applications available (free and purchasable) to tailor activities to participants' interests Can be used both with and without internet access Intuitive touchscreen	Small screens can be difficult to view for the ageing eye or for those with eyesight limitations People with dexterity challenges may find it difficult to operate Older iPads can be heavier and difficult for people to hold and interact with	A TV connector enables the iPad screen to be viewed through a television An iPad stylus, which operates like a pen, facilitates greater control when pressing the iPad screen Newer versions of the iPad such as iPad Air are lighter and easier to hold. iPad covers also provide a table support for the device so it does not need to be physically held
Microsoft Kinect	Gaming device that requires an Xbox 360 or the newer Xbox One (which can be bought together) and a TV screen Sensor technology detects a player's body, enabling them to interact with the game without the need for a hand-held controller The built-in camera function can capture videos of players as they interact with the games	The lack of a controller means players do not need to push any buttons. This makes it easier to use, as only actions are required Wide range of games that promote activity and mental and physical stimulation	Sensors can become confused if participants use wheelchairs or are supported by other people Sensors can detect other people within its vicinity, thereby hindering playability Some players may experience disconnect between themselves and the games as there is no physical object connecting them	Players can be supported to engage out of their chair Walking sticks can be used as golf clubs Ensure there is clear space surrounding the player and between them and the TV screen Practitioners can mirror required actions away from the screen to support players

Technology	Description	Benefits	Challenges	Potential solutions
Nintendo Wii	Gaming device that uses sensor technology to detect sensors with in hand-held controllers. The sensor detects the player holding the controller and then mimics their hand movements on screen	The device will only pick up the players holding the controllers. Suitable for wheelchair users as players remain seated	Players with dexterity challenges can find it difficult to press buttons while simultaneously carrying out actions. The controller may come out of a player's hand as they engage with the game. Error messages are common and are designed to encourage people to beat their score, but players may perceive them in a negative light	With practice players are likely to improve on the game mechanics. Gaming accessories such as a steering wheel can be purchased to overcome controller issues. Ensure that the controller straps are fastened around a player's hand before the game begins. Ensure that players feel supported before engaging with competitive games
Nintendo Balance Board	Gaming device that connects to the Nintendo Wii and requires players to stand on a balance board, which detects lower body movements	Provides access to additional games that will challenge a player's balance and ability to shift their weight between their feet, thereby providing both mental and physical stimulation	Games may require exaggerated lower body movements (bending knees or rotating hips), which can be challenging for some players, particularly those with walking aids. Some players may be unstable on the board (either stepping on or off it, or when engaging with the game). A change of player may disrupt the balance board settings, which can interrupt the game	Simpler games are available that do not require exaggerated movements. Practitioners should be vigilant when supporting people to use the board, and enable them to practise movements on the floor beforehand. The balance board may have to be reset when there is a change of player, during which time participants can reflect on previous players' performance
Nintendo Wii Motion	Gaming device that connects to the Nintendo Wii controller. It detects small movements in players' wrists and arms	Provides access to games that require fine motor skills	Some games require exaggerated wrist and hand movements that may be difficult for players with dexterity challenges	Over time and with practice, players are likely to improve at the game. Simpler, alternative, games are available that do not require exaggerated movements

References

ADI (Alzheimer's Disease International) (2017) *Dementia friendly communities: Global developments* (2nd edn), London: ADI.

ADI (2018) *World Alzheimer Report 2018. The state of the art dementia research: New frontiers*, London: ADI.

Australian Government (2010) *National male health policy: Building on the strengths of Australian males*, Canberra: Department of Health and Ageing, Australian Government.

Baker, P. (2015) *Review of the National Men's Health Policy and Action Plan 2008–2013*, Dublin: Health Service Executive.

Baker, S., Warburton, J., Hodgkin, S. and Pascal, J. (2017) 'The supportive network: rural disadvantaged older people and ICT', *Ageing & Society*, 37(6): 1291–309.

Bartlett, R. and Brannelly, T. (2018) *Life at home for people with a dementia*, London: Routledge.

Bartlett, R. and O'Connor, D. (2010) *Broadening the dementia debate: Towards social citizenship*, Bristol: Policy Press.

Bartlett, R., Gjernes, T., Lotherington, A.T. and Obstefelder, A. (2016) 'Gender, citizenship and dementia care: a scoping review of studies to inform policy and future research', *Health and Social Care in the Community*, 26(1): 14–26.

Bowes, A., Dawson, A. and McCabe, L. (2018) 'RemoDem: delivering support for people with dementia in remote areas', *Dementia*, 17(3): 297–314.

Bryce, H. (2013) 'Navigating multiple roles as a researcher in a Photovoice project', *Groupwork*, 22(3): 33–48.

Carone, L., Tischler, V. and Dening, T. (2016) 'Football and dementia: a qualitative investigation of a community based sports group for men with early onset dementia', *Dementia*, 15(6): 1358–76.

Clarke, C. L. and Bailey, C. (2016) 'Narrative citizenship, resilience and inclusion with dementia: on the inside or on the outside of physical and social places', *Dementia*, 15(3): 434–52.

Clarke, L.H. and Bennett, E. (2013) '"You learn to live with all the things that are wrong with you": gender and the experience of multiple chronic conditions in later life', *Ageing & Society*, 33(2): 342–60.

Clarke, L.H. and Lefkowich, M. (2018) '"I don't really have any issue with masculinity": older Canadian men's perceptions and experiences of embodied masculinity', *Journal of Aging Studies*, 45: 18–24.

Cohen-Mansfield, J., Thein, K., Dakheel-Ali, M., and Marx, M. S. (2010) 'The underlying meaning of stimuli: Impact on engagement of persons with dementia', *Psychiatry research, 177*(1): 216–22.

Connell, R. and Pearse, R. (2015) *Gender: In world perspective* (3rd edn), Cambridge: Polity Press.

Connell, R.W. (2005) *Masculinities* (2nd edn), Cambridge: Polity Press.

Connell, R.W. and Messerschmidt, J.W. (2005) 'Hegemonic masculinity rethinking the concept', *Gender & Society*, 19: 829–59.

Coston, B. and Kimmel, M. (2013) 'Aging men, masculinity and Alzheimer's: caretaking and caregiving in the new millennium', in Kampf, A., Marshall, B.L. and Petersen, A. (eds) *Aging men, masculinities and modern medicine* Abingdon and New York, NY: Routledge, pp 191–200.

Courtenay, W.H. (2000) 'Constructions of masculinity and their influence on men's well-being: a theory of gender and health', *Social Science & Medicine*, 50: 1385–401.

Cutler, C. (2018) 'Quality of life and digital gaming technology: the benefits of a technology based intervention for community dwelling people with dementia', Unpublished doctoral thesis, Bournemouth University.

Cutler, C., Hicks, B. and Innes, A. (2016) 'Does digital gaming enable healthy aging for community-dwelling people with dementia?', *Games and Culture*, 11(1–2): 104–29.

Dove, E. and Astell, A.J. (2017) 'The use of motion-based technology for people living with dementia or mild cognitive impairment: a literature review', *Journal of Medical Internet Research*, 19(1): e3.

Dupuis, S.L., Gillies, J., Carson, J., Whyte, C., Genoe, R., Loiselle, L. and Sadler, L. (2012) 'Moving beyond patient and client approaches: mobilizing "authentic partnerships" in dementia care, support and services', *Dementia*, 11(4): 427–52.

Dupuis, S., McAiney, C.A., Fortune, D., Ploeg, J. and Witt, L. (2016) 'Theoretical foundations guiding culture change: the work of the Partnerships in Dementia Care Alliance', *Dementia*, 15(1): 85–105.

Genoe, M.R. (2010) 'Leisure as resistance within the context of dementia', *Leisure Studies*, 29(3): 303–20.

Genoe, M.R. and Singleton, J.F. (2006) 'Older men's leisure experiences across their lifespan', *Topics in Geriatric Rehabilitation*, 22(4): 348–56.

Hammer, J.H., Vogel, D.L. and Heimerdinger-Edwards, S.R. (2013) 'Men's help seeking: examination of differences across community size, education, and income', *Psychology of Men & Masculinities*, 14(1): 65.

Hicks, B. (2016) 'Exploring the use of a commercial digital gaming technological initiative to enable social inclusion for community-dwelling older men with dementia in rural England', Unpublished doctoral thesis, Bournemouth University.

Hicks, B., Innes, A. and Nyman, A. (2019) 'Exploring the "active mechanisms" for engaging rural-dwelling older men with dementia in a community technological initiative', *Ageing & Society*: 1–33.

Hulko, W. (2009) 'From "not a big deal" to "hellish": experiences of older people with dementia', *Journal of Aging Studies*, 23(3): 131–44.

Joddrell, P. and Astell, A.J. (2016) 'Studies involving people with dementia and touchscreen technology: a literature review', *JMIR Rehabilitation and Assistive Technologies*, 3(2): e10.

Keating, N., Eales, J. and Phillips, J.E. (2013) 'Age-friendly rural communities: conceptualizing 'Best-Fit', *Canadian Journal on Aging*, 32(4): 319–32.

Kenigsberg, P.-A., Aquino, J.-P., Bérard, A., Brémond, F., Charras, K., Dening, T. and Innes, A. (2017) 'Assistive technologies to address capabilities of people with dementia: from research to practice', *Dementia*, doi: 1471301217714093.

Kenigsberg, P.-A., Aquino, J.-P., Berard, A., Gzil, F., Andrieu, S., Banerjee, S. and Mangialasche, F. (2016) 'Dementia beyond 2025: knowledge and uncertainties', *Dementia*, 15(1): 6–21.

Keyes, S.E., Clarke, C.L., Wilkinson, H., Alexjuk, E.J., Wilcockson, J., Robinson, L. and Cattan, M. (2016) '"We're all thrown in the same boat…": a qualitative analysis of peer support in dementia care', *Dementia*, 15(4): 560–77.

Kolanowski, A., Litaker, M., Buettner, L., Moeller, J. and Costa, J.P.T. (2011) 'A randomized clinical trial of theory-based activities for the behavioral symptoms of dementia in nursing home residents', *Journal of the American Geriatrics Society*, 59(6): 1032–41.

Levant, R.F. and Habben, C. (2003) 'The new psychology of men: application to rural men', in B. Stamm (ed) *Rural behavioural health care: An interdisciplinary guide*, Washington, DC: American Psychological Association, pp 171–80.

McParland, P., Kelly, F. and Innes, A. (2017. 'Dichotomising dementia: is there another way?', *Sociology of Health & Illness*, 39(2): 258–69.

Meiland, F., Innes, A., Mountain, G., Robinson, L., van der Roest, H., García-Casal, J. A., …, Dröes, R.-M. (2017) 'Technologies to support community-dwelling persons with dementia: a position paper on issues regarding development, usability, effectiveness and cost-effectiveness, deployment, and ethics', *JMIR Rehabilitation and Assistive Technologies*, 4(1): e1.

Milligan, C., Payne, S., Bingley, A. and Cockshott, Z. (2015) 'Place and wellbeing: shedding light on activity interventions for older men', *Ageing & Society*, 35(1): 124–49.

Nyman, S.R. and Szymczynska, P. (2016) 'Meaningful activities for improving the wellbeing of people with dementia: beyond mere pleasure to meeting fundamental psychological needs', *Perspectives in Public Health*, 136(2): 99–107.

Øksnebjerg, L., Diaz-Ponce, A., Gove, D., Moniz-Cook, E., Mountain, G., Chattat, R. and Woods, B. (2018) 'Towards capturing meaningful outcomes for people with dementia in psychosocial intervention research: a pan-European consultation', *Health Expectations*, 21(6): 1056–65.

Phinney, A., Dahlke, S. and Purves, B. (2013) 'Shifting patterns of everyday activity in early dementia experiences of men and their families', *Journal of Family Nursing*, 19(3): 348–74.

Phinney, A., Kelson, E., Baumbusch, J., O'Connor, D. and Purves, B. (2016) 'Walking in the neighbourhood: performing social citizenship in dementia', *Dementia*, 15(3): 381–94.

Ravneberg, B. (2012) 'Usability and abandonment of assistive technology', *Journal of Assistive Technologies*, 6(4): 259–69.

Roland, K.P. and Chappell, N.L. (2015) 'Meaningful activity for persons with dementia: family caregiver perspectives', *American Journal of Alzheimer's Disease and other Dementias*, 30(6): 559–68.

Sandberg, L.J. (2018) 'Dementia and the gender trouble?: theorising dementia, gendered subjectivity and embodiment', *Journal of Aging Studies*, 45: 25–31.

Sloan, C., Conner, M. and Gough, B. (2015) 'How does masculinity impact on health? A quantitative study of masculinity and health behavior in a sample of UK men and women', *Psychology of Men & Masculinities*, 16(2): 206.

Solari, C.A. and Solomons, L. (2012) 'The World Cup effect: using football to engage men with dementia', *Dementia*, 11(5): 699–702.

Spindler, E. (2015) *Beyond the prostate: Brazil's national healthcare policy for men (PNAISH)*, EMERGE Case Study 1, Promundo-US, Sonke Gender Justice and the Institute of Development Studies, Brighton: IDS.

Szymczynska, P., Innes, A., Stark, C. and Mason, A. (2011) 'A review of diagnostic process and postdiagnostic support for people with dementia in rural areas' *Journal of Primary Care and Community Health*, 2(4). 262–76.

Thompson Jr, E.H. and Bennett, K.M. (2015) 'Measurement of masculinity ideologies: a (critical) review', *Psychology of Men & Masculinities*, 16(2): 115.

Thompson Jr, E.H. and Langendoerfer, K.B. (2016) 'Older men's blueprint for "being a man"', *Men and Masculinities*, 19(2): 119–47.

Tolson, D. and Schofield, I. (2012) 'Football reminiscence for men with dementia: lessons from a realistic evaluation', *Nursing Inquiry*, 19(1): 63–70.

Twigg, J. (2018) 'Dress, gender and the embodiment of age: men and masculinities', *Ageing & Society*, pp 1–21.

Wentzell, E.A. (2013). *Maturing masculinities: Aging, chronic illness, and viagra in Mexico*: Durham, NC: Duke University Press.

White, A. (2011) 'The state of men's health in Europe: how do we compare in the UK?', *Trends in Urology & Men's Health*, 2: 12–16.

White, A., de Sousa, B., de Visser, R., Hogston, R., Madsen, S.A., Makara, P., Richardson, N. and Zatonski, W. (2011) *The state of men's health in Europe*, Brussels: European Commission.

Wiersma, E. and Chesser, S. (2011) 'Masculinity, ageing bodies, and leisure', *Annals of Leisure Research*, 14(2–3): 242–59.

Wiersma, E.C., O'Connor, D.L., Loiselle, L., Hickman, K., Heibein, B., Hounam, B. and Mann, J. (2016) 'Creating space for citizenship: the impact of group structure on validating the voices of people with dementia', *Dementia*, 15(3): 414–33.

Yousaf, O., Grunfeld, E.A. and Hunter, M.S. (2015) 'A systematic review of the factors associated with delays in medical and psychological help-seeking among men', *Health Psychology Review*, 9(2): 264–76.

9

Farm-based care: providing meaningful activities in dementia care as an alternative to 'standard day care' in the UK

Fiona Marshall

Dementia care is changing. Research on human wellbeing assumes that engaging in meaningful, purposeful activities is essential to maintain a sense of personal control, contribution and independence. Connecting with nature is thought to enhance a sense of wellbeing, although clear evidence of these benefits among those with chronic health conditions, poor mobility and cognitive capacity is less established. What makes for wellbeing among those who are involved in using and delivering rural dementia care? Experiences of ageing, having dementia and/or being a caregiver are diverse. Understanding this diversity, and especially the fluid intersections where place, personal histories and future needs all converge, is necessary. This chapter examines two forms of care that offer support and care in rural communities in England. Day care generally consists of sessional care that takes places in buildings adapted or designed to accommodate older people. By contrast, farm-based care primarily takes place in the outdoors surrounded by natural connections in mostly rural locations that are not necessarily designed to accommodate older people with dementia. By comparing these two very different contexts, this chapter discusses the possible ways each can adopt perspectives and practices from farm-based care to enhance dementia care in more standard places.

It is well documented that older people living in more rural and remote areas of the UK are vulnerable to rural specific barriers in addition to the barriers associated with declining health and living longer (Bennett et al, 2018). Health barriers in the older population tend to include lowered independence because of reduced physical mobility, chronic pain, anxiety and isolation as a consequence of multiple health conditions (BGS, 2018). Those who live in rural areas are likely to face rurality-specific issues as they age, which can exacerbate the challenges of managing to live with often multiple health issues.

Rural-specific barriers include location issues with housing, transport, digital connectivity, fuel poverty and increased isolation and associated loneliness (Keating, 2009; Alzheimer's Society, 2018). Many of these barriers are masked by attractive ideas of rurality as representative of romantic retirement idylls (Keating, 2009). While many rural regions are indeed beautiful and offer tranquility, they may also be harsh and demanding environments, which can exacerbate the challenges of living independently with a sense of wellbeing. As people age in rural and remote regions, they may find themselves facing complex multiple barriers related to place yet hold deep emotional attachment to living in these locations (Cutchin, 2018). Challenges to maintaining independence, wellbeing and remaining in place, especially as multiple chronic conditions develop, may further be exacerbated by many assumptions about rural ageing by care providers (Alzheimer's Society, 2018). Culturally, rural dwellers with dementia may find services, often urban-centric approaches to day care, alien to their own expectations and experiences of life. Rural dwellers often have a preference for being in the outdoors and keeping physically busy with everyday tasks. These preferences are likely to be rooted in earlier working or home lives, such as homemaking and farming, and so reflect individual and local community identities.

Living with dementia affects many different aspects of a person's life (including the individual's physical and mental health, cognitive function, and social and home environment). Over time, dementia disrupts and causes memory failure, personality changes, perceptual challenges and problems carrying out daily activities. Dementia progression may occur over many years with the 'early' to 'moderate' stages lasting around six to nine years. During these stages, the majority of care is provided by family, often elderly spouses, with minimal respite or formal support. Spending longer in the milder stages of dementia, rather than longer at the more severe stages, will lead to a better quality of life among families (Lewis et al, 2014). Delaying the progression of dementia and frailty may lead to longer periods of wellbeing, fewer family care demands and lowered health and social care demands (Lewis et al, 2014). Connecting with nature is thought to enhance a sense of wellbeing, although clear evidence of these benefits among those with chronic health conditions, frailty and dementia is less established (Bragg and Atkins, 2016).

The term farm-based care will be used in this chapter as an alternative to the more common terms related to this type of dementia care, such as care farming and social farming. This type of care has been established in the Netherlands, Italy, Germany and Japan for many years and in many forms (Hassink et al, 2017). Farm-based care includes a mixture of activities such as animal care, horticulture, crafts, cooking, creative arts, walking, birdwatching,- and socialising (de Bruin et al, 2010; Elings, 2012; Natural England, 2017). Care is provided, depending on the facilities, as sessional or whole-day periods, multiple days per week, or monthly and/or residential periods. In the UK, people with dementia are less likely to access such provision, although the number of attendees is on the increase and is thought to account for up to 12 per cent of all forms of beneficiaries attending farm-based care (Natural England, 2017). This is why it is timely to consider the rise of farm-based care in the UK, especially for those living and working in rural and remote locations.

This chapter aims to explore farm-based care as an exemplar of dementia care that provides an alternative to the more standard day-centred care often provided in the UK. Farm-based care will not appeal to all. This chapter focuses on the ethos of dementia care, which includes taking risks and encouraging new opportunities to take part in 'work-kind', 'being-in-nature' activities and connect with others. Drawing on international evidence, the chapter describes the types of activity available and the ways in which they can help promote wellbeing among people with dementia and their family caregivers. Additionally, it makes suggestions for transferring some of these activities into more standard settings to enable providers to consider ways of increasing opportunities for connecting with nature and the outdoors. This chapter explores some of the ways people living with dementia can continue to contribute towards maintaining their independence, learn new skills and share old ones, in a supportive manner.

Policy and organisational aspects of care in dementia care

There is an established geography to the age distribution of most countries, with variable rates of change in each country (Phillips and Feng, 2018). Worldwide the number of people living in rural and urban areas is roughly equal. Older people are over-represented in rural areas; worldwide the proportion of older people in rural areas is growing far more rapidly than that in urban areas (Keating, 2009). Concurrently, there are reduced numbers of working-age people to provide older people with paid and unpaid care. Migrations towards urban areas for employment and educational opportunities have resulted in a steady decline in the numbers of younger working-age people living in rural areas across the world. Lowered rates of childbirth in Western countries contribute towards a growing need to reconsider the current and future organisation of health and social care. Coupled with movement on retirement of older people from urban to rural areas, the age distribution in rural areas is often skewed with the greatest increases in the oldest old people (those over the age of 85) being found in some of the most remote areas (ONS, 2015).

It is not surprising that the demographics of rural ageing in the UK indicate that there are proportionally higher numbers of people aged over 65 years living in rural communities compared with urban ones. Typically, 17 per cent of the total population in the UK comprises people over 65 years of age; in rural areas, this rises to 28 per cent (Rural England 2017). At parish levels (local regions), some 52 per cent of rural populations comprise people over 65 years (Rural England, 2019). Notably, within rural areas a higher proportion of older people are living beyond 80 years compared with the proportion of urban dwellers (ONS, 2017). These rural demographics and general infrastructure challenges have implications for addressing local care needs as the supply of skilled working-age adults able to deliver care is significantly lower than in urban areas (Keating, 2009).

Living longer is often associated with diminishing health and especially the onset of multiple chronic conditions including dementia (Prince et al, 2014; BGS, 2018). Dementia is strongly associated with increased ageing and presents particular challenges for those living in rural and remote areas (Alzheimer's Society, 2018). Having multiple chronic conditions and living in a rural area are two factors likely to affect the ability to maintain independence in everyday activities, leading to a need for care and support to enable affected individuals to remain in their own homes and communities (LGA, 2018). Remaining in one's own home and maintaining connections with the local community are priorities for individuals as they age. To maintain themselves in their own homes, many older people in rural communities are reliant on spouses and other family members to provide most of the day-to-day care. However, there are many individuals living in rural communities alone without any regular or local family support, who often manage despite multiple health difficulties (Kane and Cook, 2013). In some rural and remote communities, dementia carries a stigma and so individuals are more likely to access dementia-specific support later.

Such hidden, isolated individuals may not come to the attention of formal services until a crisis occurs, such as acute hospital admission or, distressingly, a winter-associated death (Watkins et al, 2017).

Current social and community care policies in the UK, and most Western countries, aim to support as many people as possible to remain in their own homes (WHO, 2012; NHS, 2014, 2019). In the UK, the Five Year Forward View (NHS, 2014) and the more recent NHS Long Term Plan (2019) do not distinguish between geographical locations in relation to service accessibility. The geographical location of own-home care delivery, as rural and remote, is rarely considered in health and social care policy and practice, leading to heightened risk of structural social exclusion (Warburton et al, 2016). This means that older people requiring care and support for multiple health and social needs may be inadvertently disadvantaged by virtue of where they live. Rural dwellers face many challenges; in the absence of local, regular, own-home support and/or day care, people may find themselves having to move into residential care despite this being contrary to their own wishes and the UK policy directive of supporting people to remain in their own home (Lewis et al, 2014; NHS, 2014). It is known that moves into institutional care tend to be earlier and further away from their community for rural dwellers than for urban dwellers, regardless of the level of care need (Keating, 2009). Some individuals seek residential and nursing home care earlier than would normally expected given the stage of dementia (LGA, 2018). This indicates a possible lack of adequate support for families affected by dementia that matches their cultural expectations and needs in their local communities (Alzheimer's Society, 2018).

In rural communities, there is likely to be a greater reliance on family and unpaid care rather than on statutorily funded and provided care (Henning-Smith and Lahr, 2018). Care in the community has emerged as care *by* the community, meaning that the majority of care is provided not by statutory or paid workers but by local residents themselves, who are often retirees. Older people are diverse individuals who seek choice and opportunities in their care provision that match their personal preferences (Alzheimer's Society, 2018). In the UK, statutorily provided direct payments enable individuals to purchase their own care, which in theory increases choice and competition in the markets of care. While there is a growing need for greater choice and flexible forms of care, this has yet to be fully realised in rural and remote areas of the UK. Scarce statutory community care provision in the UK focuses on providing care for those with high-level needs, such as complex assistance with personal care, as in frailty states and more challenging stages of dementia (Rahman et al, 2018). This means that those with less complex, but nonetheless very real, needs may benefit from more tailored care – particularly that which encourages rehabilitation and maximisation of independence for as long as possible, given that many people live with mild to moderate dementia for eight to ten years before developing the complex care needs that typify the later stage of the condition (Lewis et al, 2014). These forms of care may include social groups, day centres, creative arts, men in sheds and farm-based care. However, in many rural areas of the UK, there is little choice in dementia care provision, with a tendency to deliver sporadic and universal models of care (Bennett et al, 2018).

Best care is often expressed by beneficiaries and family members as care that is least task-orientated and includes genuine choices and opportunities to maximise independence. In dementia care, best care is often described as person-centred (Kitwood, 1997) or relationship-centred (Rahman et al, 2018), both indicating the importance of sustained relationship building with caregivers and beneficiaries. Typically, the best dementia care is described as providing meaningful, personalised care that aims to restore function, ameliorate periods of decline and seek to delay progression of the disabling conditions associated with dementia (BPS, 2016). Characteristically, such care includes helping people to continue to live well with dementia and health needs by self-management and appropriate support to maintain a sense of control, identity and community connections.

Statutory and third sector providers, which deliver the majority of formalised care in the UK, tend to be clustered in more urban areas, such as towns and cities (Skinner and Winterton, 2018). Standard older people's care includes group sessions, day centre care, residential respite, caregiver support and information provision. While there is a thrust towards more digitalised care and support as a way towards inclusion, this can be further excluding among those living in communities with a lack of robust digital infrastructure to support technologies such as broadband and mobile signals (Rural England, 2019). More people, including working-age adults, living in these regions of sparse connectivity will be more likely to have low digital skills (Alzheimer's Society, 2017). Additionally, provider staff and volunteers may not have the resource capacity to respond to those living in rural and remote regions. In a dominant culture of target setting where care delivery effectiveness is measured by crude means such as number and length of time per contact, staff may be less inclined or able to provide equitable services to those living further from urban locations (Bennett et al, 2018). In the context of rurality and dementia care, it is clear that urban–centric models of care design and delivery are not likely to neatly fit rural contexts.

Standard forms of dementia day care in the UK tend towards sessional care and support groups, often short weekly or monthly sessions. These forms of care tend to provide social connections and the opportunities to take part in activities such as crafts, music, poetry, games and gentle exercise. While many also provide gardening and being outdoors where possible, these tend to be very passive experiences, such as sitting in the garden. Standard forms of care are not easily adaptable to include or increase opportunities for being in nature or the outdoors because of their physical locations and resources (especially staffing skills, time, equipment and facilities). Staff may feel ill equipped to deliver outdoor and nature-based activities because of their perceptions that such activities carry particular risks to their beneficiaries, self and community that outweigh the potential gains in wellbeing. These risks include increased number and severity of falls, getting lost, increased disorientation and injuries caused by being outdoors. Despite the best attempts by staff, many opportunities for being outdoors are sporadic, of short duration and irregular (de Bruin et al, 2009; Noone et al, 2015). Many activities are confined to the outdoor boundary of the care building and do not take place in the wider community or in public spaces such as allotments. There is a need to determine how these settings can be configured to transfer some of the learning from farm-based care to enable people to benefit by expanding the opportunities to engage in everyday outdoor activities within their communities (Kane and Cook, 2013; Buist et al, 2018).

Alternative forms of rural care, such as farm-based care, can potentially offer therapeutic care to families affected by dementia. Farm-based care is characterised as therapeutic care that takes place in mostly rural agricultural locations (because agriculture most often occurs in rural regions). This form of care can also take place in urban and suburban communities, although the organisational configurations and users are likely to be different from those in rural locations. Such care is also known as care farming, green care farming, social farming and, more broadly, nature-based and green care (Hassink et al, 2017). However, the term farm-based care is preferred by people with dementia, consulted as part of this enquiry, because of the derogatory historical associations with UK institutions for mentally ill people, often referred to as 'funny farms' and 'social farms' as an indication of reliance on financial aid from the state In the UK. Currently not enough is known about the ways in which farm-based care can meet the health and social needs of older adults affected by dementia in the UK.

Workforce consideration

The challenges of providing a rural workforce are complex but include a significantly lowered capacity to provide a skilled care workforce. There are proportionally fewer working-age people living in rural communities and a reluctance of urban workers to travel to rural areas to work in the lower-paid care sector (Dorling and Thomas, 2016; Rural England, 2017). More unproductive time and money are spent travelling to deliver care in rural homes, attending meetings and accessing continuing professional development for staff (Rural England, 2017). Coupled with these longstanding challenges, provision tends to be hub-based in design and located in urban areas, with decreased provision the further the location from these urban centres. The recruitment and retention of care staff in rural areas tends to be erratic, geographically patchy and more expensive to deliver than in urban areas.

The emotional motivations for working in a rural area are complex and distinctive as identified by one scoping review that examined retention of rural health workforce (Cosgrave et al, 2019). However, in some rural areas, these retention challenges have prompted the design and delivery of alternative dementia services by adding leverage to those who may otherwise not choose to work in the care sector. One such form of care is that provided by farms, which can offer the workforce diverse opportunities to work beyond the more standard forms of day care (de Bruin et al, 2010). Retention rates are highest among less institutionalised/standard forms of care (Braedley, 2018), indicating the possible gains in worker wellbeing and work satisfaction. Considering the high turnover of care staff in more standard settings (32 per cent a year in the UK), it is important that greater understanding of the characteristics of working in less standard forms of care is researched.

The ethos of therapeutic care in farm-based care

The characteristics of farm-based care include the perceived benefits of being outdoors or in nature. Being in nature is often assumed to be of benefit to humans by stimulating a sense of wellbeing through the senses (Bragg and Atkins, 2016). Green care often includes being surrounded by elements found in nature such as open sky, water, green landscapes, trees and creatures. However, there has been very little evidence to establish if and how people with dementia may benefit from being in nature for many pragmatic reasons, including the lack of research attention this attracts from major research organisations

(Noone et al, 2015). The majority of green-based dementia care has been developed on anecdotal evidence and the cultural resurgence of being in nature as a positive aspect of human wellbeing. Aligned to green care are philosophical approaches to living a life of inner growth, mindfulness and relatedness with the environment (Clark et al, 2013). While these more esoteric ideas may offer some insight into the values and practices of green care, it is important to prioritise enjoyment, continued learning and hope as key elements in dementia care. Drawing on the evidence available, it is reasonable to assume that farm-based care provides a valuable form of therapeutic care, especially among those who prefer being outdoors and like engaging in practical tasks (Steigen et al, 2016). Among individuals who are naturally more reserved and are comfortable with being alone or simply prefer animals and gardening to people, farm-based care provides much-needed personal space. It can also provide paced activities, slowly building meaningful connections with others. For some, group activities such as dementia cafés can be too demanding, and experienced as unsafe or as an overwhelming emotional bombardment. The need for personal space among people with dementia is often overlooked by providers and seen as a sign of detachment or loneliness. However, as with all forms of care, it needs to be recognised that farm-based care will not suit all people with dementia and may cause distress or even emotional harm to those who find it deeply challenging.

Therapeutic care is provided by professionals with varied backgrounds, typically in occupational therapy, physiotherapy, nursing or social care. The majority of providers also have a tendency towards interests in horticulture and/or animal care. In more rural areas, providers may also be farmers and so the development of a care facility meets the interests of the individual and complements the business needs of the farmer to diversify (Hassink et al, 2018). The models of care, often used implicitly, vary according to the professional background of the provider. There is scant explicit information about the types of models of care used, but they tend towards a hybridisation of the underlying ethos of different care professions. Occupational therapists will lean towards the idea of meaningful occupation in contrast to a more formal nursing therapist who may lean towards the more person-centred care approach commonly used with those affected by dementia (Hasselkus, 2002). Psychotherapists will employ an entirely different approach from that of occupational therapists, as will arts-based therapists. These differences in approach can harbour interesting perceptions about attitudes towards dementia. These perceptions are often expressed as rehabilitation potential, promoting wellbeing, connectedness, personal growth and expression, acceptable risk taking and delivering appropriate personalised dementia care.

Dementia care remains strongly aligned to the medicalisation of care; indeed, many services can only be accessed with a formal diagnosis of dementia (Morrisby et al, 2018). There is a growing acceptance that a diagnosis of dementia, in the absence of a cure, can offer limited remediation of the condition in the more medicalised sense of prescriptive and pharmacological approaches. As such, the majority of people with dementia seek to maximise their wellbeing and minimise the more challenging aspects of dementia. Some people may decide to resist any formal diagnosis on the basis of preferring not to know; these individuals can find themselves excluded from formal sources of support as a consequence. Collaborative responsive care, rather than intensive medical interventions, are most relevant to the care of people with dementia. Living better with dementia, as a long-term goal, can be difficult for professionals who usually seek to cure and alleviate. The often-declared, person–centred care approach can all too often be practised as *doing for* rather than *doing alongside* in dementia care. Despite more than 30 years of person-centred care, many practitioners and places of care still find delivering such care consistently as wrought with challenges and practical difficulties. Perhaps it is time to look beyond this idealised model of care and consider the need to develop *place*-responsive models of care that encompass rurality-specific cultures of community, provider, staff, volunteer and individual preferences and values in relation to flexible, responsive dementia care.

Organisations that promote wellbeing in dementia challenge the dominance of medicalised advice by seeking to mobilise local populations through initiatives such as dementia-friendly communities (Alzheimer' Society, 2018). These schemes, often devised from the ground up, recognise the need for working with the local cultures and resources. From these, especially those in Japan and Europe, evolving services have emerged (Alzheimer's Society, 2017). These are often based on human rights agendas and seek to demand minimum rights for individuals to remain as active contributors in their local communities (McGettick and Williamson, 2015; WHO, 2018). Some organisations seek to promote a rights-based agenda, often drawing on the success of other representative organisations of marginalised groups of people who have gained traction with profound societal and legal change as a consequence. Currently, the shift towards a human rights agenda among those with dementia and their caregivers is gaining pace in the UK, but for many remains disconnected. The drive towards a social model of disability as an integral part of a rights–based model can raise expectations of wider choices in care as a basic right and not an optional extra, but in the absence of local accessible services this remit can seem hollow to families providing the majority of care. However, the core determinants, many enshrined in human rights law, may prove to incentivise responsive support regardless of any disadvantage because of geographical location.

Since the majority of these initiatives are co-produced among small communities, they are more likely to be responsive and flexible enough to respond to the preferences of members of those communities. However, in rural and remote areas, there may be a need to collaborate with neighbouring communities to ensure adequate community capability to build and sustain dementia-friendly communities. The risk to these approaches is that there can be a diverse and numerous responses that may be unsustainable in economic and social viability terms. There is an urgent need to identify the most effective models of rights-based initiatives that can be transferred to similar communities (NHS, 2014).

In the UK, nursing and social worker professionals tend towards a strong risk-averse culture of working and so can find the idea of farm-based care undertaken by people with dementia as inherently high risk and challenging to manage effectively (Brown, 2010; Bates and Lymbery, 2011). Perceived risks, stated by professionals, can include increased falls, getting lost and exposure to bad weather, infections and harm by animals. Similarly, caregivers may prefer care to be contained within four walls as a way of ensuring physical and emotional safety. Underlying these genuine concerns are tensions about the novelty of, and non-familiarity with, farm-based care and the professional desire to provide dignified care. Allied healthcare professionals, such as occupational therapists, lean towards a less risk-averse perspective (Hasselkus, 2002) and towards maintaining everyday interests and activities. Occupational therapists, especially those with experience of working beyond acute hospital settings, can counter the risk-averse cultures of care by drawing on their professional expertise and personal ethos of care, and promoting engagement within environments that may be laden with potential risks. Significantly, these identified risks are managed to enable participation rather than avoided. However, one of the distinct advantages of being older is the inherent ability to circumvent risks and demonstrate adept ways of doing so. Sometimes, older people deserve more credit for their abilities and determination to succeed. Balancing risk and meaningful activity can be difficult, but is not a reason to deny a person with dementia the opportunity to take part in activities from which they may benefit, especially if they indicate that they wish to do so.

Comparative evidence between farm-based and standard day care is patchy, with many of those studies undertaken being less than robust. The exceptions to this are the contributions by de Bruin and colleagues (2009), Hassink and colleagues (2017) and de Boer (2017), who continue to develop robust work. De Bruin and colleagues' findings were inconclusive or showed no significant differences in functional status, cognition, emotional wellbeing or behaviours between the types of care (de Bruin et al, 2009). However, the authors did identify marked improvements in the nutritional and hydration status of those attending the farm-based care settings (de Bruin et al, 2009). Similarly Hassink and colleagues (2018) highlighted the need to consider the role of farm-based care as an innovative addition to care opportunities and not a replacement for more standard care, which is important.

The following discussion outlines the main characteristics of farm-based care, which include being outdoors, horticulture, animals, domestic activities and working activities. Photographic evidence is provided by the beneficiaries of a care farm in the UK and permissions for publication have been kindly provided by the members of Connection Space Community Interest Company (CIC).

Being outdoors

Living in a rural area, it is often assumed that individuals have regular access to the outdoors as an integral part of their everyday lives. However, older people with dementia can become very isolated and choose to remain within the boundaries of four walls despite living in an idyllic rural area (Kane and Cook, 2013). In the UK, the continued severance of public transport, and reduced numbers of local shops, post offices and weekly church services, may result in profound isolation and loneliness. The higher concentration in urban areas of social groups such as dementia cafés and singing for the brain makes it very easy for rural dwellers, who are less likely to access urban located groups, to feel and become disconnected from their local community. Older people and their caregivers may be limited by a lack of physical independence and difficulties accessing services.

Evidence suggests that being outdoors has significant benefits to quality of life, wellbeing and health gains (Franco et al, 2017). While the majority of evidence related to quality of life and the outdoors has taken place in urban locations, it can be assumed that rural dwellers are similarly affected by a lack of direct exposure to the outdoors.

Older rural people often hold very strong attachments to the places they live and particularly the landscapes in which they have lived and worked (Myren et al, 2017). These connections to the land and monuments are often regarded as animate rather than devoid of any meaning and connection (Cutchin, 2018). It is not uncommon for rural dwellers to hold values associated with being an integral part of the land and a guardian of the land. These views may seem romantic and spiritual, but they do nonetheless indicate the importance of connections with place.

Being in nature, or perhaps for the rural dweller, simply being out and about, exposes the person to elements such as changing colours, weathers, landscapes and experiences. These all invoke past experiences and recollections that can be harnessed in dementia care. Many skills and experiences gained over the years can be shared among providers as a part of programmes of care. The benefits to the workforce are also often overlooked, yet it is not uncommon for care staff working long shifts in standard care to rarely venture outdoors. Working in the outdoors as a regular component of a job may help to maintain a healthy workforce.

Too often, the importance of place and the environment is considered in more prescriptive forms of dementia-friendly architecture and infrastructure in the built environment; often located within four walls of a building. Farm-based care challenges these boundaries and offers ways of considering the importance of place as a wilderness of opportunities that need not be tamed to adhere to some dementia-friendly viewpoint. Confidence in those who have lived and continue to live in these places is key to understanding the contributions the land can make towards providing health and social gains among people. People with dementia can be energised by walking in the snow, resting with the sun on their faces and/or enjoying a windswept picnic.

Being with animals

Animals have been used as a form of therapy to ameliorate mental and physical health conditions for centuries (Alves and Policarpo, 2018). This includes not only domestic pets such as dogs, cats and birds, but also docile farming animals such as hens, goats, ponies, llamas, alpacas, pot-bellied pigs and sheep. Small animals such as rabbits and hamsters may also tolerate petting, and fish and garden birds may provoke a calming effect on humans. In the context of farm-based care, animals can provide numerous forms of therapeutic value (Hassink et al, 2018). These include the need for care and attention to maintain the animals'

Figure 9.1: Connecting with docile animals as part of the cleaning-up task

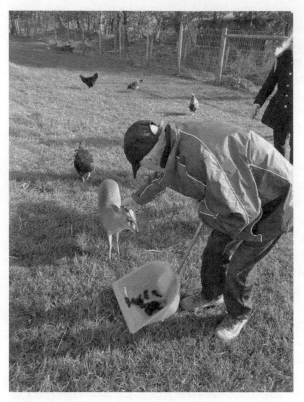

health and welfare. Structured activities such as cleaning out, feeding, watering and exercising can imbue a sense of usefulness, contribution and enjoyment among beneficiaries. Walking by leading animals across fields can give purpose to exercise and by default support the building of muscles for leg strength. Similarly, pushing a wheelbarrow full of hay engages the muscles and involves coordination of movement, with often more pleasure than gym exercises. Stroking, grooming and talking with animals can also prompt better eye–hand coordination, lower heart rate, increase engagement with others and boost verbal communication by raising confidence and motivation. Observing animals at play, such as lambs jumping for joy, can offer respite from anxiety, often associated with dementia. It is not uncommon for very deep attachments to develop between humans and animals in much the same way that household pets stimulate intense attachments.

However subtle these encounters with animals may be, they do rely for their development on the skills of the therapeutic caregiver. Often such skills remain hidden as therapists' work is so implicit that it can be very difficult to appreciate the decisions they make to maximise their approaches. A therapist may be selective with which animals can tolerate and respond best to a person who may be unable to appreciate animal nuances such as spitting llamas. Likewise a mischievous goat may draw out the laughter of a normally reserved beneficiary. The role of the therapist is dual, not only providing care towards the person but also maintaining the safety and wellbeing of the animals in their care.

Standard day care settings can consider including contact with animals by providing opportunities for 'trained therapeutic animal contact'. It is not uncommon for dogs, lambs, chickens, donkeys and small domesticated animals to visit such settings. Those with more land can consider keeping their own small group of chickens to provide outdoor activities for beneficiaries who can help with routine tasks. Research is also under way to measure the effectiveness of interactive animal-like models similar to large-eyed seals and dogs among people with dementia. These artificial animals raise issues about their use in imbuing different realities, such as owning a pet of one's own and the sense of responsibility for that pet. Further work is required to determine the perceptions of individuals with dementia about the use of such artificial pets, which is very different from connecting with a real animal. However, the use of virtual reality may offer genuine comfort especially during periods of intense anxiety among some people with dementia and the opportunity to "experience" being with animals such as dolphins which are not readily available in the real world.

For those who cannot readily engage with real animals, there are a number of resources such as the Pictures to Share Books that can promote memories and conversations about animals, agriculture and living in rural areas (Bate, 2014). Similarly, some enjoyment can be gained by watching and listening to animal life and sounds via media channels. People with dementia can also gain immense pleasure from watching wild birds and squirrels feeding near to windows.

Horticulture

Growing and cultivating plants is an activity that many people engage in as a hobby. Some growers aim to produce food while others prefer flowers or the challenge of a particular species. In the context of farm-based activities, horticulture mainly involves growing vegetables and flowers for use by the beneficiaries and/or as a commercial part of sustaining the financial costs of the farm (Leck, 2013). In the UK, the majority of farms grow herbs, vegetables and flowers. Some farms also include elements of land management such as hay making, woodland clearance and similar activities. Notably in Japan, rice farming is an integral part of one form of farm care, whereby beneficiaries engage in all aspects of rice farming as a culturally acceptable means of working towards a measurable harvest (Ura et al, 2018).

The act of growing can be deeply relaxing for people with dementia (Schmutz et al, 2014). The process of growing plants can imbue a sense of intense attention, getting into the 'zone' as described by Csikszentmihályi (1997), which can generate a sense of having done something meaningful and thus increase happiness. Seeing, over time, seedlings progress to plants, offers a tangible connection with the passage of time. This sense of time can help to support the person in the present and provide opportunities to realise the past, present and future. This contrasts with many reminiscence therapies, which can diminish the experience of the present, among people with dementia. It is important to promote the activities in the present to minimise any confusion or ideas that the beneficiaries are undertaking a job as they may previously have done.

One aspect that is perhaps often overlooked is that regular physical momentum, such as digging with a spade, can give a sense of wellbeing (Hasselkus, 2002). The digger is not simply taking part in the immediate tangible exercise of turning over soil, but also engaging in the task of preparing the ground for the next season. Undertaking a physical task, which may seem monotonous or even adverse for an older person, can provoke a sense of usefulness and contribution. This is important because such activities not only enhance conversations and cooperation with others, but also provide increased confidence in capabilities. Coupled with being in the outdoors, there can be genuine therapeutic gains in a sense of wellbeing.

Standard care settings can introduce regular horticultural activities even in the absence of outdoor spaces by growing potted plants and windowsill produce. Evidence suggests that indoor gardening can help sleep, agitation and cognition in people with dementia (Detweiler et al, 2012). However, greater gains can be gained by gardening in the outdoors as comprehensively discussed by Noone and colleagues (2015). If land is available, such settings could consider the development of an area for growing plants, sitting and taking part in activities such as gardening. People with dementia benefit most from gardens that are less formal than many designed dementia-specific spaces, and studies have shown that the latter may invoke in providers and beneficiaries a sense of anxiety and reluctance to touch the plants. More informal spaces can encourage beneficiaries and providers to connect with the soil, plants and necessary tasks more readily. Many UK organisations can provide advice in this area, including the Society of Horticultural Therapists (Thrive) as well as suppliers of gardening products. The Alzheimer's Society has produced information about accessing gardening centres as a way of enabling people with dementia to engage with horticulture, and provides extensive advice on horticulture and gardening in care settings (Alzheimer's Society, 2017).

The creative arts

In rural areas, where the majority of farm-based care is located, the arts are accessed in different ways from the more urban-centric modes of delivery. Music, dance, writing and poetry are all practised in farm-based settings and often relate to the cultural markers of rural life. These markers include the seasons, local rituals (such as well dressings, which are decorative boards made from petals, moss and seeds, often depicting religious symbolism), weather, life events and religious celebrations (such as clyping the church, in which members of a community clasp hands forming an outward-looking circle around the perimeter of a church and seek a blessing for the coming year). All these markers derive from activities such as farming, life-course events and local customs. This means that they are an important conduit for intergenerational work among beneficiaries.

Evidence suggests that older people and those with dementia enjoy taking part in the arts. Beyond enjoyment, the arts can also contribute towards increased health gains, such as nutritional intake, contentment, and lowered physical and psychosocial stress. Although the evidence is patchy, people with dementia and their caregivers value ongoing engagement with the arts rather than singular events (APPGAHW, 2017). This is understandable given that ongoing engagement can foster confidence and feelings of safety, and foster new friendships. It also provides time and opportunities for more flexible working, which is important in dementia care.

Care settings often provide activities that also reflect the seasonal and celebratory periods of the year as a cycle of events. Engaging in the creative arts requires particular measures that foster the individual contribution of the person with dementia and avoids childlike approaches. People with dementia can use tools and materials such a metal and wood to construct items in very creative ways. Suggestions for different activities that reflect rural life can be found on various websites including those focused on farming communities, such as national farming organisations, and those with a focus on therapy.

Domestic work

The majority of farm-based care includes social opportunities to eat and drink together (de Bruin et al, 2015). Domestic work can provide many opportunities for people with dementia to demonstrate their abilities and to also contribute towards the tasks necessary for the routine of the day. It is not intended to replicate or give the impression that the person with dementia has resumed previous work, before their dementia. However, the opportunity to engage in supported routines with which the beneficiary is familiar can foster a deep sense of satisfaction, contribution and connection with others.

Home makers, in particular, may value undertaking domestic tasks, as these are often familiar to them. Domestic tasks include preparing and cooking meals, washing pots, folding linen, cleaning and caring for domestic animals. Domestic tasks, carried out in previous years, such as hanging out terry nappies, can bring a sense of emotional safety and comforting contribution. They also trigger conversations and memories of past experiences that are shared in the present, such as comparing baby care and parenting with present-day approaches.

Maintaining nutritional status and hydration can be challenging among those with dementia who may be disinterested in food. Shared meals with friends provide the pleasant experience of eating together. Evidence has shown that eating and drinking in farm-based care settings raises the nutritional status and fluid intake of individuals with dementia more than attendance at more standard forms of care (de Bruin et al, 2009, 2010). This may be because of the increased exertion and the motivation of assisting with the production and preparation of the food. Anecdotal evidence from the Connection Space farm-based initiative has identified increased nutritional intake of fluids and food during the sessions. These findings suggest that the farm-based care offers an unintended but important contribution towards increasing and/or maintaining the nutritional and hydration needs of the beneficiaries. This is especially important among those with dementia.

Within standard care settings, many beneficiaries adopt a passive role and are not provided with opportunities to take part in activities they are able to undertake with support. These include making refreshments, cooking (especially own home-grown produce) and general assistance. Taking part in such activities can help with mobilisation and a sense of usefulness. They can also generate increased connections with care staff as they support and encourage beneficiaries.

For those with younger onset dementia, working in a café can add meaning and continued paid employment. This is illustrated by the

Figure 9.2: Working in the community café providing refreshments

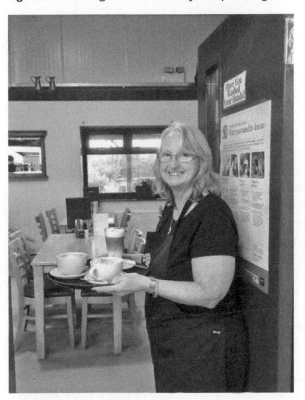

woman in the photograph in Figure 9.2, who, after attending farm-based care, secured part-time work in the café there. For the individual, the gains in returning to recognised work have been enormous in raising self-esteem and general wellbeing. This raises the issues about continuing in employment with dementia and the ways in which the workplace can adapt to more inclusive practices. Standard care settings could consider ways of providing alternative activities and work-like approaches among those with younger onset dementia who are often assimilated into groups comprising older people with dementia. More broadly, the scarcity of dedicated standard younger onset dementia services and care is in urgent need of reconfiguration, especially in rural areas.

Relevance to international care

This chapter intentionally focuses on UK care provision, using farm-based care as a possible exemplar of future rural dementia provision. However, the development of rural farm-based care potentially holds promise worldwide, especially among those countries where the ageing population resides in predominantly rural areas. It is important that those living in rural and remote areas are not disadvantaged by virtue of where they live and have access to appropriate and timely dementia care. Each country and region will have their own cultures and ways of developing and delivering farm-based dementia care. However, many face challenges in addressing the need for high-quality care and economic viability.

Pioneering countries such as the Netherlands have well-established models of farm-based care, some more than 30 years old, whereas others have no such provision. In the Netherlands, farm-based care is partly funded by the state in recognition of the need for flexible rural dementia care (Hassink et al, 2014). A few countries, such as in Japan, do not readily identify as providing farm-based care, yet in practice offer services that characterise this type of dementia care (Ura et al, 2018). In other countries, farm-based care is located primarily in regions that are identified as deprived and so attract sustainable funding based on crude measures of local demographics such as unemployment, health status and population. Many rural areas, especially in Europe, remain hidden within these indices of health measures and so fail eligibility for regeneration funding (Rural England, 2019). There are indications of a shift towards concepts with more of a public health focus on wellbeing (less medicalisation) and a recognition of the need to work collaboratively across agricultural, social and health sectors. In many rural communities, the influence of church, media and local politicians contributes towards the evolution and development of farm-based care (Hassink et al, 2014). Understanding the multiple and complex nature of the organisational aspects of farm-based care in local communities is necessary to legitimately develop and sustain such care (Di Iacovo et al, 2016).

Common to all the countries providing farm-based care are the challenges of providing sustainable services. Even in the Netherlands, the organisation of commissioning of services by health and social care continues to present challenges to maintaining long-term service provision (Hassink et al, 2018). These challenges indicate the many difficulties faced by novel and innovative provision in times of increasing demands for dementia care. In the absence of robust, evidence-based measures of wellbeing among beneficiaries and providers at the individual and small provider levels, large commissioning organisations are likely to be risk-averse to allocating funds towards this type of care. It is possible for such care to help sustain agricultural communities through the diversification of businesses and the provision of regular financial incentives to halt diminishing rural economies and communities (Bragg and Atkins, 2016; Hassink et ak, 2018). It is necessary to devise more nuanced, evidenced measures to understand the organisational and multiple perspectives to ultimately determine the models of care that provide high-quality rural dementia care.

Increased awareness and advocacy of dementia care as a human right that includes choice of dignified care and access to activities may provide the international and national drive towards flexibility, choice and more diverse forms of dementia care (WHO, 2018). In rural and remote areas, farm-based care may offer a pragmatic and economically viable way to provide local provision that is culturally acceptable to users and enables them to remain in their own locality. This would provide an alternative to the persistent challenges of travel and time required to access care provision by rural older people who often reject leaving their local communities and the demands made on professionals trying to deliver care. Farm-based care can provide care that supports people and local communities by retaining care in places readily accessible and acceptable by users.

People with dementia are living longer; care provision needs to be tailored not only to the personal interests but also the stage of dementia. Farm-based care can offer varied and meaningful activities that may also provide ongoing rehabilitation and therapy, and so delay the onset of physical and mental decline. This is important in the absence of any cure for dementia and the imperative to support families affected by dementia who provide the majority of care worldwide. Models of farm-based care, predominantly from the Netherlands, have demonstrated that people with dementia can remain in their own locality and that continued access to farm-based care provides a sense of continuity and support along the trajectory of the dementia pathway. Notably, some farms operate with residential and nursing home facilities co-located with the farm, providing connection with the farm and others regardless of the stage of dementia. These sites provide comprehensively trained workforce staff who are skilled in all aspects of dementia care. From a workforce perspective, retention is higher than that found in more urban and standard built environment locations of care (Cosgrave et al, 2019). This implies that the locus of care also matters to workforce members and that worker wellbeing may be enhanced by such a comprehensive model of care. However, more robust work focused on workforce measures would be required to determine what matters most to these providers.

Standard care providers, especially sessional and day care providers, can learn and adapt ways to enable their beneficiaries to access the outdoors and being in nature. Barriers may exist, but with some support and knowledge sharing it is possible that lives can be enhanced by adopting some of the approaches utilised by farm-based dementia care providers. This is key to ensuring the future of dementia care that is responsive to the needs of families affected by dementia and to address the challenges of sustainable robust provision. Commissioners should seek to ensure that any statutory funding meets the needs of the local community in the most economic ways while delivering high-quality accessible care. Many countries face unprecedented challenges in meeting the needs of older people with chronic health needs. More broadly, the rise of rights-based dementia care will demand the need for flexible, high-quality, responsive care that is relevant and located within rural communities for rural residents. Although often overlooked, farm-based care may provide the urgent response to increasing demands for high-quality rural dementia care.

Summary

Farm-based care provides therapeutic care underpinned by routinised, purposeful activities. Day care settings also provide activities that emphasise participation and purpose, but may find it difficult to offer the types of activity found in farm-based care because of resource and environmental limitations. The majority of activities provided in standard day care involve larger groups and there may be less choice of activity. However, despite these barriers to implementation in standard care settings, there is evidence of a growing interest and drive towards increased opportunities to include more outdoor, nature-based experiences on a routine basis. More work needs to be done to enable the more standard settings to adapt and implement opportunities as an integral aspect of their care delivery. Closer partnership across both types of provider would foster mutual knowledge sharing of respective expertise in dementia care.

Farm-based care is underpinned by an ethos of shared goals that take place as part of a routinised programme. These routines, important for achieving the necessary tasks, not only maintain the welfare of animals but also offer structure and a sense of security to the beneficiaries. Layered on to these routine tasks are more individualised and small-group activities that provide wider choice. This is important because the organisation of the care is one of flexible learning, meaningful occupation and purpose. This active participation fosters a sense of collaboration and connection with others and so reduces the isolation and loneliness often experienced with dementia. There also seems to be an acceptance of risk taking that more medicalised professions may find difficult to assimilate into their own work and organisations.

As a form of novel and innovatively designed and delivered form of dementia care in mainly rural communities, farm-based care can provide stimulus about the organisation and delivery of rural dementia care. For most, farm-based care is located within the 'edge lands' of the care sector, intersecting agricultural, health and social care organisations. There is an understandable hesitancy to harness the potential contribution of innovative care that can be viewed as risky, especially by those responsible for funding and being accountable for care. Lessons can be learnt from the pioneers of farm-based care, such as the Netherlands, where established and evidence-based work has contributed towards the development of rural dementia care. There are, for many countries, inherent political, policy and practice challenges that need to be addressed by collaborative research and knowledge sharing. Ultimately, those living in rural communities with dementia have a right to responsive, relevant and high-quality care within their localities.

As more people age well and expect to have greater choices in their care, greater consideration needs to be afforded to these alternative forms of care. Knowledge sharing and the development of aligned services that meet the diverse expectations of individuals and those who provide care is required to move dementia care towards excellence as standard. Farm-based care is potentially one of the ways forward, especially for those living in rural and remote areas.

References

All Party Parliamentary Group on Arts, Health and Wellbeing (APPG) (2017) *Creative health: the arts for health and wellbeing. Inquiry Report*. Available from: www.artshealthandwellbeing.org.uk/appg-inquiry/Publications/Creative_Health_Inquiry_Report_2017.pdf

Alves, R and Policarpo, I. (2018) 'Animals and human health: where do they meet?', in R. Alves and U. Alburquerque (eds), *Ethnozoology: Animals in our lives*, London: Academic Press, pp 233–59.

Alzheimer's Society (2017) *Dementia-friendly garden centre: A practical guide to becoming dementia-friendly*, London: Alzheimer's Society. Available from: www.alzheimers.org.uk/sites/default/files/2018-05/AS_Designing_Garden_Guide_Web.pdf

Alzheimer's Society (2018) *Dementia friendly rural communities guide: A practical guide for rural communities to support people affected by dementia*, London: Alzheimer's Society. Available from: www.alzheimers.org. uk/sites/default/files/2018-05/Dementia-friendly%20rural%20 communities%20guide.pdf

Bate, H. (2014) *Too late to learn to drive: Dementia, visual perception and the meaning of pictures*, Pictures to Share CIC. Available from: www. picturestoshare.co.uk

Bates, P. and Lymbery, M. (2011) 'Managing risk in a risk adverse society', in R. Taylor, M. Hill and F. McNeill (eds) *Early professional development for social workers*, Birmingham: Venture Press, pp 29–44.

Bennett, L., Honeyman, M. and Bottery, S. (2018) *New models of home care*, London: The King's Fund. Available from: www.kingsfund.org. uk/sites/default/files/2018-12/New-models-of-home-care.pdf

Braedley, S. (2018) 'Reinventing the nursing home: metaphors that design care', in S. Katz (ed) *Ageing in everyday life: Materialities and embodiments*, Bristol: Policy Press, pp 45–63.

Bragg, R. and Atkins, G. (2016) *A review of nature-based interventions for mental health care*, Natural England Commissioned Report NECR 204. Available from: http://publications.naturalengland.org.uk/ publication/4513819616346112

BGS (British Geriatrics Society) (2018) *Effective healthcare for older people: Position statement on primary care for older people*, London: BGS. Available from: https://www.bgs.org.uk/sites/default/files/ content/attachment/2018-08-22/Position%20Statement%20on%20 Primary%20Care%20for%20Older%20People_0.pdf

BPS (British Psychological Society) (2016) *Psychological dimensions of dementia: Putting the person at the centre of care*, Leicester: BPS. Available from: www.bps.org.uk/sites/bps.org.uk/files/Policy/Policy%20- %20Files/Psychological%20dimensions%20of%20dementia_ Putting%20the%20person%20at%20the%20centre%20of%20care.pdf

Brown, L. (2010) 'Balancing risk and innovation to improve social work practice', *The British Journal of Social Work*, 40(4): 1211–28.

Buist, Y., Verbeek, H., De Boer, B. and De Bruin, S. (2018) 'Innovating dementia care: implementing characteristics of green care farms in other long-term care settings', *International Psychogeriatrics*, 30(7): 1– 12, doi: 10.1017/S1041610217002848.

Clark, P., Mapes, N., Burt, J. and Preston, S. (2013) *Greening dementia: A literature review of the benefits and barriers facing individuals living with dementia in accessing the natural environment and local greenspace*, Natural England Commissioned Reports NECR137. Available from: http:// publications.naturalengland.org.uk/publication/6578292471627776

Cosgrave, C., Malatzky, C. and Gillespie, J. (2019) 'Social determinants of rural health workforce retention: a scoping review', *International Journal of Environmental Research and Public Health*, 16(3): 314.

Csikszentmihályi, M. (1997) *Finding flow: The psychology of engagement with everyday life*, New York, NY: Basic Books.

Cutchin, M. (2018) 'Active relationships of ageing people and places', in M. Skinner, G. Andrews and M. Cutchin (eds) *Geographical gerontology: Perspectives, concepts, approaches*, London: Routledge, pp 216–28.

de Boer, B. (2017) 'Green care farms as innovative nursing homes, promoting activities and social interaction for people with dementia', *Journal of the American Medical Directors Association*, 18(1): 40–6.

de Bruin, S., Oosting, S., Kuin, Y., Hoefnagels, E.C., Blauw, Y.H., de Groot, L. and Schols, J.M. (2009) 'Green care farms promote activity among elderly people with dementia', *Journal of Housing for the Elderly*, 23(4): 368–89.

de Bruin, S., Oosting, S., van der Zijpp, A., Enders-Slegers, M.J. and Schols, J. (2010) 'The concept of green care farms for older people with dementia: an integrative framework', *Dementia: The International Journal of Social Research and Practice*, 9(1): 79–128.

de Bruin, S., Stoop, A., Molema, C., Vaandrager, L., Hop, P.J. and Baan, C.A. (2015) 'Green care farms: an innovative type of adult day service to stimulate social participation of people with dementia', *Gerontology and Geriatric Medicine*, doi: 10.1177/2333721415607833

Detweiler, M.B., Sharma, T., Detweiler, J.G., Murphy, P.F., Lane, S., Carman, J., Chudhary, A.S., Halling, M.H. and Kim, K.Y. (2012) 'What is the evidence to support the use of therapeutic gardens for the elderly?', *Psychiatry Investigation*, 9(2): 100–10.

Di Iacovo, F., Moruzza, R. and Rossignoli, C. (2016) 'Measuring the effects of transdisciplinary research: the case of a social farming project', *Futures*, 75: 24–35.

Dorling, D. and Thomas, B. (2016) *People and places: A 21st-century atlas of the UK*, Bristol: Policy Press.

Elings, M. (2012) *Effects of care farms: Scientific research on the benefits of care farms for clients*, Wageningen: University of Wageningen. Available from: http://library.wur.nl/WebQuery/wurpubs/450976 [Accessed 2 March 2018].

Franco, L., Shanahan, D. and Fuller, R. (2017) 'A review of the benefits of nature experiences: more than meets the eye', *International Journal of Environmental Research and Public Health*, 14(8): 864.

Hasselkus, B. (2002) *The meaning of everyday occupation*, Thorofare, NJ: Slack Inc.

Hassink, J., de Bruin, S.R., Berget, B. and Elings, M. (2017) 'Exploring the role of farm animals in providing care at care rarms', *Animals: An Open Access Journal from MDPI*, 7(6): 45.

Hassink, J., Grin, J. and Hulsink, W. (2018) 'Enriching the multi-level perspective by better understanding agency and challenges associated with interactions across system boundaries. The case of care farming in the Netherlands: multifunctional agriculture meets health care', *Journal of Rural Studies*, 57: 186–96.

Hassink, J., Hulink, W. and Grin, J. (2014) 'Farming with care: the evolution of care farming in the Netherlands', *NJAS: Wageningen Journal of Life Sciences*, 68: 1–11.

Henning-Smith, C. and Lahr, M. (2018) *Perspectives on rural caregiving: Challenges and interventions*, Policy Brief: Minneapolis, MN: University of Minnesota Rural Health Research Centre. Available from: http://rhrc.umn.edu/2018/08/rural-caregiving-challenges-and-interventions

Kane, M. and Cook, L. (2013) *Dementia 2013: The hidden voice of loneliness*, London: Alzheimer's Society. Available from: www.alzheimers.org.uk/sites/default/files/migrate/downloads/dementia_2013_the_hidden_voice_of_loneliness.pdf

Keating, N. (2009) *Rural ageing: A good place to grow old?*, Bristol: Policy Press.

Kitwood, T. (1997) *Dementia reconsidered: The person comes first*, Milton Keynes: Open University Press.

Leck, C. (2013) 'The impact of care farming in the UK', Unpublished PhD thesis, University of Worcester. Avaialble from: http://eprints.worc.ac.uk/2733 [Accessed 2 March 2018].

Lewis, F., Karlsberg Schaffer, S., Sussex, J., O'Neil, P. and Cockroft, L. (2014) *Trajectory of dementia in the UK: Making a difference*, Report for Alzheimer's Research UK by OHE Consulting, London: Office of Health Economics. Available from: www.ohe.org/publications/trajectory-dementia-uk-making-difference#

LGA (Local Government Association) and PHE (Public Health England) (2018) *Health profile for England: 2018*, London: LGA and PHE. Available from: www.gov.uk/government/publications/health-profile-for-england-2018

McGettick, G. and Williamson, T. (2015) *Dementia, rights, and the social model of disability: A new direction for policy and practice?*, London: Mental Health Foundation. Available from: www.mentalhealth.org.uk/sites/default/files/dementia-rights-policy-discussion.pdf

Morrisby, C., Joosten, A. and Ciccarelli, M. (2018) 'Do services meet the needs of people with dementia and carers living in the community? A scoping review of the international literature', *International psychogeriatrics*, 30(1): 5–14.

Myren, G.E.S., Enmarker, I.C., Hellzén, O. and Saur, E. (2017) 'The influence of place on everyday life: observations of persons with dementia in regular day care and at the green care farm', *Health*, 9(2): 261–78.

NHS (National Health Service) (2014) *Five Year Forward View*, London: NHS England. Available from: www.england.nhs.uk/wp-content/uploads/2014/10/5yfv-web.pdf

NHS (2019) *The NHS Long Term Plan*, London: Department of Health and Social Care. Available from: www.longtermplan.nhs.uk

Natural England (2017) *Good practice in social prescribing for mental health: The role of nature-based interventions*, Natural England Commissioned Report NECR228. Available from: http://publications.naturalengland.org.uk/publication/5134438692814848

Noone, S., Innes, A., Kelly, F. and Mayer, A. (2015) ' "The nourishing soil of the soul": the role of horticultural therapy in promoting well-being in community-dwelling people with dementia', *Dementia*, 16(7): 897–910.

ONS (2015) 'Principal projection: England population in age groups. 2014 based dataset', [online]. Available from: https://www.ons.gov.uk/peoplepopulationandcommunity/populationandmigration/populationprojections/datasets/tablea24principalprojectionengland populationinagegroups

Phillips, D. and Feng, Z. (2018) 'Global ageing', in M. Skinner, G. Andrews and M. Cutchin (eds) *Geographical gerontology: Perspectives, concepts, approaches*, London: Routledge, pp 93–109.

Prince, M., Knapp, M., Guerchet, M., McCrone, P., Prina, M., Comas-Herrera, A., Wittenberg, R., Adelaja, B., Hu, B., King, D., Rehill, A. and Salimkumar, D. (2014) *Dementia UK: Second edition. Overview*, London: Alzheimer's Society. Available from: http://eprints.lse.ac.uk/59437/1/Dementia_UK_Second_edition_-_Overview.pdf

Rahman, S., Harrison Dening, K. and Dening, T. (2018) 'Frailty and dementia: promoting health assets and resilience', *Nursing Times*, 114(9): 52–6.

Rural England (2017) *Issues facing providers of social at home to older rural residents*, Rural England CIC. Available from: https://ruralengland.org/wp-content/uploads/2018/01/Launch-Report-Issues-Facing-Providers-Social-Care-in-Rural-England.pdf

Rural England (2019) *State of rural services 2018*, Rural England CIC. Available from: https://ruralengland.org/wp-content/uploads/2019/02/SORS18-Full-report.pdf

Schmutz, U., Lennartsson, M., Williams, S., Devereaux, M. and Davies, G. (2014) *The benefits of gardening and food growing for health and wellbeing*, Coventry and London: Garden Organic and Sustain. Available from: www.growplaces.org.uk

Skinner, M. and Winterton, R. (2018) 'Rural ageing: contested spaces, dynamic places', in M. Skinner, G. Andrews and M. Cutchin (eds) *Geographical gerontology: Perspectives, concepts, approaches*, Abingdon: Routledge, pp 136–48.

Steigen, A., Kogstad, R. and Hummelvoll, J. (2016) 'Green care services in the Nordic countries: an integrative literature review', *European Journal of Social Work*, 19(5): 692–715.

Ura, C., Okamura, T., Yamazaki, S., Ishiguro, T., Ibe, M., Miyazaki, M. and Kawamuro, Y. (2018) 'Rice-farming care for the elderly people with cognitive impairment in Japan: a case series', *International Journal of Geriatric Psychiatry*, 33: 435–7.

Warburton, J., Cowan, S., Winterton, R. and Hodgkins, S. (2014) 'Building social inclusion for rural older people using information and communication technologies: perspectives of rural practitioners', *Australian Social Work*, 67: 479–94.

Watkins, J., Wulaningsih, W., Da Zhou, C., Marshall, D.C., Sylianteng, G.D., Rosa, P.G.D., Miguel, V.A., Raine, R., King, L.P. and Maruthappu, M. (2017) 'Effects of health and social care spending constraints on mortality in England: a time trend analysis', *BMJ open*, 7(11): e017722.

WHO (World Health Organization) (2012) *Active ageing: Good health adds years to life. Policies and priority interventions for healthy ageing*, Geneva: WHO. Available from: www.euro.who.int/__data/assets/pdf_file/0006/161637/WHD-Policies-and-Priority-Interventions-for-Healthy-Ageing.pdf?ua=1

WHO (2018) *A healthier humanity: The WHO investment case for 2019–2023*, Geneva: WHO. Available from: https://apps.who.int/iris/bitstream/handle/10665/274710/WHO-DGO-CRM-18.2-eng.pdf?sequence=1&isAllowed=y

10

Transportation issues in dementia

Mark Rapoport, Andy Hyde and Gary Naglie

Introduction

Transportation is a key aspect of mobility and quality of life for older adults, and this remains true for people living with dementia who are often isolated and cut off from family, friends and social services when driving a car becomes unfeasible or unsafe. Most research on driving and other transportation options for people living with dementia is undertaken in urban settings, and services and solutions that work in urban areas may not translate into rural settings where people with dementia have particular challenges in remaining connected without a vehicle. In this chapter, we bring together perspectives from Canada and the UK on the topic of transportation for people with dementia. We review the transportation needs of older adults, the road risks that arise when people with dementia drive cars, and the risks to the quality of lives of those with dementia when they stop driving. We review the information that is available on this topic for those living in rural settings. Although there have been no universal solutions proposed to the particular challenges of transportation needs for those living in rural areas with dementia, we discuss an innovative national approach that is under way in Scotland, one of the few places to have addressed transport needs of people with dementia and other disabilities living in remote areas. This is truly a nascent area in which there are significant limitations to the literature. We hope to summarise what is known and provide some thoughts on helpful future directions.

Transportation needs in older adulthood

It is interesting to compare the Canadian and Scottish contexts since, albeit different in size, both countries have large rural populations. As we discover in this section, both countries show similar trends of increasing dependence on the car, ageing populations, and growing numbers of people living with dementia.

Canadian data

Driving is by far the primary mode of transportation for older adults in Canada. According to a recent survey, more than two thirds of adults age 65–74 years, and just less than a third aged 85 rely on driving their own vehicle as their primary means of transportation (The Conference Board of Canada, 2016). Cars accounted for 64–77 per cent of trips made by older adults in 1992, and 69–84 per cent in 2005 (The Conference Board of Canada, 2016; Turcotte, 2012). Surprisingly, 17 per cent of older adults with dementia and 7 per cent of older adults with significant visual impairment also identified driving as their primary method of transportation (The Conference Board of Canada, 2016). Reliance on the car for transportation appears to also be increasing over time in Canada.

The Canadian Longitudinal Study of Aging (CLSA) is a national prospective longitudinal study of Canadians recruited between the ages of 45 and 85 years, and the authors recently published their cross-sectional baseline data, which included over 40,000 participants (Raina et al, 2018; Vrkljan et al, 2018). This report identified a significant sex difference in driving licensure in those aged 75 years and older, with 94.1 per cent of men having an active license compared with 78 per cent of women (Vrkljan et al, 2018). Among those age 75 years and over, far fewer men than women reported never having had a driver's license (0.2 per cent versus 5.8 per cent) or no longer having a license (5.7 per cent versus 16.2 per cent). Men with licenses in this age group were more likely to drive four or more times per week than women (84.2 per cent versus 68 per cent). This gap likely represents a cohort effect that will close over time.

Other modes of transportation are much less commonly used as the primary means of mobility in older Canadians. As a primary method of transportation, public transit was endorsed by less than 8 per cent of older adults and walking and cycling were endorsed by less than 5 per cent in that survey (Vrkljan et al, 2018). Although taxis or accessible transit were only used by 1 per cent as a primary method of transportation for adults aged 65–74 years, this rose to more than 7 per cent among those 85 years and over (The Conference Board of Canada, 2016). Nonetheless, 20–30 per cent of Canadians age 85 and older endorsed walking or cycling and 14–18 per cent endorsed public transit as a type of mobility used at least once in the last month (Turcotte, 2012).

Rural Canada. In the CLSA study, slightly more Canadians in rural areas (97.2 per cent) had an active license compared with those living in urban areas (94 per cent). The study also identified that there was a particularly large sex discrepancy in driving in rural areas for older adults. For those aged 75 years and over, 91 per cent of men identified driving as their primary mode of transportation compared with 61 per cent of women. Of those who used public transportation as their primary mode of transportation, less than 3 per cent lived in rural areas, likely representing the lack of public transit in most rural areas (Vrkljan et al, 2018). Other reports have indicated that older adults in small Canadian cities, towns and rural areas are less likely than those in large urban areas to walk or cycle (Myers, 2015; The Conference Board of Canada, 2016).

Dementia and Driving in Canada. In 2009, 28 per cent of adults aged 65 years and over in Canada with diagnoses of Alzheimer's disease or other dementias had active drivers' licenses (Turcotte, 2012). These drivers do ultimately stop driving as their illness progresses, but one Canadian observational study of people with dementia found that two years after study entry, just over half of these drivers continued to drive, indicating that many drivers with dementia may continue to drive despite progression of their illness (Herrmann et al, 2006). It has been predicted that by 2028, there will be almost 100,000 drivers with dementia on the road in Ontario, which is Canada's most populous province (Hopkins et al, 2004).

Scottish data

There is no analysis of driving data available from the Scottish Longitudinal Study, but according to the English Longitudinal Study of Ageing, driving remains the most common form of transport for older people in the UK. In England, 86 per cent of adults aged 60–69 have access to a car in their households (Holley-Moore and Creighton, 2015). The Royal Automobile Club Foundation also recently reported that over five million people living in the UK, aged 70 and over, hold a full licence (Royal Automobile Club Foundation, 2018). Transport Scotland's analysis of the Scottish Household Survey reported that driving was the most popular mode of transportation across all ages in 2017 (52 per cent of journeys) (Transport Scotland, 2018), while 27 per cent of those aged 70–79 and 15 per cent of those aged 80 and over drove everyday (Scottish Government, 2017a).

Public transport in Scotland. While driving remains the most popular mode of transport in Scotland, public transport plays a significant role in mobility, although there is a complex and mixed picture of public transport usage. Between 2006 and 2014, public transport passenger journeys declined by 6 per cent (Douglas et al, 2018). Domestic air and ferry services also play a vital role in keeping people connected, particularly between islands and the mainland where they provide 'lifeline' services. Some routes are subsidised by the Scottish Government to ensure that isolated communities retain links with medical and other services (Transport Scotland, n.d. a). Community transport plays an important role in the mobility mix, providing accessible and inclusive transport where public transport is unavailable (Canning et al, 2015).

Although bus passenger journeys in Scotland are declining, the bus remains the dominant form of public transport in Scotland, accounting for 77 per cent of public transport journeys, while rail journeys are increasing (Douglas et al, 2018). The National Entitlement Card scheme provides free travel ('concessionary travel') for those aged 60 and over, as well as eligible disabled people under age 60, on registered bus services throughout Scotland, at any time of day for any number of journeys. Card holders resident in Orkney, Shetland and the Western Isles receive two free return ferry journeys each year to the Scottish mainland (Transport Scotland, n.d. b). The aim of the scheme is to improve access to services, facilities and social networks, promoting social inclusion for older and disabled people. It also aims to improve health by promoting a more active lifestyle. There are currently around 1.2 million cardholders, and 142 million concessionary travel journeys were taken in 2016–17 (36 per cent of all bus journeys in that year) (Transport Scotland, 2018). Others suggest, however, that despite the fact that mobility of older people by bus appeared to have increased after the scheme was introduced in 2006, the car remains important for the mobility of older people, particularly for older men (Houston and Tilley, 2016).

While Scotland has remote and rural areas, its population of around 5.4 million is concentrated in a few urban centres. Around 2 per cent of people live on one of 93 inhabited islands. A little under a quarter (24 per cent) of the population in remote rural areas is aged 65 years and over, compared with 17 per cent in the rest of Scotland (Scottish Islands Federation, 2011). Projections indicate that by 2041, 25 per cent of the overall population in Scotland will be aged 65, increasing from 19 per cent in 2017, and the fastest-growing age group will be those aged 75 and over, increasing by 79 per cent from 2016 to 2041 (National Records of Scotland, 2018). There are currently approximately 90,000 people living with dementia in Scotland and just over 3,000 of these are under the age of 65 (Alzheimer Scotland, 2017). Scottish Government research in 2016 found that, compared with urban areas, vehicle ownership per person and licence possession was higher in rural areas in Scotland, where 82 per cent of adults had a full driving licence compared with 61 per cent in large urban areas (Scottish Government, 2017c), which is a much larger gap than was found in the Canadian context (Vrkljan et al, 2018).

Driving risks in dementia

Driving with dementia is associated with a decrement in driving ability. Alzheimer's disease is the most common form of dementia, and it progresses from a mild stage, to a moderate stage, and finally to a severe stage. The stages of dementia are categorised by the degree to which the person has deficits in cognition and ability to function independently. Cognition refers to neurological skills involved in thinking and relating to the world, including attention, memory, language, visuospatial skills and problem solving. In the mild stage, people with dementia have mild cognitive difficulties and some difficulty managing independently. In the moderate stage, cognition worsens, and people have substantial difficulty managing independently and some difficulty managing their own self-care. In the severe stage of dementia, cognition deteriorates to the point that communication is very difficult, memory is extremely poor, and the person cannot manage even the basics of self-care. The decrement in driving abilities is present even in mild stages of dementia, and worsens significantly as the dementia progresses through the moderate and severe stages (Carr et al, 2010; CMA, 2012; Austroads, 2013). Diagnosis of dementia ideally would be at the earliest stages, which would best allow people to prepare proactively for driving cessation, but in reality, the initial diagnosis of dementia is often made at moderate or severe stages, by which point driving skills will have substantially deteriorated.

Risks of driving impairment and collisions associated with dementia

In our recent systematic review of studies published from 2005 to 2015 comparing people with dementia to those without dementia (healthy controls), we found medium to large effects of dementia on driving abilities in six of the seven studies that examined driving impairment. When we combined the four studies that included road tests in a meta-analysis, we found that people with dementia were almost 11 times more likely to fail a road test than healthy controls (Chee et al, 2017).

In that review, we found only two studies comparing the risk of motor vehicle collisions in those with and without dementia, and they provided contradictory results. One of the studies showed an increased risk in a retrospective analysis (that is, those with dementia were more than four times as likely to have a collision in the three years prior to the study), but the reverse was true in their prospective analysis (that is, those without dementia were 11 times more likely to have a collision than those with dementia in the three years of study follow-up) (Ott et al, 2008). It is possible that the control group increased their driving exposure over time, in contrast to the dementia group, and that this may have accounted for the increased collisions in controls. The other study showed no association between dementia and risk of motor vehicle collisions (Davis et al, 2012). Our findings were similar to a prior systematic review that incorporated studies published from 1996 to 2006 (Man-Son-Hing et al, 2007). In that prior systematic review, only one of three studies that ascertained collision risk using official state-recorded collisions showed that those with dementia had higher risk than controls, but all three studies that assessed collisions based on family report found a higher crash risk in drivers with dementia. Thus, the limited body of literature on actual crash risk to date shows conflicting results, in contrast to consistent evidence that the skills of driving deteriorate over time.

Establishing that dementia is associated with an increased risk of collision above and beyond controls without dementia has been challenging, likely in some part due to the exposure to road situations being reduced in people with dementia who often restrict their driving. In addition, There are significant limitations to the literature on driving with dementia – little data on drivers with moderate dementia, lack of screening for cognitive impairment in controls, inclusion of those with questionable dementia among the cases, variability in assessments and diagnostic criteria, age and gender mismatch between groups, and a lack of data on at-fault status among those with collisions (Rapoport et al, 2008). Regardless of the conflicting evidence, collisions in people with dementia are not rare. In a cohort of 210,550 people with dementia observed from 1997 to 2005 in Ontario, Canada, we found that of those with an active driver's licence, 24.1 per cent were involved in a collision, usually before the diagnosis was made, and they were usually found to be at fault for the collision (Rapoport et al, 2008).

Although dementia itself is not a contraindication to driving, people with mild dementia who continue to drive should have an assessment of their driving abilities that should be repeated every six to 12 months as the dementia progresses (Carr et al, 2010; CMA, 2012; Austroads,

2013; Rapoport et al, 2018). This is particularly important as it is challenging for physicians and other healthcare practitioners to know when driving has become unacceptably risky in people with dementia, and cognitive tests that are typically used in-office to assess the severity of the dementia are imprecise in predicting individual road risk (Molnar et al, 2006; Hird et al, 2016).

Risks associated with driving cessation in older adulthood

Many older adults consider driving to be vital to preserving their quality of life and their sense of independence, and this may be especially true for individuals living in rural areas where transportation options are often scarce (Rebok et al, 1994). Freund described driving cessation as a 'painful, awkward, difficult, embarrassing, sad, frustrating, tearful, ugly experience' (Freund, 2003). Driving generally means considerably more to individuals than simply providing a means of transportation to allow them to get from point A to point B. For most, driving represents convenience and autonomy, and it may also bestow a sense of competence (Yassuda et al, 1997; Byszewski et al, 2010). For some, driving may be integrally connected to their self-esteem and identity (Eisenhandler, 1990). Because driving holds such importance to older adults, they may be reluctant to give up driving, and driving cessation is associated with many adverse consequences (Byszewski et al, 2010).

Some older persons are accepting of the need to give up driving and some may even be relieved when the decision is made, but others may be angry about having to stop driving, especially if they feel a lack of control and of ownership of the driving cessation decision (Liddle et al, 2008). The lack of insight that often accompanies dementia makes it less likely that older people with dementia will appropriately self-restrict or stop driving compared with older adults who are cognitively intact, but have other health issues such as vision loss or heart disease (Wild and Cotrell, 2003). Byszewski and colleagues (2010) noted that 40 per cent of older persons with dementia who were counselled by healthcare professionals to stop driving rejected the recommendation and insisted that they were still safe to drive (Byszewski et al, 2010). A survey of physicians, nurse practitioners and physician assistants about counselling older adults about driving showed that for both urban and rural healthcare providers, second only to time constraints, the biggest barrier to counselling about driving was the resistance of the person with dementia to discuss driving issues or outright denial of driving concerns (Huseth-Zosel et al, 2016). When drivers with dementia resist giving up driving, it poses a major challenge for family caregivers and healthcare providers, putting them in the difficult situation of trying to balance being supportive of the emotional impact associated with driving cessation and the responsibility to protect the safety of the person with dementia and the public (Byszewski et al, 2010).

Chihuri and colleagues published a systematic review and meta-analysis including 16 studies pertaining to the various consequences of driving cessation in adults aged 55 and over that included a comparison group of current drivers (Chihuri et al, 2016). That study did not specifically address the impact of driving cessation in individuals with dementia, but the results almost certainly also apply to drivers with dementia who stop driving. Driving cessation was found to be associated with numerous negative consequences, including declines in general health and physical, social and cognitive functioning. Data pooled from five studies regarding the association of depression with driving cessation revealed that driving cessation increased the risk of depressive symptoms by a factor of 1.9 (95 per cent confidence interval = 1.6–2.3). Studies also showed that former drivers participated less in outside activities, had less social engagement and a reduction in the size of their social network, and had greater dependency and loss of control. Former drivers also had a faster cognitive decline over a ten-year period than active drivers after adjusting for baseline cognitive status and general health (Choi et al, 2014). The one study that looked at entry into a nursing home, assisted living community or retirement home found that former drivers compared with current drivers had a hazard ratio of 4.8 (confidence interval = 3.3–7.2) for long-term care admission (Freeman et al, 2006). Two studies that looked at the risk of mortality both found an increased mortality risk associated with driving cessation. One found that non-drivers were four to six times more likely to die than current drivers after adjusting for baseline factors (Edwards et al, 2009). The other found a 68 per cent higher five-year mortality risk for non-drivers (O'Connor et al, 2013).

Driving cessation also results in an increase in the caregiver burden for family caregivers who need to help the person they are caring for cope with their new non-driver status (Azad et al, 2002). If the family caregiver drives, this may mean becoming the main provider of transportation for the person they are caring for (Byszewski et al, 2010). If the family caregiver does not drive, they may need to identify alternative sources of transportation for themselves as well as for the person they are caring for. Family members also need to deal with the emotional aspects that driving cessation has on the person that they are caring for, as the realisation that they have to stop driving can have a huge emotional impact on older drivers who are extremely dependent on driving to meet their transportation needs (Byszewski et al, 2010).

Literature on older adults' driving in rural areas

A recent informal review of the literature that we carried out regarding driving cessation in rural areas revealed that there is a paucity of studies on this topic, with none focusing specifically on individuals with dementia. Studies on driving in rural areas highlight some distinct features compared with driving in urban areas. Rural areas tend to have a higher proportion of older adults compared with urban areas (Rosenbloom, 2003), which suggests that rural populations likely have a higher prevalence of age-related comorbidities, including dementia, that may negatively affect driving fitness. Relative to urban drivers, rural older drivers generally need to drive more frequently and longer distances to access needed services and participate in social activities (Rosenbloom, 2003).

Rural drivers are more likely than urban drivers to continue driving despite health conditions such as dementia (Ross et al, 2009). The accessibility, suitability and cost of alternative transportation options are important factors in the decision of older adults to stop driving (Donorfio et al, 2009). In urban areas, various alternatives to driving may exist, but in rural areas, driving may be the only available means for transportation and socialisation (Johnson, 1999, 2008), which poses an important barrier for older rural dwellers to give up driving. The social role of volunteering and providing care to others may be highly valued by older adults, especially women, and a lack of alternative transportation options may affect decisions about driving cessation (Byles and Gallienne, 2012). In rural communities, other important factors that may influence driving cessation decision making include long distances to needed services and community activities, the fear of social isolation and loneliness, and the lack of availability of family and friends (Johnson, 2002). Social support from families and friends in one report was found to be a critical factor in rural older adults' decision to stop driving because it assured them of social connectedness and of a dependable source of transportation (Johnson, 1998).

Similar factors that affect the decision making of urban older adults to give up driving influence the consequences of driving cessation in rural drivers. Older persons living in rural areas may experience a greater impact from driving cessation than urban seniors. Limited alternative transportation sources result in reduced access to grocery and other shopping, healthcare, religious services, social activities and family and friends, as well as access to larger communities that offer health and social services to support driving cessation, which may contribute to even greater risks of social isolation, loneliness, and declines in health with driving cessation in rural communities (Johnson, 1998).

Johnson conducted three qualitative studies highlighting important aspects of the driving cessation process for older adults in rural areas. In one study of 75 rural older adults who had decided to stop driving, more than three quarters expressed regret about their decision, and indicated that they would not make the same decision again, largely because of a sense of isolation (Johnson, 1995). In a second study of 45 rural older adults who continued driving despite contrary advice from family members, friends or healthcare providers, rationales for ignoring the advice included a disagreement with the advice, a high value placed on independence, and concerns about isolation and access to medical care and religious services (Johnson, 2002). In a third study of 75 older rural women who voluntarily stopped driving an average of five years earlier, almost half started driving again within six to nine months of stopping. Those who maintained driving cessation indicated that they did so because they perceived adequate support from family and friends to maintain their transportation needs. Several of those who resumed driving did so in order to assist others who they felt had greater needs than their own (Johnson, 2008).

The dementia and driving group of the Canadian Consortium on Neurodegeneration and Aging conducted a qualitative study of healthcare providers working with people with dementia, representatives of organisations that provide support services for those with dementia, and family caregivers of drivers and former drivers with dementia, in order to explore their process of making decisions about driving cessation, and coping with this transition (Sanford et al, in press). In that study, the participants emphasised the loss of independence that happens with driving cessation and consequent disruption to one's sense of identity. Driving cessation is perceived as one of a series of losses that occurs during the course of dementia. The particular losses of independence and identity with driving cessation were felt to be crucial targets to address in the healthcare setting, and participants felt that it was important to have support for these people to maintain their sense of purpose in life beyond cessation of driving. Although only four of the 30 participants interviewed were from rural areas, they provided an interesting perspective. These participants were from four different disciplines, and comprised an occupational therapist, a geriatrician, a nurse, and a nurse practitioner. Their comments revealed that the biggest challenge facing individuals in rural communities was a lack of transportation options. They had long distances to travel, and the primary alternate form of transportation was taxis, which many were unable to afford. The participants commented on a lack of social resources to help people stay connected and active. These healthcare providers commented on the fear of isolation that often prevents people with dementia from making the decision to stop driving. On a positive note, there was discussion that living in a smaller community often means that people watch out for and support each other. The main suggestions were to encourage networking to facilitate finding transportation alternatives, advocacy for a greater system awareness and supports, and subsidies for alternatives to transportation. Table 10.1 contains selected quotations from the rural participants highlighting some of these themes.

Another study used a survey methodology with a larger sample of healthcare providers. Huseth-Zosel and colleagues compared mobility counselling by rural (n = 157) and urban (n = 107) healthcare providers, including physicians, nurse practitioners and physician assistants (Huseth-Zosel, et al 2016). They found that rural healthcare providers were significantly less likely to discuss driving fitness or safe driving habits with patients aged 75–84 (odds ratio 0.45; 95% confidence interval = 0.25–0.80) and 85 years and over (odds ratio 0.50; 95% confidence interval = 0.28–0.89). Rural healthcare providers were also less likely to agree or strongly agree with statements about knowledge of and behaviours related to referring patients to fitness–to–drive assessments. In addition, rural healthcare providers were significantly less likely to agree that they had adequate resources to refer patients for fitness–to–drive assessments, and they were more likely to note the distance to the nearest driving assessment centre as an obstacle to addressing driving concerns. Rural healthcare providers were also significantly more likely to be concerned about the emotional consequences of their patients if they were to raise the issue of driving cessation and they were three times as likely as urban healthcare providers to identify not wanting to contribute to their patients' loss of independence as a barrier to providing counselling about driving.

Alternatives to driving in dementia: the Scottish context

According to the UK Alzheimer's Society, while about one in every three people with dementia continues to drive, most people diagnosed with Alzheimer's disease stop within about three years of the first symptoms (Alzheimer's Society, 2016). With other types of dementia, early symptoms may require people to stop driving sooner (Alzheimer's Society, 2016). Research indicates that mobility and travel is related to wellbeing in old age and that reduction in mobility and access to transport may result in an increase in isolation, loneliness and depression (Musselwhite et al, 2015). Indeed, one report describes it as having a 'devastating effect' on wellbeing (Royal Voluntary Service, 2013). It is imperative, then, to develop accessible and inclusive transport alternatives to driving if people with dementia are to remain independent and socially connected. One particular challenge in Scotland is that the only driving assessment service is based in Edinburgh. This means that drivers with dementia in rural areas and areas far from Edinburgh have to travel to, and drive in, a busy city to be assessed. The advantages and disadvantages associated with this have not been analysed.

The Chartered Institute of Logistics and Transport UK notes that while people with conditions such as dementia, autism, ADHD, dyslexia, anxiety and other invisible disabilities may have difficulties navigating travel services, the focus has remained on improving accessibility for those disabilities that are visible (CILT UK, 2017). However, in practice this is changing. For example, in 2016, Anxiety UK held a Mental Health and Transport Summit to highlight the issues associated with invisible disabilities (Mental Health Action Group and Anxiety UK, 2016). More recently, the UK's Civil Aviation Authority has published a guidance document that outlines steps that airports can take to improve their services for passengers with hidden disabilities (CAA, 2018).

A picture is emerging then, of ageing populations, widespread and continued rise in car usage, and an increasing number of people living with dementia and retiring from driving, with public transport that needs to focus on accessibility for people with hidden disabilities.

With this complex set of challenges in mind, a proposal was developed to explore the travel challenges for people living with dementia in more detail, with a view to turning insights into action, helping transport service providers to make travel experiences more enabling. Supported by the Life Changes Trust, early qualitative research was undertaken by a project called Upstream (Life Changes Trust, 2017), with the aim of understanding travel challenges from the perspective of people with dementia and exploring the use of these insights to develop a process to influence transport service improvement. The name was derived from the need to consider the experience and expertise of people living with conditions such as dementia during the initial design phase, upstream of delivery, to ensure that services are inclusive and enabling from the beginning.

Early work involved developing relationships with groups of people with dementia, such as those hosted by Alzheimer Scotland

and the Dementia Engagement Empowerment Project (DEEP) Network (Dementia Voices; website in reference list), and facilitating conversations about getting out and about. Work was focused in three areas initially: the Isle of Lewis, the largest island of Scotland's Western Isles archipelago; Aberdeen, Scotland's third largest city; and East Lothian, a large rural area to the east of Edinburgh, Scotland's capital. Using creative workshop techniques such as drawing and picture prompts, conversations explored the complexity and detail of journeys, including and beyond the transport. Most discussions focused on public transport although driving cessation was a common topic (Hyde and Garner, 2017).

A wide range of issues emerged including journey planning, purchasing and using different types of tickets, the provision and design of toilets on journeys, wayfinding, signage, the challenges of noisy environments and many more. Services can be inconsistent and complicated, and many environments and experiences can cause anxiety. While the issues pointed to a need for product and service redesign, there may also be a lack of service provider awareness and understanding about dementia. Upstream's response was to develop a process that provides an opportunity to bring transport service providers and people with dementia together to learn, develop ideas and design new services together. At the centre of this process is the concept of a 'Shared Journey', in which service providers experience a service with people with dementia, using their shared understanding of dementia and travel, to design new solutions together (Hyde and Cassidy, 2017). This work is being taken forward by Go Upstream, a social enterprise emerging from the project.

Implications in the rural setting in Scotland

The Scottish Government analyses evidence around social inequalities and its *Review of equality evidence in rural Scotland* noted that contemporary research in rural matters was relatively scarce (Scottish Government, 2015). It found that 'few people' in rural areas feel that they have good access to public transportation facilities: Scottish Government research in 2012 reported that just over half (55 per cent) of residents in remote rural areas considered that they had access to good public transport facilities, compared with 91 per cent in the rest of Scotland, and 12 per cent of remote rural respondents reported that they did not have access to a bus service (Scottish Government, 2015).

While many of the issues raised in Go Upstream's work apply in both rural and urban settings, some of them might have more of an impact in more remote areas. For example, a lack of access to public toilets during a journey has been highlighted as a significant factor in planning a journey and recent BBC research has shown that, in most rural areas of Scotland, there has been a reduction in the number of public toilets (Jones and Schrarer, 2018). It should be noted, however, that our experience in the Western Isles has highlighted the beneficial characteristics of services developed within a rural context. For example, stories were told of bus drivers who ensured that regular passengers requiring extra assistance reached home safely. Due to the relatively small size of the Stornoway Airport team, staff tended to 'multitask', potentially creating better communication between staff in different departments, leading to more personalised assistance services (Upstream meeting at Stornoway Airport, 2016).

National transport policy in Scotland

The Go Upstream approach, involving people with dementia in discovery and design, fits with national policies and strategies that have emerged in the UK in recent years. Scotland's Accessible Travel Framework (Transport Scotland, 2016) is a ten-year plan to make transport more accessible, developed with disabled people who identified a list of 48 issues and areas to address. One of the four outcomes it aims to achieve is 'disabled people are more involved in the design, development and improvement of transport policies, services and infrastructure'. Similarly, the UK government's 2018 Inclusive Transport Strategy called for better training to ensure that transport staff have a greater understanding of the needs of disabled people, leading to better assistance. It also indicated a need for change of approach from developing 'accessible transport' to 'inclusive travel', where services are designed through dialogue with disabled people from the start (Department for Transport, 2018). Additionally, the Scottish Government's National Dementia Strategy (2017–20) included, for the first time, a commitment to improve transport for people with dementia, recognising that training and service design can only be meaningfully developed and delivered with and by people with dementia (Scottish Government, 2017c).

Practical suggestions

There are limitations to the available research on the topic of dementia, driving and transportation, particularly when it comes to meeting the complex needs of older adults living in rural areas. The major theme that emerges is that accessible alternatives to driving are critical in order to ensure that people living with dementia can successfully retire from driving and continue to enjoy their lives. The work identified in this chapter highlights some practical suggestions that are worthy of consideration.

Public policy, advocacy and education

There needs to be an appreciation among policy makers that if one lives long enough, one will live several years without driving privileges (Foley et al, 2002). There is therefore a need to develop services and resources that support people living in rural areas through the transition of driving cessation, helping them plan alternative forms of transportation, facilitate their use of public transportation, and nurture availability of alternative modalities such as car sharing and community transport.

Policy makers and the public need to understand that dementia is associated with inevitable impairment in driving skills and all drivers with dementia will need to give up driving once it progresses beyond the mild stage, and even some in the mild stage will be unsafe to drive.

It will be important to engage with transport operators and other transportation service providers to raise awareness and enhance understanding of the challenges that travel can pose for people with dementia, and to appreciate their role in providing vital 'lifeline' services, particularly in rural areas. Training should be combined with opportunities for change and for service improvements in a way that enhances the mobility and quality of life for this vulnerable population. Awareness and understanding of the challenges of travelling with dementia and other invisible disabilities needs to be incorporated into early and continuing education for transport professionals.

More broadly speaking, it will be important to initiate conversations about the challenges of rural transportation among policy makers involved in designing housing, planning healthcare services, and other aspects of civic planning.

Healthcare providers

Much remains to be done about improving the education of healthcare providers so that they are comfortable with how to assess and counsel people about driving, and about improving the access to driving assessments in remote areas via remote videoconferencing or telehealth access. In the meantime, clinicians should be encouraged to routinely ask older adults if they drive and about any restrictions, crashes, infractions, or safety concerns. These conversations should be supplemented by information from objective observers such as family members, especially since a caregiver's rating of the driving ability of a relative with dementia as marginal or unsafe has been shown to be useful in identifying unsafe drivers (Iverson et al, 2010).

Healthcare providers also have an important role in initiating discussions about the impact of medical conditions and medications on driving safety. At the first sign of cognitive impairment, discussions must be initiated about the ultimate need to stop driving if the cognitive impairment progresses, and recommendations made to begin trying alternative forms of transportation. As much as possible, the person living with dementia should be actively involved in such discussions about driving cessation and alternative forms of transportation.

For people with mild dementia whose driving skills are questionable, increased access is needed to specialised on-road driving assessments that are reasonably priced or heavily subsidised. On-road driving assessment routes may need to be modified for rural drivers. An evaluation of characteristics of on-road driving assessment test routes used by occupational therapist driver assessors in Victoria, Australia found that there were restricted opportunities to include some types of road features in rural testing sites that would be considered compulsory in most jurisdictions for a comprehensive assessment of fitness to drive (Di Stefano and Macdonald, 2012). In light of this, they suggested that some driving assessment routes, such as those in some rural areas, should be recognised as 'low demand', and that these routes should only be used to assess drivers who would be willing to accept a restricted license to drive exclusively in the local area where the driving test was completed.

People with dementia and their family caregivers

There is a great need to increase the availability of tools, resources and support groups for people with dementia and their family caregivers. These should optimise proactive planning of driving cessation and enhance quality of life and mobility after cessation. Family caregivers need encouragement to have early discussions about driving safety with their relative with dementia, and to enlist the help of healthcare providers regarding driving assessment and cessation. Since these matters are of particular importance for those with dementia living in rural areas that have unique challenges in alternate transportation, the tools, resources and support groups need to be tailored to the rural context.

Partnerships

Several projects have emerged from Go Upstream's approach involving people with dementia in partnership with organisations for discovery and design. Project Onwards is working with people with dementia in Scotland to design and develop a service to support people through the transition of retiring from driving as a result of their diagnosis. Early findings from this indicated that key elements of support should include: understanding and navigating interactions with the national licencing agency and medical professionals; planning and preparing for travelling without a car; and exploring the benefits that a car-free life can bring (Life Changes Trust, 2018). Other projects involve working with people with dementia to explore the accessibility of toilets during a journey (Wilkinson et al, 2018) and the role of technology to enhance assisted rail travel (Go Upstream, 2018). Go Upstream's aim is to inform the design of new products and services, but also to influence policy, highlighting the importance of mobility and the experiences and expertise of people with dementia. This approach is attracting attention beyond Scotland.

People with dementia and their family caregivers need to be involved in planning alternative transportation that works for them. It is important to create opportunities for transportation and healthcare service providers to work together with people with dementia so that solutions reflect their real-life needs. This may take the form of workshops, training courses, events or conferences. Opportunities need to be created for involvement of people with dementia so that they can share their experience and expertise and create immediate and tangible benefits. The opportunities need to align with national strategies and policies and be backed up with evidence that strengthens arguments for developing inclusive processes. The hope is that this will ultimately lead to an inclusive, holistic approach to transportation.

Research

Clinical research on assessment of driving risk in dementia in rural areas should include novel strategies that allow for observation of driving skills in the naturalistic environment that includes the restrictions of driving made adaptively by this population. A different set of skills is needed to navigate the complex traffic congestion and hectic driving environments common in urban areas that may not be necessary in rural areas, and drivers with dementia tend to restrict driving more than their age peers. However, drivers with very low mileage may have particularly high risks when they do drive (Langford et al, 2013; Antin et al, 2017). Novel assessment strategies include adapted specialised on-road tests (Di Stefano and Macdonald, 2012) or the use of instrumented vehicles that allow for the observation of real-world driving (Charlton et al, 2013; Marshall et al, 2013; Guo et al, 2015).

Interventions used to support drivers with dementia in their process of cessation need to be tested in rural contexts to ensure that what works in cities still applies (Rapoport et al, 2017). Similarly, the use of autonomous vehicles, which has been touted as a potential panacea for meeting the transportation needs of people with dementia, will require careful study because of the potential need for drivers to take over the operation of the vehicle due to environmental or technical factors, which would likely be very challenging for people with dementia (Shergold et al, 2016).

Research is also needed to establish whether restricted licences are associated with a reduction or an increase in collision risk for rural drivers with dementia. A study from Saskatchewan, a Canadian province with large rural areas, showed mixed results about the safety impact of licences restricted for medical reasons. Those with restricted licences tended to be older, male, and living in rural areas. Once adjusting for age, sex and location (rural versus urban), those with licence restrictions were modestly at higher risk of at-fault collisions compared with those without restrictions. However, for those with restrictions, there was a modest reduction of collisions after the implementation of the restriction (Marshall et al, 2002). That study, however, did not restrict its analysis to rural drivers or examine licence restrictions related to dementia.

Conclusion

A United Nations representative wrote a hard-hitting report on the effects of poverty after a tour of the UK in late 2018. The author wrote:

> Despite the idyllic traditional image of the English countryside, poverty in rural areas is particularly harsh. Rural dwellers are particularly impacted by cuts to

transportation and public services, are at a higher risk of loneliness and isolation, and often face higher fuel costs. (Alston, 2018)

The conclusion of the report was that transportation in rural areas should be considered:

> ... an essential service, equivalent to water and electricity, and the government should regulate the sector to the extent necessary to ensure that people living in rural areas are adequately served. Abandoning people to the private market in relation to a service that affects every dimension of their basic well-being is incompatible with human rights requirements. (Alston, 2018)

Although driving is a privilege and not a right, access to transportation is a fundamental right and need of all people. If we are to respond to a call to ensure that access to transportation is met, we must act at various levels.

At the strategic level, policy and education could include:

- funding and undertaking more research into driving skills and licence restrictions that can enable safety and autonomy;
- raising awareness of the challenges of travelling with dementia among policy makers, healthcare professionals, transport professionals and the wider public;
- initiating conversations about rural transportation among those who design housing, healthcare and other aspects of civic planning;
- engaging with transport operators to improve education and enhance understanding of the role that services play in maintaining the independence of people with dementia;
- nurturing the availability of public transportation as well as new alternatives such as car sharing and community transport.

Locally, at a grass-roots level, measures could include:

- enabling healthcare providers to routinely initiate conversations about driving safety, the ultimate need to stop driving and alternative forms of transportation;
- supporting families to proactively plan for driving cessation and future mobility – discovering and trying alternative transportation that works for them;

Table 10.1: Selected perspectives of rural healthcare practitioners on driving with dementia in rural areas

Theme	Selected quotes
Lack of transportation options	"... does have a taxi system. It does have a bus system. Buses are affordable, but they don't go everywhere ... and the taxis can be 10 bucks a pop one way. The mobility van service is $10 one way.... So, for someone on a fixed income that can be, um, very challenging.... So – affording, uh, transportation, means of transport is absolutely one that can be quite a barrier for people."
	"It's not like there's a bus every 10 minutes, or, like a cab here, it costs about 60 bucks just to get down."
Lack of social resources	"We're a small town.... And so, you know, we're not able to provide or offer the same social supports, obviously, that a city is ... going to have, of course."
Fear of isolation	"Locally in this, in the more rural communities, it absolutely defines independence."
	"For some, it can be as dramatic as they can no longer live at home. If they are in a completely rural community with no ability to get out ... a client['s] ... brother, who, who was in his 90s. Still driving. And said to his sister, 'If I can't drive, I don't want to live anymore. Because that means I can no longer live where I'm living'."
Strategies to help with transportation	"Like, so culturally, developmentally in terms of communities –... how do you make transportation affordable and, and a reliable option? ... whole issue around community and how you make networks happen within communities.... We have a great, we have a great network for cancer care, right. So everybody that needs cancer treatments and through us, they get a free ride.... By volunteers. Um, it doesn't happen in the world of dementia."
	"... where are communities investing themselves in terms of creating that infrastructure that allows options for alternatives to driving.... If our elderly population ... is no longer safe to drive .... How do we ensure that we still give them the option for food, getting out for socialisation, getting their needs met? So ... some communities do. Smaller communities can do really well at that. By virtue of churches and community organisations that will support, look after each other and we do, that is part of what we call Share the Care concept ... it can happen on a one-on-one basis. Share the Care ... where families need to say, 'Okay. All of us don't need to be in there to see Mom and Dad on the same day. How do we work that out so we can support them by being there on different days?'. But it's also a community ... effort as well. How do we ... deal with our isolated seniors?"

Source: Sanford et al (in press)

- providing tools, resources and support specifically tailored to the rural context;
- actively involving people with dementia in discussions about driving cessation;
- creating opportunities for people with dementia to work directly together with transportation and healthcare service providers to develop solutions that truly reflect real-life needs;
- evaluating the implementation of these strategies.

The motor vehicle is more than a tool to get around vast rural areas – it is a symbol of identity embedded with rich meanings. Drivers with dementia need access to services that can help them retire from driving before safety concerns make this imperative and ensure that they do not stop living after they stop driving. These drivers and their family caregivers need to be actively involved in the design, implementation and evaluation of the creative solutions that will be necessary.

References

Alston, P. (2018) 'Statement on visit to the United Kingdom, by Professor Philip Alston, United Nations Special Rapporteur on extreme poverty and human rights', [online]. Available from: www.ohchr.org/Documents/Issues/Poverty/EOM_GB_16Nov2018.pdf

Alzheimer Scotland (2017) 'Statistics', [online]. Available from: www.alzscot.org/campaigning/statistics

Alzheimer's Society (2016) *Driving and dementia*, Factsheet 439LP, London: Alzheimer's Society. Available from www.alzheimers.org.uk/sites/default/files/2018-10/439LP%20Driving%20and%20dementia.pdf

Antin, J.F., Guo, F., Fang, Y., Dingus, T.A., Perez, M.A. and Hankey, J.M. (2017) 'A validation of the low mileage bias using naturalistic driving study data', *Journal of Safety Research*, 63: 115–20.

Austroads (2013) *Assessing fitness to drive for commercial and private vehicle drivers: Medical standards for licensing and clinical management guidelines*, Sydney: Austroads. Available from: http://www.austroads.com.au/images/stories/assessing_fitnes-s_to_drive_2013_rev2.pdf

Azad, N., Byszewski, A., Amos, S. and Molnar, F. (2002) 'A survey of the impact of driving cessation on older drivers', *Geriatrics Today: Journal of the Canadian Geriatric Society*, 5: 170–4.

Byles, J. and Gallienne, L. (2012) 'Driving in older age: a longitudinal study of women in urban, regional, and remote areas and the impact of caregiving', *Journal of Women & Aging*, 24(2): 113–25.

Byszewski, A.M., Molnar, F.J. and Aminzadeh, F. (2010) 'The impact of disclosure of unfitness to drive in persons with newly diagnosed dementia: patient and caregiver perspectives', *Clinical Gerontologist*, 33: 152–63.

Canning, S., Thomas, R. and Wright, S. (2015) *Research into the social and economic benefits of community transport in Scotland*, Glasgow: Transport Scotland. Available from: www.transport.gov.scot/media/32402/j368247.pdf

Carr, D., Schwartzberg, J.G., Manning, L. and Sempek, J. (2010) *Physician's guide to assessing and counseling older drivers* (2nd edn), Washington, DC: NHTSA. Available from: http://www.ama-assn.org/ama/pub/physician-resources/public-health/promoting-healthy-lifestyles/geriatric-health/older-driver-safety/assessing-counseling-older-drivers.page

Charlton, J.L., Catchlove, M., Scully, M., Koppel, S. and Newstead, S. (2013) 'Older driver distraction: a naturalistic study of behaviour at intersections', *Accident Analysis and Prevention*, 58: 271–8.

Chee, J.N., Rapoport, M.J., Molnar, F., Herrmann, N., O'Neill, D., Marottoli, R., Mitchell, S., Tant, M., Dow, J., Ayotte, D. and Lanctôt, K.L. (2017) 'Update on the risk of motor vehicle collision or driving impairment with dementia: a collaborative international systematic review and meta-analysis', *The American Journal of Geriatric Psychiatry*, 25(12): 1376–90.

Chihuri, S., Mielenz, T.J., DiMaggio, C.J., Betz, M.E., DiGuiseppi, C., Jones, V.C. and Li, G. (2016) 'Driving cessation and health outcomes in older adults', *Journal of the American Geriatrics Society*, 64(2): 332–41.

Choi, M., Lohman, M.C. and Mezuk, B. (2014) 'Trajectories of cognitive decline by driving mobility: evidence from the Health and Retirement Study', *International Journal of Geriatric Psychiatry*, 29(5): 447–53.

CILT UK (Chartered Institute of Logistics and Transport UK) (2017) *Guidance note: Understanding and meeting the needs of travellers with hidden disabilities*, Corby: CILT UK. Available from: https://ciltuk.org.uk/LinkClick.aspx?fileticket=rmsmac-7NHg%3D&portalid=0&timestamp=1512121645759

CAA (Civil Aviation Authority) (2018) *Supporting people with hidden disabilities at UK airports*, CAP 1629, London: CAA. Available from: https://publicapps.caa.co.uk/docs/33/CAP1629%20HD%20-%20FINAL%2007JUN2018.pdf

CMA (Canadian Medical Association) (2012) *CMA driver's guide: Determining medical fitness to operate motor vehicles*, Ottawa: CMA.

Davis, J.D., Papandonatos, G.D., Miller, L.A., Hewitt, S.D., Festa, E.K., Heindel, W.C. and Ott, B.R. (2012) 'Road test and naturalistic driving performance in healthy and cognitively impaired older adults: does environment matter?', *Journal of the American Geriatrics Society*, 60(11): 2056–62.

Dementia Voices UK www.dementiavoices.org.uk

Department for Transport (2018) *The Inclusive Transport Strategy: Achieving equal access for disabled people*, London: Department for Transport. Available from: www.gov.uk/government/publications/inclusive-transport-strategy

Di Stefano, M. and Macdonald, W. (2012) 'Design of occupational therapy on-road test routes and related validity issues', *Australian Occupational Therapy Journal*, 59: 37–46.

Donorfio, L.K., D'Ambrosio, L.A., Coughlin, J.F. and Mohyde, M. (2009) 'To drive or not to drive, that isn't the question: the meaning of self-regulation among older drivers', *Journal of Safety Research*, 40(3): 221–6.

Douglas, M., Higgins, M., Austin, H., Armour, G., Jepson, R., Thomson, H. and Hurley, F. (2018) *Health and transport: A guide, 2018*, Scottish Health and Inequality Impact Assessment Network Report, Glasgow: Scottish Health and Inequality Impact Assessment Network. Available from: www.scotphn.net/wp-content/uploads/2015/11/Transport-Guide-2018-Final-Formatted.pdf

Edwards, J.D., Perkins, M., Ross, L.A. and Reynolds, S.L. (2009) 'Driving status and three-year mortality among community-dwelling older adults', *Journals of Gerontology Series A: Biomedical Sciences and Medical Sciences*, 64(2): 300–5.

Eisenhandler, S.A. (1990) 'The asphalt identikit: old age and the driver's license', *International Journal of Aging and Human Development*, 30(1): 1–14.

Foley, D.J., Heimovitz, H.K., Guralnik, J.M. and Brock D.B. (2002) 'Driving life expectancy of persons aged 70 years and older in the United States', *American Journal of Public Health*, 92(8): 1284–9.

Freeman, E.E., Gange, S.J., Muñoz, B. and West, S.K. (2006) 'Driving status and risk of entry into long-term care in older adults', *American Journal of Public Health*, 96(7): 1254–9.

Freund, K. (2003) 'Mobility and older people' *Generations*, 27(2): 68–9.

Go Upstream (2018) ' "Welcome" Aboard!', Go Upstream [Blog]. Available from: www.upstream.scot/blog/2018/10/12/welcome-aboard

Guo, F., Fang, Y. and Antin, J.F. (2015) 'Older driver fitness-to-drive evaluation using naturalistic driving data', *Journal of Safety Research*, 54: 49–54.

Herrmann, N., Rapoport, M.J., Sambrook, R., Hebert, R., McCracken, P. and Robbilard, A. (2006) 'Predictors of driving cessation in mild-to-moderate dementia', *Canadian Medical Association Journal*, 175(6): 591–5.

Hird, M.A., Egeto, P., Fischer, C.E., Naglie, G. and Schweizer T.A. (2016) 'A systematic review and meta-analysis of on-road simulator and cognitive driving assessment in Alzheimer's disease and mild cognitive impairment', *Journal of Alzheimer's Disease*, 53(2): 713–29.

Holley-Moore, G. and Creighton, H. (2015) *The future of transport in an ageing society*, London: International Longevity Centre UK. Available from: https://ilcuk.org.uk/the-future-of-transport-in-an-ageing-society

Hopkins, R.W., Kilik, L., Day, D.J.A. and Rows, C. (2004) 'Driving and dementia in Ontario: a quantitative assessment of the problem', *The Canadian Journal of Psychiatry*, 49: 434–8.

Houston, D. and Tilley, S. (2016) 'Fare's fair? Concessionary travel policy and social justice', *Journal of Poverty and Social Justice*, 24(2): 187–207.

Huseth-Zosel, A., Sanders, G., O'Connor, M., Fuller-Iglesias, H. and Langley, L. (2016) 'Health care provider mobility counseling provision to older adults: a rural/urban comparison', *Journal of Community Health*, 41: 1–10.

Hyde, A. and Cassidy, S. (2017) *Travelling well with dementia*, Glasgow: Life Changes Trust. Available from: www.lifechangestrust.org.uk/sites/default/files/Upstream%20Final%20Report.pdf

Hyde, A. and Garner, B. (2017) 'Travelling well with dementia, Paper presented at the Scottish Transport Applications Research 2017 conference. Available from: www.starconference.org.uk/star/2017/Hyde.pdf

Iverson, D.J., Gronseth, G.S., Reger, M.A., Classen, S., Dubinsky, R.M. and Rizzo, M. (2010) 'Practice parameter update: evaluation and management of driving risk in dementia. report of the Quality Standards Subcommittee of the American Academy of Neurology', *Neurology*, 74(16): 1316–24.

Johnson, J.E. (1995) 'Rural elders and the decision to stop driving', *Journal of Community Health Nursing*, 12(3): 131–8.

Johnson, J.E. (1998) 'Older rural adults and the decision to stop driving: the influence of family and friends', *Journal of Community Health Nursing*, 15(4): 205–16.

Johnson, J.E. (1999) 'Urban older adults and the forfeiture of a driver's license', *Journal of Gerontological Nursing*, 25(12): 12–18.

Johnson, J.E. (2002) 'Why rural elders drive against advice', *Journal of Community Health Nursing*, 19(4): 237–44.

Johnson, J.E. (2008) 'Informal social support networks and the maintenance of voluntary driving cessation by older rural women', *Journal of Community Health Nursing*, 25(2): 65–72.

Jones, L. and Schrarer, R. (2018) 'Reality check: public toilets mapped', BBC News, [online], 15 August. Available from: www.bbc.co.uk/news/uk-45009337

Langford, J., Charlton, J.L., Koppel, S., Myers, A., Tuokko, H., Marshall, S., Man-Son-Hing, M., Darzins, P., DiStefano, M. and Macdonald, W. (2013) 'Findings from the Candrive/Ozcandrive study: low mileage older drivers, crash risk and reduced fitness to drive', *Accident Analysis and Prevention*, 61: 304–10.

Liddle, J., Turpin, M., Carlson, G. and McKenna, K. (2008) 'The needs and experiences related to driving cessation for older people', *British Journal of Occupational Therapy*, 71: 379–88.

Life Changes Trust (2017) *Life Changes Trust progress report: October 2016 – September 2017*, Glasgow: Life Changes Trust. Available from: www.lifechangestrust.org.uk/sites/default/files/publications/PROGRESS%20REPORT%202017%20WEB%20UPDATED.pdf

Life Changes Trust (2018) *Onwards: Designing a mobility service with people affected by dementia*. Available from: www.lifechangestrust.org.uk/projects/transport-and-dementia

Man-Son-Hing, M., Marshall, S.C., Molnar, F.J. and Wilson, K.G. (2007) 'Systematic review of driving risk and the efficacy of compensatory strategies in persons with dementia', *Journal of the American Geriatrics Society*, 55(6): 878–84.

Marshall, S.C., Man-Son-Hing, M., Bedard, M., Charlton, J., Gagnon, S., Gélinas, I., Koppel, S., Korner-Bitensky, N., Langford, J., Mazer, B., Myers, A., Naglie, G., Polgar, J., Porter, M.M., Rapoport, M., Tuokko, H., Vrkljan, B. and Woolnough, A. (2013) 'Protocol for Candrive II/Ozcandrive: a multicentre prospective older driver cohort study', *Accident Analysis and Prevention*, 61: 245–52.

Marshall, S.C., Spasoff, R., Nair, R. and van Walraven, C. (2002) 'Restricted driver licensing for medical impairments: does it work?', *Canadian Medical Association Journal*, 167(7): 747–51.

Mental Health Action Group and Anxiety UK (2016) *Mental Health and Transport Summit report*, Manchester: Anxiety UK. Available from: www.anxietyuk.org.uk/wp-content/uploads/2016/05/Mental-Health-Transport-Summit-Report.pdf

Molnar, F.J., Patel, A., Marshall, S.C., Man-Son-Hing, M. and Wilson, K.G. (2006) 'Clinical utility of office-based cognitive predictors of fitness to drive in persons with dementia: a systematic review', *Journal of the American Geriatrics Society*, 54(12): 1809–24.

Musselwhite, C.B.A., Holland, C. and Walker, I. (2015) 'The role of transport and mobility in the health of older people', *Journal of Transport & Health*, 2(1): 1–4.

Myers, A. (2015) 'Mobility in later life: addressing safety concerns and the needs of older Canadians', Paper presented at the Transportation and Healthy Aging: Issues and Ideas for an Aging Society conference, Toronto, Ontario, 30 April to 1 May.

National Records of Scotland (2018) *Scotland's population 2017: Infographic report*, Edinburgh: National Records of Scotland. Available from: www.nrscotland.gov.uk/files//statistics/nrs-visual/rgar-2017/rgar-2017-infographic-booklet.pdf

O'Connor, M., Edwards, J. and Waters, M. (2013) 'Mediators of the association between driving cessation and mortality among older adults', *Journal of Aging and Health*, 25(8 Suppl): 249S-269S.

Ott, B.R., Heindel, W.C., Papandonatos, G.D., Festa, E.K., Davis, J.D., Daiello, L.A. and Morris, J.C. (2008) 'A longitudinal study of drivers with Alzheimer disease', *Neurology*, 70(14): 1171–8.

Raina, P., Wolfson, C., Kirkland, S. and Griffith, L. (eds) (2018) *The Canadian Longitudinal Study on Aging (CLSA) report on health and aging in Canada: Findings from baseline data collection 2010–2015*, Hamilton: CLSA. Available from: www.clsa-elcv.ca/doc/2639

Rapoport, M.J., Cameron, D.H., Sanford, S. and Naglie, G. (2017) 'A systematic review of intervention approaches for driving cessation in older adults', *International Journal of Geriatric Psychiatry*, 32(5): 484–91.

Rapoport, M.J., Chee, J.N., Carr, D.B., Molnar, F., Naglie, G., Dow, J., Marottoli, R., Mitchell, S., Tant, M., Herrmann, N., Lanctôt, K.L., Taylor, J.P., Donaghy, P.C., Classen, S. and O'Neill, D. (2018) 'An international approach to enhancing a national guideline on driving and dementia', *Current Psychiatry Reports*, 20(3): 16.

Rapoport, M.J., Herrmann, N., Molnar, F., Rochon, P.A., Juurlink, D.N., Zagorski, B., Seitz, D., Morris, J.C. and Redelmeier, D.A. (2008) 'Psychotropic medications and motor vehicle collisions in patients with dementia', *Journal of the American Geriatrics Society*, 56(10): 1968–70.

Rebok, G.W., Keyl, P.M., Bylsma, F.W., Blaustein, M.J. and Tune, L. (1994) 'The effects of Alzheimer disease on driving-related abilities', *Alzheimer Disease & Associated Disorders*, 8: 228–40.

Rosenbloom, S. (2003) 'The mobility needs of older Americans', in B. Katz and R. Puentes (eds) *Taking the high road: A metropolitan agenda for transportation reform*, Washington, DC: Brookings Institution Press, pp 227–54.

Ross, L.A., Anstey, K.J., Kiely, K.M., Windsor, T.D., Byles, J.E., Luszcz, M.A. and Mitchell, P. (2009) 'Older drivers in Australia: trends in driving status and cognitive and visual impairment', *Journal of the American Geriatrics Society*, 57(10): 1868–73.

Royal Automobile Club Foundation (2018) 'Hundreds over 100 hold driving licence', [online]. Available from: www.racfoundation.org/media-centre/hundreds-over-100-hold-driving-licence

Royal Voluntary Service (2013) *Going nowhere fast: Impact of inaccessible public transport on wellbeing and social connectedness of older people in Great Britain*, Cardiff: Royal Voluntary Service. Available from: www.royalvoluntaryservice.org.uk/Uploads/Documents/Reports%20and%20Reviews/Trans%20report_GB_web_v1.pdf

Sanford, S., Rapoport, M.J., Tuokko, H., Crizzle, A., Hatzifilalithis, S., Laberge, S. and Naglie, G. (in press) 'Independence, loss, and social identity: perspectives on driving cessation and dementia', *Dementia*, doi: 1471301218762838.

Scottish Government (2015) *Review of equality evidence in rural Scotland*, Edinburgh: Scottish Government. Available from: https://www.gov.scot/Resource/0046/00469898.pdf

Scottish Government (2017a) *Age and transport and travel, 2016*. Available from: https://www.transport.gov.scot/media/39692/sct09170037961.pdf?

Scottish Government (2017b) *Scotland's National Dementia Strategy 2017–2020*, Edinburgh: Health and Social Care Integration Directorate, Scottish Government. Available from: www.gov.scot/publications/scotlands-national-dementia-strategy-2017-2020/

Scottish Government (2017c) 'Scottish transport statistics, No 36, 2017 edition', [online]. Available from: www.transport.gov.scot/publication/scottish-transport-statistics-no-36-2017-edition/chapter-1-road-transport-vehicles

Scottish Islands Federation (2011) 'Island statistics', [online]. Available from: www.scottish-islands-federation.co.uk/island-statistics

Shergold, I., Wilson, M. and Parkhurst, G. (2016) *The mobility of older people, and the future role of Connnected Autonomous Vehicles: A literature review, Sept 2016*, Bristol: University of the West of England. Available from: http://eprints.uwe.ac.uk/31998/1/User%20Needs%20Review_Repository.pdf

The Conference Board of Canada (2016) *Managing mobility: Transportation in an aging society*, Ottawa: The Conference Board of Canada. Available from: www.conferenceboard.ca/e-library/abstract.aspx?did=8293&AspxAutoDetectCookieSupport=1

Transport Scotland (2016) *Going further: Scotland's Accessible Travel Framework*, Edinburgh: Transport Scotland. Available from: www.transport.gov.scot/publication/going-further-scotland-s-accessible-travel-framework

Transport Scotland (2018) *Transport and travel in Scotland 2017*, A National Statistics Publication for Scotland, Edinburgh: Transport Scotland. Available from: www.transport.gov.scot/publication/transport-and-travel-in-scotland-2017

Transport Scotland (n.d. a) 'Lifeline air services', [online]. Available from: www.transport.gov.scot/public-transport/air-travel/lifeline-air-services [Accessed 29 October 2019].

Transport Scotland (n.d. b) 'Concessionary travel', [online]. Available from: www.transport.gov.scot/concessionary-travel/60plus-and-disabled [Accessed 29 October 2019].

Turcotte, M. (2012) 'Profile of seniors' transportation habits', Statistics Canada Catalogue No. 11-008, Canadian Social Trends, [online]. Available from: www150.statcan.gc.ca/n1/pub/11-008-x/2012001/article/11619-eng.pdf

Upstream meeting at Stornoway Airport (2016) https://dfclanntair.wordpress.com/2016/05/03/upstream-meeting-at-stornoway-airport/

Vrkljan, B., Cammarata, M., Marshall, S., Naglie, G., Rapoport, M., Sangrar, R., Stinchcombe, A. and Tuokko, H. (2018) 'Transportation mobility', in P. Raina, C. Wolfson, S. Kirkland and L. Griffith (eds) *The Canadian Longitudinal Study on Aging (CLSA) report on health and aging in Canada: Findings from baseline data collection 2010–2015*, Hamilton: CLSA, pp 180–93.

Wild, J., and Cotrell, V. (2003) 'Identifying driving impairment in Alzheimer disease: a comparison of self and observer reports versus driving evaluations', *Alzheimer Disease and Associated Disorders*, 17: 27–34.

Wilkinson, H., Hyde, A., Houston, A., Miller, J. and Marshall, M. (2018) 'Transport and toilets: finding solutions which maximize the design and findability of accessible toilets when travelling', University of Edinburgh.

Yassuda, M., Wilson, J. and von Mering, O. (1997) 'Driving cessation: the perspective of senior drivers', *Educational Gerontology*, 23: 525–38.

11

Considerations in dementia care for Indigenous populations in Canada

Kristen M. Jacklin and Jessica M. Chiovitte

Introduction

It is well known that population aging is occurring at a global scale. This trend is expected to continue in coming decades, but not all demographic cohorts are affected in the same way. Over the past two decades, age-related dementias have surfaced as a growing health concern in Indigenous[1] populations globally (Henderson, 2002, 2009; Smith et al, 2008; Jacklin et al, 2013a, 2015a; Radford et al, 2015), yet data on incidence and prevalence remain limited (Warren et al, 2015). Recent research suggests the increase of dementia in Indigenous communities may be attributable to a combination of complex causes, such as changing perceptions of the illness, demographic transitions, impacts resulting from the social determinants of health, exposure to risk, increased vulnerability, and co-morbidities (Jacklin et al, 2013a).

The emergence of dementia as a health disparity in Indigenous populations is set among a backdrop of health inequities experienced by Indigenous populations worldwide (Gracey and King, 2009; Sequist, 2017). Increasingly in recent years, scholars are acknowledging the need to explicitly address the underlying structures within health systems and policies that perpetuate health inequities for Indigenous and ethnic minority populations by incorporating frameworks such as structural violence, social justice, and health equity into research strategies (Farmer et al, 2006; Dilworth-Anderson et al, 2012; Bailey et al, 2017; Stanley et al, 2017). Along with this, there is growing acknowledgement that a careful consideration of Indigenous culture and context is necessary to develop appropriate frameworks for the delivery of equitable healthcare strategies (Browne et al, 2017; Jacklin et al, 2017b; Crowshoe et al, 2019).

This chapter provides an overview of what is known about the experience of dementia in Indigenous populations in North America and examines this knowledge using a cultural safety and health equity lens for rural and remote Indigenous communities in Canada. We construct a health equity argument by first establishing the dementia disparity in Indigenous peoples within the context of complex social determinants of health unique to this population. We then provide a brief overview of how both cultural and systemic forces affect the dementia experience and access to care. Cultural safety is used as a framework to understand how to respond and how to create more equitable dementia outcomes.

We draw on our team's experience of conducting qualitative ethnographic research with Indigenous populations in Ontario, Canada over the past ten years, and published studies concerning Indigenous experiences with dementia and dementia care in North America. We suggest that developing Indigenous-specific care tools and adapting best-practice mainstream approaches to care in close partnership with Indigenous community organisations and leaders can address some of the disparities. Close attention is needed to address Indigenous cultural frameworks for dementia and the impacts of colonialism in addition to the many systems barriers facing rural and remote Indigenous populations. Such an approach is a necessary step in providing culturally safe care for Indigenous patients and is fundamental to improving health equity.

The dementia disparity

Current available research findings suggest that Indigenous people in Canada, the United States (US) and Australia experience higher rates of dementia compared with their non-Indigenous counterparts (Smith et al, 2008; Jacklin et al, 2013a; Li et al, 2014). Research among First Nations in Alberta Canada shows the prevalence of dementia is 34 per cent higher and increasing at a faster rate than in non-First Nations Canadians ((Jacklin et al, 2013a). This research also revealed that the average age of onset was ten years younger, and there are a greater proportion of males diagnosed (Jacklin et al, 2013a). No national prevalence data are yet available for American Indian/Alaskan Native (AI/AN) populations in the US (Garrett et al, 2015; Browne et al, 2017); however, a study of incidence of dementia among ethnic populations in a northern California American clinic population found dementia incidence to be highest in African American (26.60 per 1,000 person-years) and American Indian and Alaska Native (22.18

per 1,000 person-years) populations. This can be compared with the White majority population incidence of 19.35 per 1,000 person-years in the same study (Mayeda et al, 2016).

While the data are limited for North America (Jacklin et al, 2013a; Mayeda et al, 2014), studies with Indigenous populations in Australia support the notion that Indigenous populations may be at increased risk for dementia (Smith et al, 2008; Li et al, 2014). The prevalence of dementia among Indigenous Australians in the Kimberley region was 12.4 per cent for those over 45, compared with the age-standardised rate of 2.4 per cent for the overall Australian population, making the Indigenous rate in Kimberly 5.2 times higher (Smith et al, 2008) than the rate for non-Indigenous Australians. Research from Australia's Northern Territories (NT) indicates that the age-standardised prevalence of dementia is 6.5 per cent in Indigenous Australians, compared with 2.6 per cent in non-Indigenous Australians in the NT (Li et al, 2014), making the Indigenous rate of dementia in the NT 2.5 times higher. In this same population, the age-adjusted incidence for those 45 years of age and older was 27.3 per 1,000 person-years, compared with 10.7 per 1,000 person-years, making the incidence rate 2.6 time higher (Li et al, 2014).

Age-related dementias arise from a combination of risk factors that may disproportionately affect Indigenous peoples when compared with majority populations. The Alzheimer Society of Canada describes two categories of risk factors: modifiable factors that may be influenced by individuals' behaviours or life circumstances, and non-modifiable factors that cannot be changed. The primary non-modifiable risk factors for dementia are age and genetics (Alzheimer Society of Canada, 2010). Genetic factors in the development of dementia have not been extensively researched among Indigenous populations in North America. One study documented a case of early onset familiar Alzheimer's disease in an Indigenous extended family in British Columbia (Butler et al, 2010), and one published research note suggests lower frequencies of Apolipoprotein E among Choctaw populations in Oklahoma (Henderson et al, 2002).

While ageing contributes to increasing rates and risk for the development of dementia, it has been shown that ageing alone does not account for the recent increasing incidence of dementia in First Nations populations (Jacklin et al, 2013a). Instead, it is suggested that Indigenous people have a markedly increased risk for dementia associated with related health disparities such as high rates of multiple, complex health conditions at younger ages compared with other populations (Gracey and King, 2009; Reading, 2009; Goins and Pilkerton, 2010; Mayeda et al, 2014), and a disproportionate share of individual, community, social, historical and colonial risk factors (King et al, 2009; Jacklin et al, 2013a; US Department of Health and Human Services, 2017). Petrasek MacDonald and colleagues (2015) explored the risk prevalence of Alzheimer's disease among Indigenous Canadians and found that modifiable risk factors may account for more than 75 per cent of cases of Alzheimer's disease among this population, suggesting a portion of the cases may be preventable (Petrasek MacDonald et al, 2015).

The *World Alzheimer Report 2014*, which examined modifiable risk factors for dementia, found probabilistic causation associated with low educational attainment in early life, hypertension in mid-life, and smoking and diabetes across the life span (Prince et al, 2014, 2016). Among Indigenous populations, many of the risks that are most often labelled 'modifiable' include disproportionate rates of smoking, obesity and associated diseases such as diabetes, hypertension, stroke and heart disease (Reading, 2009; Dyck et al, 2010; Mayeda et al, 2014). These risks are combined with increased vulnerability to the impacts of social determinants of health, including poverty, lower levels of formal educational attainment, low rates of health literacy, and potentially increased rates of post-traumatic stress disorder (PTSD) caused by residential school and Indian boarding school trauma (King et al, 2009; Jacklin et al, 2013a; Sequist, 2017). For Indigenous populations, many of these modifiable risks are intergenerational, and stem from the history of colonialism and government policy that devalued Indigenous knowledge and traditions, resulting in Indigenous peoples being marginalised, disenfranchised and oppressed (Kirmayer et al, 2003; Aguiar and Halseth, 2015; Truth and Reconciliation Commission of Canada, 2015).

Those in the field call on scholars to collaborate on dementia research in partnership with Indigenous populations in North America (Mehta and Yeo, 2017), and to embed social science approaches and perspectives (Whitehouse et al, 2005). Of urgent need are population-based studies to determine incidence and prevalence, the design and implementation of culturally relevant interventions, and the development of policy that addresses health inequities, disparities and intergenerational trauma. Research in these areas has the potential to generate new knowledge that may result in a reduction of risk factors for dementias among Indigenous peoples.

Several factors potentially influence equitable access to dementia care for Indigenous peoples, including Indigenous-specific cultural understandings and interpretations of the symptoms of dementia (Henderson, 2002; Hulko et al, 2010; Jacklin and Warry, 2012; Jacklin et al, 2015a), structural barriers to care including access to primary healthcare and specialist services (Griffin-Pierce et al, 2008; Jacklin et al, 2015a), the appropriateness of cognitive screening tools (Hendrie, 1999; Jervis and Manson, 2002; Jervis et al, 2006; LoGiudice et al, 2006; de Souza-Talarico et al, 2016), and patients' and caregivers' relationship with their healthcare provider (Cammer, 2006; Finkelstein et al, 2012).

Indigenous communities in Canada are often geographically isolated, and located in rural and remote locations, resulting in limited access to formalised health care. Although many Indigenous people reside in urban centres, 44.2 per cent of the registered First Nations population lives on reserves primarily located in rural and remote locations. Overall, approximately 60 per cent of the registered First Nations population lives in rural or small population centres (Statistics Canada, 2017). Federal and provincial policies related to health have resulted in inaccessibility to healthcare providers and a geographic maldistribution of services. Healthcare services are frequently provided off-reserve, in urban centres, often requiring that jurisdictional boundaries be crossed, which is compounded by the added burden of lengthy travel or finding appropriate transportation. Complex system navigation brings additional challenges associated with who pays – the federal or provincial government – for which services. These jurisdictional issues create confusion, gaps and barriers to accessing care, resulting in further marginalisation and inequities (Jacklin and Warry, 2011a).

The lasting effects of colonial policies affecting Indigenous peoples in Canada have been widely documented in the literature (Adelson, 2005; Jones, 2006; Truth and Reconciliation Commission of Canada, 2015). The historical assimilation that occurred included seizure of land and creation of the reserve system, in which entire settlements were uprooted and forcibly relocated to unfamiliar, resource-poor locations (Adelson, 2005). Subsequently, children were forcibly removed and institutionalised in residential schools located at great distances away from their family members and communities, resulting in entire families being stripped of their homes, personal autonomy, language, culture and traditions. Spiritual practices, customs, ceremonies and Indigenous medical systems were subjected to oppressive measures by the government and churches in an attempt to further assimilate cultural norms and beliefs. While the majority of these policies have been discontinued, the government of Canada has only recently publicly acknowledged their lasting effects (Truth and Reconciliation Commission of Canada, 2015).

The historical trauma caused by these government-led colonial assimilation policies have resulted in PTSD and long-lasting intergenerational trauma, which have been linked to fear and lack of trust when it comes to formalised healthcare (Jacklin et al, 2017a). Undeniably, healthcare institutions are regarded as a powerful symbol of a traumatic colonial history (O'Neil, 1989).

Intersections of Indigenous culture, context and dementia

Culture organises 'our conventional common sense about how to understand and treat illness; thus we can say the illness experience is always culturally shaped' (Kleinman, 1988: 5). The relationship between culture and health is such that illness symptoms vary across different cultural and ethnic groups and are often at odds with the culture of Western biomedicine, significantly affecting diagnosis, treatment and care.

Cultural understandings of dementia among Indigenous populations are embedded within a unique cultural framework that shapes beliefs and experiences related to the illness, including differences and similarities across Indigenous populations, nationally and internationally. Research on this topic has found that Indigenous populations place less emphasis on the Western, diagnostic labels and biomedical perspectives associated with cognitive decline. A qualitative evidence synthesis recently explored culture and Indigenous experiences of dementia or dementia caregiving in Canada (Jacklin and Walker, 2019). Drawing on available literature, the authors described how Indigenous culture influences peoples' understandings of dementia, theories of causation, interpretation of symptoms, caregiving practices and treatment choices.

Most research with Indigenous peoples to date has found that the biomedical construct of dementia, in which dementia is perceived as a disease, is not well understood and that often the illness is not viewed as problematic. Published research describes an Indigenous framework for understanding dementia. Participants in multiple studies described dementia as a 'natural' part of the 'circle of life'. Elders from the Secwepemc communities in British Columbia, Canada held understandings that included Secwepemc beliefs that dementia was a part of 'going through the full circle of life' (Hulko et al, 2010: 308). In Saskatchewan, grandmothers described dementia as going 'back to the baby stage' and part of the 'circle of life' (Lanting et al, 2011: 109, 110). Similarly, in a study among Ojibwe in northern Minnesota, female caregivers explained 'part of her life was just part of the circle of life; she became a little child again' (Boss et al, 1995: 8). The cultural understanding of dementia as 'normal' and as part of 'the circle of life' was consistent among diverse Indigenous communities in Ontario,

Canada including the Haudenosaunee people of Six Nations of the Grand River Territory in southern Ontario, and the seven rural Ojibwa, Odawa and Pottawatomi First Nations of Manitoulin Island in north-eastern Ontario (Jacklin et al, 2013b, 2014b, 2014d; Pace, 2013). In the studies involving Indigenous peoples cited earlier, the cultural framework of the medicine wheel and the circle of life provide context for Indigenous understandings. For instance, the understanding of the connections between the spirit world and the physical world at the intersection of old age, death, birth and infancy help explain 'childlike' behaviour and communication with the deceased.

Research in Canada reveals conflicting disease models during discussions of dementia causation. While dementia is generally accepted and understood as part of the circle of life, there is also evidence that Indigenous people see the rise in dementia as being related to colonisation and the influence of Western ways of living. In a study with First Nations communities in British Columbia, Secwepemc participants felt that changes to a Western diet, Western medicines, addictions, pollution, interruptions to cultural traditions and residential schools all influenced the onset of dementia (Hulko et al, 2010). Our work in Ontario with six Indigenous communities revealed that participants saw dementia as being related to physiological changes such as ageing, genetics and diseases; psychosocial issues including historical trauma, grief and stress; and disruptions to Indigenous ways of living and land-based activities (Jacklin and Warry, 2012).

Very little has been reported concerning Indigenous interpretations and understandings of symptoms of dementia. A detailed case study of an American Indian woman described by Henderson (2002) demonstrates how an American Indian family living in a reservation community interprets their mother's Alzheimer's disease. For this family, the hallucinations associated with the illness are viewed as a mechanism by which their mother was able to communicate with the 'other side'. In this case, her illness was not normalised; rather it was viewed as 'supernormal'. The interpretation of symptoms as expressions of culture and as part of the lifecycle was also found in Ontario where some Indigenous research participants expressed great concern, if not anger, that physicians and others labelled these behaviours as being associated with a disease (Jacklin and Warry, 2011b).

Caregiving is also rooted in cultural values. In Indigenous communities, the family is often viewed as the primary or sole provider of care (Hennessey and John, 1996; John et al, 1996; Buchignani and Armstrong-Esther, 1999; Jervis and Manson, 2002; Chapleski et al, 2003; Cammer, 2006; Jacklin et al, 2015a). In some cases, this arises from necessity, but more often it is grounded in a cultural emphasis on familial interdependence (Hennessy and John, 1995; Jervis and Manson, 1999), and the cultural values of reciprocity (Jervis et al, 2010) and respect (Jacklin et al, 2015a).

Despite dementia being viewed by some people as normal, the diagnosis could still be feared by many, and caring for someone with dementia was sometimes viewed as extremely difficult (Hulko et al, 2010). Family caregivers in Indigenous communities report that caregiving to their loved one is rewarding, but they also experience stress in the form of anxiety related to the quality of care they are providing (Jervis et al, 2010; Jacklin et al, 2015a), the psychosocial aspects of care, strains on family relations, and negative effects on personal wellbeing (Hennessey and John, 1996). Caregivers and community health services have reported feeling unprepared and poorly equipped to deal with someone with dementia, especially in the later stages of the illness (Sutherland, 2007; Hulko et al, 2010; Jacklin et al, 2015a).

In Ontario, Indigenous people shared how specific historical policies of the federal government, such as the residential school policy, child welfare policies and the 'Sixties Scoop', have led to PTSD in the older Indigenous population, and intergenerational trauma in the younger generations (Jacklin et al, 2015a). This trauma greatly affects the ability of families to function in a caregiving role without a healing process (Forbes et al, 2013).

Considerations in the provision of appropriate and equitable care for Indigenous peoples

Cultural safety served as a lens in the brief review of disparities and cultural context of dementia in Indigenous populations we have offered. Cultural safety is a concept originally defined by New Zealand Maori nurse educators to acknowledge and address structural inequalities and power relationships between healthcare providers and Indigenous patients that influence equitable access to care, and produce inappropriate healthcare encounters (Ramsden, 1990). Cultural safety retains but expands the cultural domains previously associated with cultural competence and sensitivity, allowing for more critical awareness of residual structural violence in our healthcare systems; that is, the way health institutions may harm people by preventing them from attaining appropriate, safe healthcare, and positive health outcomes (Farmer, 2004; Bailey et al, 2017; Jacklin, 2018). Cultural safety and culturally safe care are approaches that have emerged as important components in strategies to address disparities in Indigenous peoples' health and healthcare, and are promising approaches in addressing the dementia disparities described earlier.

Cultural safety inherently accepts that culture influences an individual's understandings and behaviours around illness and thus must be considered rather than dismissed in care practices. This includes what an individual believes has caused their illness, how they think it should be treated, healthcare-seeking behaviours, decision-making models, and what are considered appropriate models of care (Kleinman et al, 1978; Kane, 2000;Whitehouse et al, 2005; Coe et al, 2010).

With this in mind, we see a starting point for determining how equitable care may be achieved. With cultural safety as a guiding model, we see opportunity to address these key elements of health equity at various points in the care trajectory: health promotion and prevention, diagnosis, and care.

We emphasise the important point that there is no one-size-fits-all approach for the provision of appropriate safe dementia care with Indigenous populations. Assumptions and generalisations that beliefs and understandings are shared among diverse Indigenous populations should be avoided. We instead suggest that community-based approaches to the development and delivery of dementia care is essential to ensure services are delivered in a culturally relevant manner, respecting the values, beliefs and traditions of the individual (Smith et al, 2011; Jacklin et al, 2016; Jacklin, 2018).

Health promotion and prevention

It is established that a disproportionate burden of modifiable and non-modifiable risk factors and the social determinants of health play a critical role in the prevention of dementias among Indigenous peoples; likewise, a multitude of structural, socioeconomic and clinical barriers significantly affect prevention across the life span as well. There are far too many variables contributing to the onset of dementia in Indigenous populations to tackle here.

Research in rural First Nations communities in north-eastern Ontario found that meaningful dementia prevention strategies must be created in equal partnership with Indigenous communities and be tailored to address the unique risk factors that influence the health of Indigenous people. They must focus on incorporating cultural activities that help individuals achieve 'whole' health by tending to physical, mental, emotional, spiritual and relational aspects of the self (Jacklin et al, 2017d; Pace et al, 2019).

As an example, one place to start is health literacy. In Canada, it is reported that Indigenous persons with dementia and informal care providers often lack knowledge about dementia, including information about risk factors, symptoms, progression and treatments (Finkelstein et al, 2012; Jacklin et al, 2015a). Patients and caregivers report a discomfort with mainstream services, and a reliance on cultural teachings and spirituality (Jacklin et al, 2015a). An environmental scan of published and unpublished literature accessible via the internet found a dearth of Indigenous-specific dementia resources worldwide and just one effort in Canada (Webkamigad, 2017). The Canadian resource arose from ethnographic research and community partnerships led by Jacklin and Warry. The culturally grounded resources include a series of Indigenous specific dementia health promotion and awareness materials (fact sheets) on the Indigenous Cognition and Aging Research Exchange website, www.I-CAARE.ca (Jacklin et al, 2015b, 2015c, 2017c, 2017d, 2017e, 2017f, 2017g).

The series of fact sheets includes information on Indigenous understandings of dementia, signs and symptoms, what to expect, and healthy brain ageing, all from the perspective and experiences of Indigenous peoples who were interviewed for the research (Jacklin et al, 2017f). These resources are designed to bridge Western and Indigenous knowledge systems concerning ageing, health and dementia as opposed to the more common approach that tends to medicalise Indigenous conceptions of disease. Two-eyed seeing was used as a model to guide the development of the resources that privilege Indigenous ways of knowing and Indigenous experiences (Bartlett et al, 2012).

While these resources begin to fill a gap, there is much more to be done. We encourage researchers to partner with communities to develop local teaching tools that respond to various potential intervention points in the disease's development and progression, for example to prevent dementia, promote healthy ageing, encourage early diagnosis, improve dementia literacy, delay the progression of symptoms, improve quality of care and life, support caregivers and prevent caregiver burnout. We suggest this be done within frameworks that allow Indigenous knowledge to be placed on equal footing with biomedical knowledge.

Diagnosis

Timely, accurate and appropriate diagnosis is an issue for many Canadians living in rural communities across the country. Indigenous populations experience additional barriers to diagnosis that affects when or even if they receive a diagnosis. Dementias may be regularly undiagnosed or underdiagnosed in Indigenous populations for various reasons, including poor understanding in the non-Indigenous clinical population of the culturally grounded beliefs and understandings of dementia held by many Indigenous peoples. Indigenous explanations of dementia include reference to the process of memory loss and confusion as being a normal, accepted and expected part of ageing (Hulko et al, 2010; Lanting et al, 2011; Jacklin et al, 2015a). There may also be denial associated with behavioural changes (Jacklin et al, 2014d), fear of diagnosis or diagnosis repercussions, and an overall mistrust of healthcare providers (Cammer, 2006; Finkelstein et al, 2012).

In a study with Indigenous peoples living in rural and remote areas of Ontario (Pace et al, 2013), there was a shared perception among care workers that dementia was underdiagnosed in their community. The research found that there were 'likely many more community members experiencing memory loss than they were aware of' (Pace et al, 2013: 31). Normalisation and acceptance of the illness were one factor, but this was coupled with poor access to family physicians and in some cases culturally unsafe healthcare encounters in the past. Misdiagnosis also remains a significant issue in establishing accurate estimates of the dementia burden in Indigenous populations (Griffin-Pierce et al, 2008) and may be attributable to the lack of formal and consistent diagnosis procedures in rural and remote Indigenous communities (Pace et al, 2013; Jacklin et al, 2014c, 2014d).

Accurate diagnosis is inextricably linked to effective dementia care and access to services for people and families. Indigenous people in Canada, particularly First Nations peoples in rural and remote communities, are faced with inequitable access to healthcare throughout their lifetime. Access to physicians varies by location, but geographic isolation results in an underabundance of geriatric care specialists and dementia-specific services, which are rare to non-existent (Jacklin, 2018). Access to care affects the accuracy and timeliness of diagnosis. Particularly for rural and remote Indigenous populations, clinical encounters often require lengthy travel to unfamiliar urban centres. During the medical visit, time with practitioners is limited; chronic conditions or other urgent health issues take precedence (Pace et al, 2013). These issues may result in delayed diagnoses, late-stage diagnoses, postponed dementia services, and an overall reduction in quality of life (Health Council of Canada, 2013; Pace et al, 2013; Jacklin et al, 2015a).

Further, the diagnosis of dementia is reliant on the administration of cognitive assessments, which have been shown to be less accurate and reliable in Indigenous contexts (Jervis and Manson, 2002; Hendrie, 2006; Jervis et al, 2007; Morgan et al, 2009; Lanting et al, 2011).

Although there is no single test to determine if an individual has dementia, neuropsychological tools such as screening interviews and cognitive assessment tests play a significant role in the accuracy of diagnosis. Culturally appropriate cognitive assessment tests with validated psychometric properties of sensitivity and specificity may improve diagnostic accuracy for Indigenous people experiencing cognitive decline. Cognitive assessments, therefore, represent one place in the diagnosis journey where cultural safety can affect outcomes and foster equity. To date, only a limited number of such cognitive assessment tests have been developed in North America and none has been validated for use (Hall et al, 1993; Lanting et al, 2011).

Recognising the lack of culturally safe assessment tools, researchers have focused efforts on the creation of a culturally appropriate diagnostic tool for use with Indigenous peoples in Canada. This instrument has been called the Canadian Indigenous Cognitive Assessment (CICA) (Canadian Institutes of Health Research, 2018), and is an adaptation of the Kimberley Indigenous Cognitive Assessment (KICA-cog) developed in response to similar needs among Indigenous populations in Australia (LoGiudice et al, 2006, 2011). The adaptation process involved intensive community involvement in the linguistic and cultural translation and back translation of each chapter of the KICA-cog over 18 months and eventual piloting and fine tuning of the CICA (Jacklin et al, 2016; Blind et al, 2017). The validation of the CICA was again conducted in partnership with the Anishinaabe communities it is intended to serve. The validated CICA is one example of how disparities can be addressed, although much remains to be done. For example, in Australia researchers have developed a suite of adapted tools for Indigenous clients to support the KICA-cog, including KICA-Carer, KICA-Behaviour, CICA-ADL, KICA-Screen, and a modified version of the KICA-cog for urban Indigenous people (Western Australia Centre for Health and Aging, 2019).

Supportive care

Care encompasses formal and informal sectors. As has been stated, much of the care along the dementia journey for Indigenous peoples is reported to be delivered by family caregivers. Efforts in better education and training for family care providers is one way to support culturally appropriate care. Health information, as previously described, is one way to support family caregivers. Additionally, innovative and appropriate practices are needed for support group activities and respite.

Previous research has shown that informal care in Indigenous contexts may also include community care. Research with a remote First Nations community in British Columbia found that community members participated in dementia caregiving in two distinct ways: first, elders from the community became involved in decision making in cases where the person with dementia had no family; and second, community members participated in monitoring people with dementia who were known to wander. In the latter case, caregivers sent letters to other community members to alert them to the person's behaviour (Lombera et al, 2009). The role of community members in locating wandering elderly people was also mentioned in an Ontario study where one caregiver explained how everyone in her community knew where she worked and knew that her loved one wandered, so those who located her always knew where to bring her (Jacklin et al, 2015a). This may suggest that Indigenous communities are well suited to the creation of dementia-friendly spaces. However, the culture of community caring is also affected by inequitable distribution of resources; that is, at every point in the system, Indigenous communities do not have sufficient resources to support community caregiving. Suggestions to strengthen community care include sustainable programming, improved home care, supporting traditional caregiving values, more culturally congruent and safe care from service providers, and nursing homes that more closely resemble assisted living facilities under the ownership and operation of the tribe or First Nations community that better reflect Indigenous culture, language and values (Chapleski et al, 2003; Graves et al, 2004; Brown and Gibbons, 2008; Smith et al, 2011).

Formal care is fraught with the systemic barriers and impacts of the colonial past. Appropriate delivery of dementia care in a culturally safe way requires that care providers be trained on the colonial and sociohistorical factors affecting Indigenous Peoples as a first step. Training healthcare providers in cultural competency is a specific call to action of the Truth and Reconciliation Commission of Canada (Truth and Reconciliation Commission of Canada, 2015). Such training has become more accessible to healthcare providers in Canada (Ward and Varley, n.d.) and medical students (Jacklin et al, 2014a) in recent years. However, dementia-specific cultural safety training needs to involve additional information, including Indigenous explanatory models of dementia, appropriate approaches to the clinical encounter with older Indigenous adults, and how to access appropriate supports and services.

Conclusion

Dementia has recently been added to the long list of health inequities facing Indigenous populations. While data on prevalence and incidence are extremely limited, taken together, they support the conclusion that dementia is elevated in Indigenous populations, age of onset is younger, and rates are rising more quickly. Like other disparities, the elevated risk of dementia is multifactorial and intimately tied to historical and contemporary government policies that affect the social determinants of health uniquely among this population. While there are obviously causes of inequity that fall outside the reach of healthcare providers, there are many opportunities to address equity in clinical and public health approaches.

We have proposed cultural safety as one frame of reference that may assist healthcare providers, institutions and communities to respond in appropriate and effective ways to the increasing dementia needs across the illness trajectory for Indigenous populations. Cultural safety asks us to consider real systems barriers facing Indigenous people as they try to access services for dementia care. Some of the barriers we have highlighted in our discussion include those common to rural communities such as geography, transportation and access to clinical care, but also include Indigenous specific barriers such as approaches to care that are culturally unsafe or unfair. Providers and organisations can address some of these through cultural safety education for staff and healthcare providers and through advocacy for Indigenous patients. Improved approaches to care should also involve creating partnerships with Indigenous communities and organisations to counteract tools and approaches to care that may be inappropriate.

Cultural safety also asks us to consider culture in our care; that is, seeing and reflecting on culture instead of ignoring it. We have presented several ways in which culture is a factor in dementia and dementia care for Indigenous populations. A view of dementia as natural and part of the circle of life provides an explanatory framework of the illness that is accepted. There is much utility to this framework in that it reduces stigma and facilitates family and community caring. However, this understanding may also mean medical interventions are delayed and family caregivers become overwhelmed due to limited knowledge of the illness. We suggest approaches that honour and respect culture and avoid medicalisation of the illness. Two-eyed seeing is one way to achieve this. To do this, providers must examine their own beliefs and biases – those that are personal as well as embedded in their professional culture. They must also seek out information and learning on Indigenous cultures and reach out to local resources to help guide their understandings. This is not to say one can become an expert in another culture, but some understanding and good connections to Indigenous community organisations and resources will improve approaches and understandings when providing services to Indigenous patients and families.

Health equity involves interventions across the spectrum of the social determinants of health. For Indigenous people, this includes the unique distal determinant of colonialism. We suggest adopting culturally safe dementia care practices as one way in which healthcare providers and organisations can have an impact on health equity.

Notes

1 'Indigenous' refers to the original inhabitants of the lands. In this chapter, we use the term 'Indigenous' to refer to the first peoples of Canada.
2 'Sixties Scoop' refers to a period from the 1960s to the mid-1980s in which thousands of Aboriginal children were removed from their birth parents and adopted into non-Aboriginal homes in Canada, the United States or outside of North America.

References

Adelson, N. (2005) 'The embodiment of inequity: health disparities in Aboriginal Canada', *Canadian Journal of Public Health*, 96: S45–S61.

Aguiar, W. and Halseth, R. (2015) *Aboriginal peoples and historic trauma: The processes of intergenerational transmission*, Prince George: National Collaborating Centre for Aboriginal Health.

Alzheimer Society of Canada (2010) *Rising tide: The impact of dementia on Canadian society*, Toronto: Alzheimer Society of Canada. Available from: https://alzheimer.ca/sites/default/files/files/national/advocacy/asc_rising_tide_full_report_e.pdf [Accessed 28 August, 2019].

Bailey, Z.D., Krieger, N., Agenor, M., Graves, J., Linos, N. and Bassett, M.T. (2017) 'Structural racism and health inequities in the USA: evidence and interventions', *The Lancet*, 389: 1453–63.

Bartlett, C., Marshall, M. and Marshall, A. (2012) 'Two-eyed seeing and other lessons learned within a co-learning journey of bringing together Indigenous and mainstream knowledges and ways of knowing', *Journal of Environmental Studies and Sciences*, 2: 331–40.

Blind, M., Pitawanakwat, K., Jacklin, K., O'Connell, M., Walker, J., McElhaney, J. and Warry, W. (2017) 'Piloting the adapted Kimberly Indigenous Cognitive Assessment tool with Indigenous seniors in Canada', *Innovation in Aging*, 1(Suppl.1): 1286–7.

Boss, P., Kaplan, L. and Gordon, M. (1995) 'Accepting the circle of life: lessons for the Anishinabe about caring for elders', *Center for Urban and Regional Affairs Reporter*, 25: 7–11.

Brown, C.M. and Gibbons, J.L. (2008) 'Taking care of our elders: an initial study of an assisted-living facility for American Indians', *Journal of Applied Gerontology*, 27(4): 523–31.

Browne, C.V., Ka'opua, L.S., Jervis, L.L., Alboroto, R. and Trockman, M.L. (2017) 'United States Indigenous populations and dementia: is there a case for culture-based psychosocial interventions?', *Gerontologist*, 57: 1011–19.

Buchignani, N. and Armstrong-Esther, C. (1999) 'Informal care and older native Canadians', *Ageing & Society*, 19(1): 3–32.

Butler, R., Beattie, B.L., Thong, U.P., Dwosh, E., Guimond, C., Feldman, H.H., Hsiung, G.Y.R., Rogaeva, E., St. George-Hyslop, P. and Sadovnick, A.D. (2010) 'A novel PS1 gene mutation in a large Aboriginal kindred', *The Canadian Journal of Neurological Sciences*, 37(3): 359–64.

Cammer, A. (2006) 'Negotiating culturally incongruent healthcare systems: the process of accessing dementia care in northern Saskatchewan', Unpublished thesis, University of Saskatchewan.

Canadian Institutes of Health Research (2018) 'Sharing knowledge will help Indigenous dementia patients face their disease', [online]. Available from: https://cihr-irsc.gc.ca/e/50792.html

Chapleski, E.E., Sobeck, J. and Fisher, C. (2003) 'Long-term care preferences and attitudes among Great Lakes American Indian families: cultural context matters', *Care Management Journals*, 4(2): 94–100.

Coe, K., Attakai, A., Papenfuss, M., Giuliano, A., Martin, L. and Nuvayestewa, L. (2010) 'Traditionalism and its relationship to disease risk and protective behaviors of women living on the Hopi reservation', *Health Care for Women International*, 25(5): 391–410.

Crowshoe, L., Henderson, R., Jacklin, K., Calam, B., Walker, L. and Green, M. (2019) 'Educating for Equity Care Framework: addressing social barriers of Indigenous patients with type 2 diabetes', *Canadian Family Physician*, 65(1): 25–33.

De Souza-Talarico, J.N., De Carvalho, A.P., Brucki, S.M.D., Nitrini, R. and Ferratti-Rebustini, R.E.D. (2016) 'Dementia and cognitive impairment prevalence and associated factors in Indigenous populations: a systematic review', *Alzheimer Disease and Associated Disorders*, 30: 281–7.

Dilworth-Anderson, P., Pierre, G. and Hilliard, T.S. (2012) 'Social justice, health disparities, and culture in the care of the elderly', *Journal of Law, Medicine & Ethics*, 40: 26–32.

Dyck, R., Osgood, N., Hsiang, T., Gao, A. and Stang, M.R. (2010) 'Epidemiology of diabetes mellitus among First Nations and non-First Nations adults', *Canadian Medical Association Journal*, 182(3): 249–56.

Farmer, P. (2004) 'An anthropology of structural violence', *Current Anthropology*, 45: 305–25.

Farmer, P.E., Nizeye, B., Stulac, S. and Keshavjee, S. (2006) 'Structural violence and clinical medicine', *PLoS Medicine*, 3(10): e449.

Finkelstein, S.A., Forbes, D.A. and Richmond, C.A. (2012) 'Formal dementia care among First Nations in southwestern Ontario', *Canadian Journal on Aging*, 31(3): 257–70.

Forbes, D., Blake, C., Thiessen, E., Finkelstein, S., Gibson, M., Morgan, D.G., Markle-Reid, M. and Culum, I. (2013) 'Dementia care knowledge sharing within a First Nations community', *Canadian Journal on Aging*, 32(4): 360–74.

Garrett, M.D., Baldridge, D., Benson, W., Crowder, J. and Aldrich, N. (2015) 'Mental health disorders among an invisible minority: depression and dementia among American Indian and Alaska native elders', *The Gerontologist*, 55(2): 227–36.

Goins, R. and Pilkerton, C. (2010) 'Comorbidity among older American Indians: the Native Elder Care Study', *Journal of Cross-Cultural Gerontology*, 25(4): 343–54.

Gracey, M. and King, M. (2009) 'Indigenous health part 1: determinants and disease patterns', *The Lancet*, 374(9683): 65–75.

Graves, K., Smith, S., Easley, C. and Kanaqlak, G.P.C. (2004) *Our view of dignified aging. National Resource Center for American Indian, Alaska Native, and Native Hawaiian Elders.* Paper presented at Conferences of Alaska Native Elders, Anchorage, Alaska.

Griffin-Pierce, T., Silverberg, N., Connor, D., Jim, M., Peters, J., Kaszniak, A. and Sabbagh, M.N. (2008) 'Challenges to the recognition and assessment of Alzheimer's disease in American Indians of the southwestern United States', *Alzheimer's & Dementia. The Journal of the Alzheimer's Association*, 4(4): 291–9.

Hall, K.S., Hendrie, H.C. and Brittain, H.M. (1993) 'The development of a dementia screening interview in two distinct languages', *International Journal of Methods in Psychiatric Research*, 3: 1–28.

Health Council of Canada (2013) *Canada's most vulnerable: Improving health care for First Nations, Inuit, and Metis seniors*, Toronto: Health Council of Canada. Available from: https://healthcouncilcanada.ca/files/Senior_AB_Report_2013_EN_final.pdf

Henderson, J.N. (2002) 'The experience and interpretation of dementia: cross-cultural perspectives', *Journal of Cross-Cultural Gerontology*, 17(3): 195–6.

Henderson, J.N. (2009) 'American Indian family caregiving: cultural context and dementia patient care', *Anthropology News*, 50: 13–15.

Henderson, J.N., Crook, R., Crook, J., Hardy, J., Onstead, L., Carson-Henderson, L., Mayer, P., Parker, B., Petersen, R. and Williams, B. (2002) 'Apolipoprotein E4 and tau allele frequencies among Choctaw Indians', *Neuroscience Letters*, 324(1): 77–9.

Hendrie, H.C. (1999) 'Alzheimer's disease: a review of cross cultural studies', in R. Mayeux and Y. Christen (eds) *Epidemiology and Alzheimer's disease: From gene to prevention*, Berlin: Springer, pp 87–101.

Hendrie, H.C. (2006) 'Lessons learned from international comparative crosscultural studies on dementia', *The American Journal of Geriatric Psychiatry: Official Journal of the American Association for Geriatric Psychiatry*, 14(6): 480.

Hennessy, C.H. and John, R. (1995) 'The interpretation of burden among Pueblo Indian caregivers', *Journal of Aging Studies*, 9: 215–29.

Hennessey, C.H. and John, R. (1996) 'American Indian family caregivers' perceptions of burden and needed support services', *Journal of Applied Gerontology*, 15(3): 275–93.

Hulko, W., Camille, E., Antifeau, E., Arnouse, M., Bachynski, N. and Taylor, D. (2010) 'Views of First Nation elders on memory loss and memory care in later life', *Journal of Cross-Cultural Gerontology*, 25(4): 317–42.

Jacklin, K. (2018) *Current evidence on Alzheimer's disease and its related dementias (ADRD) and Indigenous populations in Canada: A report prepared for the Expert Panel on Evidence and Best Practices in Dementia*, Duluth, Minnesota: Canadian Academy of Health Sciences, University of Minnesota.

Jacklin, K. and Walker, J. (2019) 'Cultural understandings of dementia in Indigenous peoples: a qualitative evidence synthesis', *Canadian Journal on Aging*, Special Issue, 1–15.

Jacklin, K. and Warry, W. (2011a) 'Decolonizing First Nations health', in J.C. Kulig and A.M. Williams (eds) *Health in rural Canada*, Vancouver: UBC Press, pp 373–89.

Jacklin, K. and Warry, W. (2011b) 'Diverse experiences: perspectives on Alzheimer's disease and dementia in Aboriginal communities in Ontario, Canada', Paper presented at Alzheimer's Disease International 26th Annual Conference, Toronto, Canada.

Jacklin, K. and Warry, W. (2012) 'Forgetting and forgotten: dementia in Aboriginal seniors', *Anthropology and Aging Quarterly*, 33(1): 13.

Jacklin, K., Henderson, R., Green, M., Calam, B. and Crowshoe, L. (2017a) 'Healthcare experiences of Indigenous people living with Type 2 diabetes in Canada: sequential focus group findings from diverse Indigenous contexts', *Canadian Medical Association Journal*, 183(9): 106–12.

Jacklin, K., Pace, J. and Warry, W. (2015a) 'Informal dementia caregiver among Indigenous communities in Ontario, Canada', *Care Management Journals*, 16(2): 106–20.

Jacklin, K., Strasser, R. and Peltier, I. (2014a) 'From the community to the classroom: the Aboriginal health curriculum at the Northern Ontario School of Medicine'. *Canadian Journal of Rural Medicine*, 19(4): 143–50.

Jacklin, K., Walker, J. and Shawande, M. (2013a) 'The emergence of dementia as a health concern among First Nations populations in Alberta, Canada', *Canadian Journal of Public Health*, 104: e39–e44.

Jacklin, K., Warry, W. and Blind, M. (2013b) *Perceptions of Alzheimer's disease and related dementias in Aboriginal peoples in Ontario*, Moose Cree First Nation Community Report.

Jacklin, K., Warry, W. and Blind, M. (2014b) *Perceptions of Alzheimer's disease and related dementias in Aboriginal peoples in Ontario*, Ottawa Community Report.

Jacklin, K., Warry, W. and Blind, M. (2014c) *Perceptions of Alzheimer's disease and related dementias in Aboriginal peoples in Ontario*, Six Nations Community Report.

Jacklin, K., Warry, W. and Blind, M. (2014d) *Perceptions of Alzheimer's disease and related dementias in Aboriginal peoples in Ontario*, Sudbury Community Report.

Jacklin, K., Warry, W., Blind, M., Jones, L. and Webkamigad, S. (2017c) 'A medicine wheel model for preventing dementia in Indigenous people by aging well: advice from older Indigenous peoples', Indigenous Cognition and Aging Awareness Research Exchange, [online]. Available from: https://docs.wixstatic.com/ugd/27ba04_4fbf621143c741ee9fa3cafaa3b74874.pdf [Accessed 2 April 2018].

Jacklin, K., Warry, W., Blind, M., Jones, L. and Webkamigad, S. (2017d) *Preventing dementia in Indigenous peoples by aging well: Advice from older Indigenous peoples*, Indigenous Cognition and Aging Awareness Research Exchange, [online]. Available from: https://docs.wixstatic.com/ugd/27ba04_3a49b97afde14d7aba5dee9e8355c09e.pdf [Accessed 2 April 2018].

Jacklin, K., Warry, W., Blind, M., Jones, L. and Webkamigad, S. (2017e) *What to expect after a diagnosis of dementia: An Indigenous persons' guide*, Indigenous Cognition and Aging Awareness Research Exchange, [online]. Available from: https://docs.wixstatic.com/ugd/27ba04_63357f59e3584b1da17ed8e3e5ec95d3.pdf [Accessed 2 April 2018].

Jacklin, K., Warry, W., Blind, M., Jones, L., Webkamigad, S. and Otowadjiwan, J. (2017f) *Developing educational materials for community based dementia care: Methodology report*, Sudbury: Indigenous Cognition and Aging Awareness Research Exchange. Available from: https://docs.wixstatic.com/ugd/27ba04_472fa677a166482dad000f0daf98abeb.pdf

Jacklin, K., Warry, W., Blind, M., Webkamigad, S. and Jones, L. (2015b) *Signs and symptoms of dementia: An Indigenous guide*, Indigenous Cognition and Aging Awareness Research Exchange, [online]. Available from: https://docs.wixstatic.com/ugd/27ba04_63f11dcd595a49edb3a07469d107c03c.pdf [Accessed 2 April 2018].

Jacklin, K., Warry, W., Blind, M., Webkamigad, S. and Jones, L. (2015c) *What is dementia? Indigenous perspectives and cultural understandings*, Indigenous Cognition and Aging Awareness Research Exchange, [online]. Available from: https://docs.wixstatic.com/ugd/27ba04_7042c9f81bf946feba37b90d9db5261d.pdf [Accessed 2 April 2018].

Jacklin, K., Warry, W., Blind, M., Webkamigad, S. and Jones, L. (2017g) 'The path of dementia', Indigenous Cognition and Aging Awareness Research Exchange, [online]. Available from: https://docs.wixstatic.com/ugd/27ba04_8390fb60914441d2a9f5df5ac17e84a5.pdf [Accessed 28 August 2019].

Jacklin, K., Warry, W., Pitawanakwat, K. and Blind, M. (2016) 'Considerations in culturally safe care for Indigenous people with dementia in Canada', *Alzheimer's & Dementia: The Journal of the Alzheimer's Association*, 12(7): 270–1.

Jervis, L.L. and Manson, S. (1999) 'Native elder component – major themes and emerging questions', in *Redefining retirement: Research directions for successful aging among America's diverse seniors*, Washington, DC: SPRY Foundation.

Jervis, L.L. and Manson, S.M. (2002) 'American Indians/Alaska natives and dementia', *Alzheimer Disease & Associated Disorders*, 16(Supplement 2): S89–S95.

Jervis, L.L., Beals, J., Fickenscher, A. and Arciniegas, D.B. (2007) 'Performance on the Mini-Mental State Examination and Mattis Dementia Rating Scale among older American Indians', *Journal of Neuropsychiatry and Clinical Neurosciences*, 19(2): 173–8.

Jervis, L.L., Boland, M. and Fickenscher, A. (2010) 'American Indian family caregivers' experiences with helping elders', *Journal of Cross-Cultural Gerontology*, 25(4): 355–69.

Jervis, L.L., Cullum, C.M. and Manson, S.M. (2006) 'American Indians, cognitive assessment, and dementia', in *Ethnicity and the dementias* (2nd edn), New York, NY: Routledge, pp 87–101.

John, R., Hennessey, C.H., Roy, L.C. and Salvini, M.L. (1996) 'Caring for cognitively impaired American Indian elders: difficult situations, few options', in G. Yeo and D. Gallagher-Thompson (eds) *Ethnicity and the dementias* (1st edn), Washington, DC: Taylor & Francis, pp 187–203.

Johnston, P. (1983). *Aboriginal children and the child welfare system*, Toronto: Canadian Council on Social Development.

Jones, D.S. (2006) 'The persistence of American Indian health disparities', *American Journal of Public Health*, 96(12): 2122–34.

Kane, M.N. (2000) 'Ethnoculturally-sensitive practice and Alzheimer's disease', *American Journal of Alzheimer's Disease and Other Dementias*, 15(2): 80–6.

King, M., Smith, A. and Gracey, M. (2009) 'Indigenous health part 2: the underlying causes of the health gap', *The Lancet*, 374(9683): 76–85.

Kirmayer, L.J., Simpson, C. and Cargo, M. (2003) 'Healing traditions: culture, community and mental health promotion with Canadian Aboriginal peoples', *Australasian Journal of Ageing*, 11(S1): S15–S23.

Kleinman, A. (1988) *The illness narratives: Suffering healing and the human condition*, New York, NY: Basic Books.

Kleinman, A., Eisenberg, L. and Good, B. (1978) 'Culture, illness, and care: clinical lessons from anthropologic and cross-cultural research', *Annals of Internal Medicine*, 88: 251–8.

Lanting, S., Crossley, M., Morgan, D. and Cammer, A. (2011) 'Aboriginal experiences of aging and dementia in a context of sociocultural change: qualitative analysis of key informant group interviews with Aboriginal seniors', *Cross Cultural Journal of Gerontology*, 26(1): 103–17.

Li, S.Q., Guthridge, S.L., Eswara Aratchige, P., Lowe, M.P., Wang, Z., Zhao, Y. and Krause, V. (2014) 'Dementia prevalence and incidence among the Indigenous and non-Indigenous populations of the Northern Territory', *Medical Journal of Australia*, 200(8): 465–9.

LoGiudice, D., Smith, K., Thomas, J., Lautenschlager, N.T., Almeida, O.P., Atkinson, D. and Flicker, L. (2006) 'Kimberley Indigenous Cognitive Assessment tool (KICA): development of a cognitive assessment tool for older indigenous Australians', *International Psychogeriatrics*, 18(2): 269–80.

LoGiudice, D., Strivens, E., Smith, K., Stevenson, M., Atkinson, D., Dwyer, A., Lautenschlager, N., Almeida, O.A. and Flicker, L. (2011) 'The KICA Screen: the psychometric properties of a shortened version of the KICA (Kimberley Indigenous Cognitive Assessment)', *Australasian Journal on Ageing*, 30(4): 215–19.

Lombera, S., Butler, R., Beattie, B.L. and Illes, J. (2009) 'Aging, dementia and cognitive decline: perspectives of an Aboriginal community in British Columbia', paper presented at Canadian Association of Neuroscience Annual Meeting, Vancouver, Canada.

Mayeda, E.R., Glymour, M.M., Quesenberry, C.P. and Whitmer, R.A. (2016) 'Inequalities in dementia incidence between six racial and ethnic groups over 14 years', *Alzheimer's & Dementia: The Journal of the Alzheimer's Association*, 12(3): 216–24.

Mayeda, E.R., Karter, A.J., Huang, E.S., Moffet, H.H., Haan, M.N. and Whitmer, R.A. (2014) 'Racial/ethnic differences in dementia risk among older type 2 diabetic patients: The Diabetes and Aging Study', *Diabetes Care*, 37(4): 1009.

Mehta, K.M. and Yeo, G.W. (2017) 'Systematic review of dementia prevalence and incidence in United States race/ethnic populations', *Alzheimer's & Dementia: The Journal of the Alzheimer's Association*, 13(1): 72–83.

Morgan, D.G., Crossley, M., Kirk, A., D'arcy, C., Stewart, N.J., Biem, J., Forbes, D., Harder, S., Basran, J., Dal Bello-Haas, V. and Mcbain, L. (2009) 'Improving access to dementia care: development and evaluation of a rural and remote memory clinic', *Aging & Mental Health*, 13(1): 17–30.

O'Neil, J.D. (1989) 'The cultural and political context of patient dissatisfaction in cross-cultural clinical encounters: a Canadian Inuit study', *Medical Anthropology Quareterly*, 3(4): 325–44.

Pace, J. (2013) 'Meanings of memory: understanding aging and dementia in First Nations communities on Manitoulin Island, Ontario', Unpublished doctoral thesis, McMaster University.

Pace, J., Jacklin, K. and Warry, W. (2013) *Perceptions of Alzheimer's disease and related dementias in Aboriginal peoples in Ontario*, Manitoulin Island Report.

Pace, J., Jacklin, K., Warry, W. and Pitawanakwat, K. (2019) 'Perceptions of dementia prevention among Anishinaabe living on Manitoulin Island', in W. Hulko, D. Wilson and J. Balestrery (eds) *Indigenous peoples and dementia: New understandings of memory loss and memory care*, Vancouver: UBC Press, pp 86–106.

Petrasek MacDonald, J., Barnes, D.E. and Middleton, L.E. (2015) 'Implications of risk factors for Alzheimer's disease in Canada's Indigenous population', *Canadian Geriatrics Journal*, 18(3): 152–8.

Prince, M., Albanese, E., Guerchet, M. and Prina, M. (2014) *World Alzheimer Report 2014. Dementia and risk reduction: An analysis of protective and modifiable risk factors*, London: Alzheimer Disease International.

Prince, M., Ali, G.-C., Guerchet, M., Prina, A.M., Albanese, E. and Wu, Y.-T. (2016) 'Recent global trends in the prevalence and incidence of dementia, and survival with dementia', *Alzheimer's Research & Therapy*, 8(1): 23.

Radford, K., Mack, H.A., Draper, B., Chalkley, S., Daylight, G., Cumming, R., Bennett, H., Delbaere, K. and Broe, G.A. (2015) 'Prevalence of dementia in urban and regional Aboriginal Australians', *Alzheimer's & Dementia: The Journal of the Alzheimer's Association*, 11(3): 271–9.

Ramsden, I. (1990) 'Cultural safety', *The New Zealand Nursing Journal. Kai Tiaki*, 83(11): 18–19.

Reading, J. (2009) *The crisis of chronic disease among Aboriginal peoples: A challenge for public health, population health and social policy*, Victoria: Centre for Aboriginal Health Research, University of Victoria. Available from: www.uvic.ca/research/centres/circle/assets/docs/Publications/chronicdisease-cahr.pdf

Sequist, T.D. (2017) 'Urgent action needed on health inequities among American Indians and Alaska natives', *The Lancet*, 389(10077): 1378–9.

Smith, K., Flicker, L., Lautenschlager, N.T., Almeida, O.P., Atkinson, D., Dwyer, A. and Logiudice, D. (2008) 'High prevalence of dementia and cognitive impairment in Indigenous Australians', *Neurology*, 71(19): 1470–3.

Smith, K., Flicker, L., Shadforth, G., Carroll, E., Ralph, N., Atkinson, D., Lindeman, M., Schaper, F., Lautenschlager, N.T. and Logiudice, D. (2011) '"Gotta be sit down and worked out together": views of Aboriginal caregivers and service providers on ways to improve dementia care for Aboriginal Australians', *Rural and Remote Health*, 11(2): 1650.

Stanley, L.R., Swaim, R.C., Keawe'aimoku Kaholokula, J., Kelly, K.J., Belcourt, A. and Allen, J. (2017) 'The imperative for research to promote health equity in Indigenous communities', *Prevention Science*: 1–9

Statistics Canada (2017) 'Focus on Geography Series, 2016 Census', Catalogue No. 98-404-X2016001, Statistics Canada, [online].

Sutherland, M.E. (2007) 'Alzheimer's disease and related dementias (ADRD) in Aboriginal communities: new visions and understandings', Alzheimer's Disease and Related Dementias within Aboriginal Individuals – Roundtable Forum, Sudbury, Ontario, Canada.

Truth and Reconciliation Commission of Canada (2015) *Truth and Reconciliation Commission of Canada: Calls to action*, Winnipeg: Truth and Reconciliation Commission of Canada.

US Department of Health and Human Services (2017) 'Indian health disparities', Indian Health Service Fact Sheet, [online]. Available from: www.ihs.gov/newsroom/factsheets/disparities

Ward, C. and Varley, L. (n.d.) 'San'yas Indigenous Cultural Safety Training', British Columbia Provincial Health Services Authority, [online]. Available from: www.sanyas.ca [Accessed 28 August 2019].

Warren, L.A., Shi, Q., Young, K., Borenstein, A. and Martiniuk, A. (2015) 'Prevalence and incidence of dementia among Indigenous populations: a systematic review'. *International Psychogeriatrics*, 27(12): 1959–70.

Webkamigad, S. (2017) 'Developing dementia health promotion materials for Indigenous people in an urban Northern Ontario community', Unpublished thesis, Laurentian University.

Western Australia Centre for Health and Aging (2019) 'Kimberly Indigenous Cognitive Assessment', [online]. Available from: www.perkins.org.au/wacha/our-research/indigenous/kica [Accessed 28 August 2019].

Whitehouse, P.J., Gaines, A.D., Lindstrom, H. and Graham, J.E. (2005) 'Anthropological contributions to the understanding of age-related cognitive impairment', *The Lancet Neurology*, 4(5): 320–6.

PART IV

Lived experiences

12

Living with dementia in rural Ireland

Helen Rochford-Brennan

Introduction

They say it takes a village to raise a child. I think it takes a village (or in my case a town) to support a person living with dementia. My town is called Tubbercurry; the town and its hinterland comprise approximately 5,000 people. We are 37 km from the nearest hospital; however, some of our medical centres of excellence are in Galway. That is where my consultant doctor is located and it is 105 km from where I live.

Living in rural Ireland my town is of critical importance. The people, the place and the feeling when walking in the beautiful Sligo countryside have a huge impact on my wellbeing.

I was born in the middle of the Ox Mountains, in Lough Talt, Tubbercurry, County Sligo in 1950. We were a traditional Irish family. I was one of nine; my brothers and sisters were my first 'town'.

I emigrated like many others in rural Ireland to the United States, and I had a wonderful career in Ohio and Kentucky. While home on holidays I met my husband in Tubbercurry. We wrote and telephoned – no emails then!

After getting married in 1982 in Cincinnati, we moved to the UK where my husband Sean worked and I embarked on a new career. Four years later, our son Martin arrived and thoughts turned to returning home. In 1994, we settled in Tubbercurry and Martin found 40 cousins on his first day at school!

Coming home was a great decision for all of us. I think our life was like any family; there was hard work in our café and bed and breakfast business, ups and downs, and health difficulties, but we were happy. I became an activist locally, joining committees and taking an active part in welcoming refugee families to Tubbercurry.

Age 52, I returned to university to study community development, and this led me to working in the disability sector. I was President of the Chamber of Commerce, and Chair of a state agency – very unique for a woman in Ireland at that time. I was living a life of my choosing, in a rural part of Ireland, that was fulfilling.

Diagnosis

Following a head injury and a diagnosis of mild cogitative disorder, for which I had strategies that were not working, I was worried about my memory. At the age of 57, I got my first diagnosis of Alzheimer's. I did not accept this – I wanted to believe my memory problems were due to my head injury. I struggled at work: sitting in meetings, the words would not come; things never seemed to leave the in-tray; I was failing to manage my diary and feeling constantly stressed.

At home, my relationship with Sean and Martin was strained because I found myself forgetting important events and conversations. It seemed like I didn't care and instead of being open I covered up. Those men are my heart and my greatest supporters, but admitting that I could not remember recent conversations was very difficult.

After years of tests, I finally got my formal diagnosis aged 62 in Galway, and because I live in a rural area, far from services, I had a two-hour drive home alone. I couldn't imagine how to tell my family. I stopped at the Knock Shrine (a Roman Catholic pilgrimage site in County Mayo) on the way home and went into a church where I met an African priest. Saying out loud for the first time that I had Alzheimer's made it a tiny bit more manageable.

I can still remember the priest's kindness; he gave me a calm and peaceful space and I began to realise that at least I had a diagnosis, I wasn't going mad. The shock of diagnosis began to be replaced with a sense of relief; my symptoms were real, I was not imagining this.

However, telling Sean and Martin was the hardest thing I have ever done and I believe no matter how my dementia progresses I will never forget their pain. The solace I found in Knock was quickly gone. Telling them was unbearable and I felt helpless.

A cloud descended on our life after diagnosis. I was too ashamed to mention my illness to my friends and there were many dark nights.

I had resigned from my job prior to diagnosis due to an inability to cope; the offer of early retirement had come up and I jumped at it without telling anyone why. I didn't even tell Sean; I just knew I could not continue working.

And I now withdrew from my public activities. My professional life was over and my work as a community activist finished abruptly. Whereas before I had a full life, one of active citizenship, I now sat at home, depressed and isolated.

Stigma

For a long time I couldn't find the courage to tell anyone. Living in a rural area, everyone knows everyone. I had owned a business and lived on the main street of the town. The only people I knew with Alzheimer's lived in the nursing home and they were not active members of the community. Back then, I thought my situation was worse because I lived in rural Ireland. However, through my advocacy work I see people living with dementia across Europe facing stigma.

There were not the resources to educate and support people to understand what Alzheimer's was. I believed the community would think I was mentally ill and I had no tools to communicate my diagnosis.

I believed there was more help and understanding available to people living in urban areas and from my work in the disability sector I was familiar with the extreme lack of services in rural areas.

I worried about the reaction of my town. Would they think I was mad? I remembered the words I heard both as a child and an adult about people living with dementia – 'away with the fairies', 'doting'. These were not labels I could wear and so I took what I believed was the easier path and hid my diagnosis.

Grief

There was a lot of grief in those early days. I was grieving for the life I had planned for my family in retirement. I envisaged Sean and myself travelling and had planned to see every theatre show under the sun. We had agreed Martin would come to the musicals because Sean isn't a fan!

I was fearful of losing my memories of our family life. We have banked some wonderful memories and the idea that a day will come when those are gone was frightening and upsetting.

I was also grieving for Helen pre-diagnosis – the woman about town, the person who put on her makeup and went for her daily walks, chatting to neighbours and knowing what was happening in the community.

I remember lying awake at night staring into the blackness and wondering where I was going to go from here. I felt isolated and lonely; I couldn't see any way forward.

Sharing my diagnosis and becoming an advocate

Eventually, I found the courage to share my diagnosis. There were tears and misunderstanding, but my town community supported me, and life began to improve.

I engaged with local services, I went to Western Alzheimers, an organisation that supports families affected by Alzheimer's and dementia in the west of Ireland, which brought me to a research project at Trinity College Dublin, which in turn led me to the Alzheimer Society of Ireland and ultimately the Irish Dementia Working Group (an advocacy group of people living with dementia).

It is hard to explain the joy I felt to finally meet people who were just like me.

With the support of the Alzheimer Society of Ireland, I made a decision to speak publicly about my diagnosis. I was the first Irish person with the illness to appear on television and share my diagnosis. I spoke on national radio and appeared in newspapers. I encouraged others to do the same and became Chair of the Irish Dementia Working Group.

I experienced considerable lack of understanding. My community found it hard to reconcile the traditional view of a person with Alzheimer's with me. I hadn't changed on the outside. I put on my lipstick and went about my business. I didn't look like someone with a cognitive impairment; my husband would be told, "I saw Helen, she looks great, ah sure there is nothing wrong with her".

The first campaign which I did with the Alzheimer Society of Ireland was called 'Forget the Stigma'. My picture was in the paper, on bus shelters and even on the back of a bus, much to the amusement of family and friends!

In this campaign, I spoke about the fact that I was a wife, a mum, a friend, a sister and an aunt. I was still me.

However, I started to be considered a bit of an anomaly – "It's okay for you", "I could never do that". I worked very hard to try to be what I considered 'normal' and not ask for help. But I began to realise that in order to truly foster understanding, I had to speak about how dementia affected my life. I had to share how much work and effort private Helen undertook to become public Helen.

When I am at home in Tubbercurry, I lose my keys, I get frustrated, and I burn my hands when cooking because I forget to use the oven gloves. I worry a lot and an immense amount of planning and support is required to enable me to engage in my advocacy work. Organising my clothes, my makeup, my meals, my home and daily life is tiring and much more difficult than before I lived with dementia. But I am still me and I hope that by being open I can show that even though I have those symptoms of the disease I am still a person who has a lot to give to her community.

I am currently Chair of the European Working Group of People with Dementia, supported by Alzheimer Europe. I speak about living with dementia across Europe. I raise awareness, take part in research and work to influence public policy. But to do this successfully, I need help and support.

Carmel Geoghegan (a Galway woman who cared for her mother who had dementia and is now a powerful advocate), travels with me in a voluntary capacity. I need Carmel because air travel is very stressful as airports across Europe are not set up to support people living with dementia to travel independently.

The Alzheimer Society of Ireland supports me to review documents, prepare speeches and research topics so I have the information necessary to be the best possible advocate. The organisation is now part of the town!

Being part of this organisation spurs me on; it encourages me to speak up about human rights and to have my voice heard. I feel that through the Alzheimer Society I can champion everyone's human rights, not just mine.

Because I live in rural Ireland, any journey to an Alzheimer Europe meeting is long and arduous. I either have a four-hour bus journey to Dublin, sometimes having to stay overnight, or I fly from my local airport via London and wait for hours for a connection.

It takes a lot of work not to be isolated from my international colleagues; I take part in live, web-based video conferences and telephone conference calls, and try not to let my location influence my ability to participate.

And it takes work not to be isolated in my community. I go to the Alzheimer Café in Sligo, which is a 74-km round trip (luckily, I can still drive). I take my driving assessment each year, but I do worry about what will happen when I cannot drive. I go to the Alzheimer Café to help support the initiative – but I go for me too. It has taken some time to view myself as someone who needs these services, who doesn't just pop in as a guest speaker.

I have neighbours and friends living with dementia, people I meet in the supermarket and the pub. It is comforting to know I am not alone, to know that when the time comes when I go to a day care centre, I will have someone to sit beside while I advocate for red wine or champagne (because apparently they may cure Alzheimer's!).

Recommendations

I am an advocate because I want to change the culture around living with dementia and improve the experience for others who are diagnosed. My experience has been difficult and in some ways exacerbated by where I live.

I am not an expert on human rights or dementia policy and practice. I am, however, an expert on Helen Rochford-Brennan. I am an expert on my lived experience and I hope that my expertise can be valued in the same way as academic and clinical expertise, and that this combined knowledge can create an improved landscape of dementia care.

Support at the moment of diagnosis

When I was told I had early onset Alzheimer's disease, I was alone, and I had to get into my car and drive alone for two hours afterwards. I did not have an informal or comforting chat with a healthcare professional. Nobody asked if I was okay to drive, or whether I need some time to absorb the news.

I felt like a patient, not a person. I was a collection of symptoms and I believed those symptoms would severely limit my quality of life in a short space of time. At my moment of diagnosis, there was no hope, no optimism for how I could live with dementia.

I did not get advice about how to tell my family. Like any wife and mother, I was concerned about my husband and son, as their wellbeing is intrinsically linked with mine. There was a lack of information for Sean and Martin, for them to understand the illness. Access to information is a powerful comfort and should the right of any person and family facing a diagnosis.

I believe that support must begin at the moment of diagnosis and that support must be tailored to the circumstance of each individual.

I also want to be sure that every person diagnosed will get information. I was completely dependent on 'Dr Google', and that brought fear and unnecessary anxiety, both for me and for my son. Dr Google filled the void where quality information should have been available.

Post-diagnostic support

Getting a diagnosis felt like falling off a cliff. There was no pathway of care or signposting to support and services. There appeared to be an acceptance by healthcare professionals that my decline was inevitable and would be swift.

There were no suggestions for non-pharmacological interventions, so I had to create those myself – going for regular walks, planting my rose garden, staying socially active. My rose garden was a turning point; a new rosebud gives me great enjoyment and hope – hope that like the mystery of a new rose a cure for my illness will soon appear. Someone once said: 'Do not watch the petals fall from the rose with sadness; know that, like life, things sometimes must fade, before they can bloom again'. I hung on to this.

Had I not found my way to cognitive rehabilitation therapy and advocacy, I imagine my life would be very different now. Cognitive rehabilitative therapy is hard work, but it helps me manage my life. I have to use the skills and tools I have been given, a quality of life I could not have imagined.

Many people with dementia are diagnosed when their dementia has progressed significantly, and the interventions they need are very different from those I needed when diagnosed.

I consider my advocacy work to be therapeutic, to be an integral part of my post-diagnosis journey. I hope that in time such engagement and occupation will be the foundation of post-diagnostic care for everyone diagnosed with dementia, and I challenge healthcare professionals to think creatively and consider social prescribing.

I believe that a bespoke pathway of care that includes information, peer support, input from multidisciplinary healthcare professionals and the provision of a variety of services is critical.

I also want to see medical professionals offer hope. When diagnosed aged 62, I think I was viewed by medical professionals as a person with a hopeless illness, not a person with a disability needing support to live as well as possible.

When I turned 65, I changed from being a person with a cognitive issue to an older person. I thought being an 'official' older person would bring a certain amount of access to additional support, but it didn't because older people are traditionally encouraged to accept their fate and not offered rehabilitation.

That is not acceptable. I want post-diagnostic care to take a hopeful, rehabilitative view. I know dementia is a progressive illness, but surely we can work to slow down that progression in every way possible. I wish to see an investment in psychosocial support while we are waiting for a cure, a change of mindset so that I am viewed as an active citizen and not someone simply waiting to die.

Care in my community

I recently joined Instagram and I notice that 'finding your tribe' is very fashionable at the moment. How lucky am I that I already have my tribe! I want to live at home in my community, surrounded by that tribe.

Dementia villages are becoming more popular, and while I understand their value, I do not want to move to a specially constructed village when I already live in a real one. It seems strange that we think it is acceptable to gather together all the people with dementia and put us in a village when we want to be fully integrated into our community. I do not believe that would be considered for a group of people with any other chronic illness.

Many care facilities and dementia villages are homely, person-centred places that offer high-quality care. I know of many such care facilities in my town. My doubts are not a criticism of those facilities, but rather a criticism of a system that offers no other choice.

I want to see robust investment in home care – appropriate pay and conditions for staff, high-quality training, and an acceptance that the provision of home care in a rural location creates unique challenges. Care workers often have to travel long distances but are not remunerated for that time; this is something that must change. I believe that to support another human being in their home, to honour their choices and empower them to live as well as possible is important work. I would like to see society place a real and tangible value on this career.

Social health

I have regular medical check-ups with a variety of medical professionals. They measure my blood pressure, and check my sight and my hearing (things that are easy to measure), and then they make a pronouncement on my health.

I wish medical professionals would also measure my empowerment, my sense of wellbeing and my independence, because they are equally important. I believe these more complex needs are a reflection of my overall health and wellbeing.

Tom Kitwood wrote about person-centred dementia care in the 1990s, setting out needs such as inclusion, attachment, comfort and occupation. His work still informs dementia care today, and yet, more than 20 years later, these needs are still not adequately measured. I have certainly never been asked by a medical professional about comfort or attachment, about what brings me joyful occupation in my life.

Social health focuses on relationships. When I think about social health, I am reminded of the Sligo poet W.B. Yeats, who wrote, 'Think where man's glory most begins and ends and say my glory was I had such friends'. To have good social health, I must interact with my community.

But my human right to life in my community is infringed because I do not have a statutory right to home care in Ireland, and my right to participate in social and cultural activities is infringed because not all cultural institutions are aware of the challenges that dementia brings.

If I were in a wheelchair, you would not think it unreasonable for me to look for a ramp. Yet a cognitive ramp is still not available to many people living with dementia. I want to see that metaphorical cognitive ramp available throughout rural communities and a recognition that with support people living with dementia can achieve good social health.

Human rights and participation

I am passionate about the human rights of people living with dementia. I believe it is one of the most pressing human rights issues of our time and change is coming very slowly.

People living with dementia may be denied their human rights from the time of diagnosis. We are not always respected or informed. As we live with the disease, we navigate systems and structures that are not person-centred or rights-based. As a result, either deliberately or by omission, our human rights are denied.

To counteract this, people living with dementia must be actively involved in all aspects of the disease. From research to healthcare, legislation to awareness, the lived experience, no matter where one lives, must be valued and have the power to influence.

But, critically, this engagement must be non-tokenistic, come with appropriate supports and place a value on experts by experience. The lived experience is in vogue, it's trendy. Everybody wants a person living with dementia on their board, their policy group or research panel.

Researchers are often granted funding on the basis that they will consult with people living with dementia. But this engagement is only worthwhile if the person with dementia is empowered, and if there is shared power and decision making. I don't simply want to answer questions; I would like to set the research question. I want to see co-design from the beginning, not a last-minute invitation.

And if I take part in policy and research work, I want to know the outcomes. Too often, people living with dementia are asked for their opinion or to share the lived experience, and have no idea where this input goes. What happened next? Did public policy or care practice change? Is there a next step?

I also want to consider the diversity of the voice of people living with dementia. We must acknowledge and amplify the diverse voices of people living with dementia. Living in rural locations is one part of that diverse experience.

There are so many types of dementia, and people living with the condition vary in age, ethnicity and socioeconomic circumstances. We live in a diverse, multicultural society, and research and policy must reflect that.

My dementia does not exist in a vacuum and neither does anyone else's. It is influenced by my economic circumstances, where I live (rural Ireland), my family situation, my general health, my access to interventions such as cognitive stimulation therapy and the availability of post-diagnostic supports. If research and policy work does not examine that context, I believe the work is compromised.

Conclusion

I do my best to think positively and remain active, but I worry about how I will live as my dementia progresses. Living in rural Ireland means I am a considerable distance from dementia-specific services and healthcare professionals. Transport links are poor, and it is my experience that care innovations tend to centre around urban areas.

In the 1600s, the English general Oliver Cromwell gave the Irish a choice – 'to hell or to Connaught'. They would either be killed or sent to Connaught (a province in the west of Ireland), which would result in death because they could not survive there.

However, I think I am surviving pretty well, in County Sligo in Connaught!

Despite the challenges that living in rural Ireland brings, I choose to stay and do my best to live well in this community because it is home. It has my husband, my family, my friends and the most beautiful countryside, which I cherish every day. I open the door every morning and hear the birds singing. In the midst of my grief, soon after my diagnosis, I couldn't hear the birds.

I urge health and social care practitioners to listen to people living with dementia, uphold our human rights and understand that my needs may be different from those of my family. Prescribe hope, support me to be me as my dementia progresses. I want to try to live as joyfully as possible and I hope professionals will support me to find moments of joy in each day. My medical health may not improve, but my social health certainly can.

I ask researchers to work harder to hear the voice of people living with dementia in rural areas. Being involved in research gives me hope and a sense of purpose, but it is not easy. Recently I took an eight-hour round trip on a bus to be part of a research project. I am working hard to participate, and I want researchers to work hard to place a value on that participation; to share power, involve me from the beginning and think 'co-design'.

To people with dementia, I say: "Be brave, stay in your employment, don't walk away, don't withdraw and give in to the fear. Stay active – for me, it's community development and it will be different for you, but do what you love, what brings you joy. Your voice is important, use it to advocate for yourself so you can live a life of your choosing".

References
Kitwood, T. (1998) *Dementia reconsidered: the person comes first.* Buckingham: Open University Press.

'The Municipal Gallery Revisited', from *The Collected Poems of W.B. Yeats* (1996).

13

Living with dementia in rural Scotland

Nancy McAdam

I am a gardener who happens to have dementia. I live on the Black Isle of Scotland, on a remote croft 44 km from the nearest city, Inverness. I moved to the Black Isle for health reasons around 2002, which coincided with the time of receiving a diagnosis of dementia. I rented properties in the first instance and then met someone interested in gardening and got the 'gardening bug'. I went on to buy a property with 1.7 hectares of land. I began to grow vegetables – amazing, lovely produce – and ate what I grew.

In my early days living on the Black Isle, I had two short-lived romances. One was with someone who did not make me happy, so I had to end the relationship – not much more to say on that! The other was with a younger man, a 'toy boy', if you will, which was fun while it lasted. But one part of that relationship has a legacy with me still, as it was he who introduced me to gardening, and to his father, who was also a great gardener and from whom I learnt a lot. I now live alone and I am very happy about this. I can do what I want when I want. It is quiet. But I have my family in the Glasgow area and my friends on the Black Isle to turn to and meet when I need to. I have the best of both worlds! Happiness is a state of mind and I no longer worry about my life and my dementia. I try to practise mindfulness and live in the moment.

This is not how it always was for me. When I was first diagnosed, I did not cope very well. Vascular dementia, two years to live, both things I really didn't expect at the ripe age of 58. But those were the words said to me nearly 16 years ago in 2003. At this point in my life, I was young and independent, and then dementia came along and threatened both my way of life and life itself. I had begun to prepare myself for death. I was scared. I felt as if I was the most isolated I had ever been.

Figure 13.1: Nancy's garden

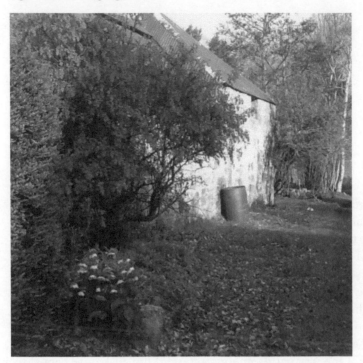

For two years, I felt everything was a bit foggy. The stroke I had caused that feeling. I worried, I thought about death and dying. I found life difficult. After those years, I thought to myself, 'Okay, I have dementia but I still have a life, I can go out and enjoy the world'. So that is exactly what I have been doing. I started going to groups and committees – trying to connect myself with other people going through the same condition as me. The Scottish Dementia Working Group (SDWG) was one of the first committees I joined back in 2005. I started to build up from there, and ended up getting involved with dozens of projects. In 2015, I received a British Empire Medal for services in connection with the Inverness Dementia Memory Group, the first Scottish Highland involvement group for people with a diagnosis of dementia.

With dementia I have learnt not to be afraid to ask for help, and my community is more than willing to give it. 'Getting to know your Techno' is a class I have been going to for the past five years. Almost every Wednesday, I go to the local library in the nearby town of Fortrose and get help with my iPad from the pupils at the academy (secondary school). This might seem quite trivial – an older person coming to ask for help on technology – but I love the classes, and the young people help me connect with others through email and sometimes Facebook. Even if it's just helping me with little things like sharing photos or making sure my email has sent, it can be a big help.

On my birthday, I like to celebrate with a big party in my barn with my family and friends. It takes place in the summer each year, but this is not my real birthday. I was born on Boxing Day, 26 December, but a party on that day doesn't really work, so I have a celebration in the middle of the year. My family is very important to me; we are a large clan and we meet up regularly, not just at my birthday. But sometimes the noise that comes with a big group is too much for me, and I return to the peacefulness of my home. My family know this and it is okay. They support me to live in the way that works for me.

I am a member of a walking group; we meet once a week, and there are three walks we do often. The views of the Scottish countryside are stunning. I love the outdoors and also having some company to enjoy it with. I am a member of a community wood and enjoy visiting it and being in nature, although getting there can be difficult due to the lack of public transport and because I can no longer drive on public roads. I do still drive, though, on my privately owned track, down to a local farm just over a kilometre away, where I can park the car and then walk another ten minutes to the bus stop. I love my little car and without it I would find it harder to get to public transport and to access the beautiful places near where I live and the groups I attend, and to get to Inverness where I still go shopping on a regular basis. But I also like online shopping. I do a supermarket order to get deliveries and the iPad class helps me do my ordering. This is a great thing for me!

I have no time to be lonely. I like living on my own, I have a strong internal life. I love to read and work in my garden. A real lifesaver for me is my garden; growing vegetables gives me a sense of purpose and of course eating something that I have grown gives me great satisfaction. It's like you are involved in the circle of life and are helping to progress that cycle. My neighbour helps me out, sending over horse manure to fertilise the soil and help my plants grow. My house faces up a hill; the landscape faces down the hill to the track. At the bottom of the track is my mail box. I walk down to get the mail every morning, if there is any. It is very scenic – I love the peace and quiet. No neighbours to see or hear me!

And I attend so many group activities in the local community, which provides me with friendship and practical support. It takes a bit of effort and planning to attend the activities. I drive down to the farm, park the car and walk the ten minutes to the bus stop. There is

Figure 13.2: Nancy's car

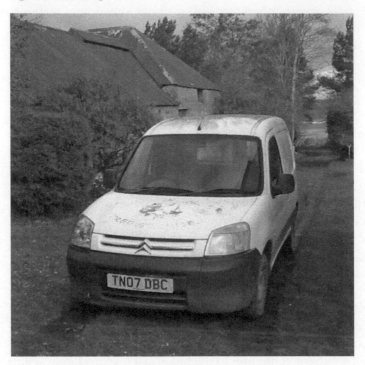

one bus an hour and this gives me some flexibility to attend different activities, including yoga, mindfulness, tai chi, my walking group, choir and my iPad class. My friend and supporter at the iPad class helps me plan my transport each week. He suggested that each Monday I book transport through the community car scheme, so I get the bus to the class (the bus is free for older people living in Scotland) and get the community car back. It's a great resource and costs about five times less than a taxi would. It was started by a local councillor and local people volunteer to do the driving. As long as there are volunteers, I can book a car. It's only harder, say, during public holidays, like Christmas or Easter, when volunteers might be on holiday or have other family commitments.

I've taken part in different research projects. One of these, 'Reimagining Life with Dementia', involved a residential holiday where I met another person with dementia who has become a great friend. I've also had a holiday through a company called Dementia Adventures, which runs holidays specifically for people living with dementia. But the best one was an adventure holiday in the Highlands of Scotland with a great friend of mine, who also has dementia. This involved various outdoor activities in rural Scotland, including white water rafting. It had been my lifelong dream to try it, and I loved it!

What helps me most about living in a rural area is having friends, people I can ask for favours – I am now 74 and need help to do things. One of my friends from the mindfulness class will help me with anything. I also attend a 'Sangha' group – a supportive, contemplative gathering, where members practise 'deep listening and sharing' and everyone knows that their stories won't go any further. It's a safe environment in which to share what is on our minds, and what is going on in our lives. All my activities keep me active. I have retired from the SDWG but still go to my local Dementia Friendly Community initiative in the town of Helmsdale each month. I also go to the Scottish Dementia Alumni meetings in Glasgow – we are working on a project about self-management. That's what I do – I self-manage; I have a range of activities that keep me involved and live in a quiet place that I love.

It's peaceful living alone – I don't have to worry about other people. I enjoy my own company. But I have good access to other places and people. I can go to Glasgow and see the family; we have strong, loving relationships. Sometimes, though, it's just too noisy and I need to leave. I love the peace and silence of the Black Isle.

What difficulties does living in a rural place create for me? Sometimes there are power cuts – not always for too long, maybe two hours – but I have lots of candles. And if I've had enough, I go to bed and sleep.

When I first got diagnosed with dementia, I thought, 'I am going to die'; then you think, 'I am still here'. I used to look forward to a good death without pain. Now I don't even think about it. Mindfulness helps keep me on an even keel. The weather can create difficulties – when I get snowed in, for example. But I have a friend who comes over to check I am okay. He has to walk as it's not possible to drive in snowy conditions. And I need to remember to keep turning the engine of my car over each day, so I can drive again when the track is safe. If my car doesn't work, or breaks down, it's a problem, since, apart from using it to park near the bus stop, I have to drive my rubbish to a collection point for the refuse men. If I had no 'wheels', I would have to call a taxi, but taxis are costly. But the community car scheme is great – we are lucky to have this in my area.

The main thing that needs to be improved in rural areas is transport. I chaired the transport group when I was involved with the SDWG, and I know that not everyone has as many options as I do where I live. I love being outdoors, but to access places such as the community woods, I need to plan my trip very carefully. I need to book a lift there through the community car scheme, and arrange to be collected two hours later. An extension of this scheme would be great. I would like to go on more outings further afield – I like to visit places and see things – but the lack of transport makes it difficult. I have friends I would like to visit in Stornoway, on the island of Lewis and Harris in the Outer Hebrides; I can do this with a bit of planning, but it takes me time. When I visited France last year with my family, they planned the whole trip for me. I am lucky to live in a beautiful place that I love, but I also like to travel a lot. I have a lot of people to thank for the help they give me to function well. I have one life and I am living it the best I can.

14

Conclusion: navigating 21st-century remote and rural dementia care and a future research agenda

Jane Farmer, Debra Morgan and Anthea Innes

> Even though the intention is to offer the whole population services of comparable quality regardless of where they live, there are some challenges with living in rural areas....
> (Kirkevold and Kristiansen, from Chapter 4 in this book)

Drawing across the material in this book, in this chapter we raise and discuss the emergent themes as highlighted by the contributions of leading experts and commentators from around the world. In terms of **policy** we consider systems issues and between–countries similarities and differences; for **practice**, we examine the relevance of culture and the importance of heeding the central human experience of dementia within the current healthcare system; and in respect of key emergent **research** topics, we feature the relevance of place-based planning and the role of technology. We end with a collated research agenda, drawing from topics suggested by authors across the chapters.

Policy and systems

Dementia is a costly issue for governments as people with dementia can live for a long time following their diagnosis, variably requiring different health and social care inputs (Prince et al, 2015). The World Health Organization (WHO) has taken a lead in establishing the need for coordinated national policy and planning approaches (2018), and has provided a toolkit for planning, education and community engagement (WHO, 2017), an online training programme for dementia carers (iSupport for Dementia) (WHO, 2020), and a knowledge exchange platform with access to key dementia data and indicators so that progress in meeting global dementia targets can be evaluated (Global Dementia

Observatory) (WHO, 2019). The mhGAP toolkit can be adopted by individual countries and adapted to local systems and contexts.

The chapters in this book highlight the relevance of countries' health systems and the contexts in which services are provided, as well as the characteristics of such services. By one interpretation, chapters depict health systems with features across a wide spectrum, from those with atomised services provided by a mixture of public, private and non-governmental organisations (in Australia), through those that have become depleted (in Ireland), to apparently more coordinated and adaptive social welfarist models (such as those in Austria and Norway).

Bearing out this interpretation, Chapter 7 depicts a 'weak and fragmented' Irish rural service landscape. The authors note that, while much of the care 'model' depends on people living at home and in their own communities, there are few, and sometimes no, social services to support them. This challenge is exacerbated by considerable out-migration of people from rural communities, resulting in a lack of family support for those left behind. Chapter 3 depicts rural dementia services in Victoria, Australia as a 'complex network of health and aged care services delivered variously through funding and services from Commonwealth (that is, national federal) government, state and territory governments, and local governments as well as private and not-for profit service providers'. Where there is place-based innovation, it seems emergent from time-limited research projects such as HelpDem rural dementia volunteers and Verily Connect, a technology platform to connect carers and provide dementia service information. Similarly, individual health services offer examples of innovation built on the efforts of inspired local health leaders such as the Wattle House initiative in an Australian rural town four hours' drive from the state capital. In contrast, Austria's Dementia Service Centres, as depicted in Chapter 6, appear to have developed incrementally since 2001, originating with a process that systematically gathered evidence from people with lived experiences and community members. These centres are located in rural areas and provide a 'multicomponent, low-threshold, "one-stop shop" psychosocial support model'. Similarly, Norway's commitment to equitable services can be traced back to 2007, as depicted in Chapter 4. A feature is the Norwegian Dementia ABC programme targeted at health and social care practitioners and aiming to 'increase workers' awareness of their own values and approaches to people with dementia'. In Norway's publicly funded and operated health system, the authors depict a system that aims for equitable care and services across the country driven by two national dementia plans and national guidelines.

Highlighting different health system features, Chapters 9 and 10 provide hints of the UK's incorporation of social enterprise as part of a service provision solution for rural areas. The depiction of farm-based care in Chapter 9, whereby some income is generated through activities of people with dementia such as the sale of vegetables grown on the farm, and the story in Chapter 10 behind Go Upstream, an initiative providing rural social enterprise transport solutions in Scotland, suggest social enterprise can be built on rural inclinations to social solidarity as well as entrepreneurialism. Chapter 7 picks up on the idea that social entrepreneurialism could have a role to play in generating a rural social care sector and a community movement. The authors call for training and funding to be made available to assist growth of rural social enterprise.

Chapter 2 highlights that, although the WHO's frameworks are having an impact in some countries, for example Cuba and Togo, in low- and middle-income countries (LMICs), much responsibility for care still lies solely with families and communities that have few resources. In these settings, the emerging challenge of dementia as societies age vies with planning and funding more acute challenges that affect young people, women and children. Adding to the challenge of pursuing national dementia strategy and planning, understanding of dementia can be contested between ideas of the condition as 'a natural part of ageing' and understandings of it as a health condition requiring intervention and treatment. In LMICs, much national emphasis is on the growing cities that are absorbing young, able people who move out of rural areas for economic reasons. It would be understandable, therefore, if there is less emphasis on addressing dementia care in rural areas and on measures to stimulate workers to invest in their own rural careers. Where high-income countries find considerable challenges in addressing rural dementia, these challenges are multiplied many-fold in resource-depleted developing country scenarios.

Issues at the heart of practice

In terms of practice, we have chosen here not to focus on workforce, a well-worn issue of rural health service provision that we touch on in the next section considering place-based planning. Rather, we highlight two issues that emerged across chapters: culture and humanity. Chapter 11 raises a set of issues in the Canadian Indigenous setting that are of primary importance to Indigenous health equity. We go further, however, suggesting that the issue of cultural safety should be widely and deeply considered across health and social care provision more generally. That is, we recognise the importance of understanding how different people, ethnic and social groupings see the world; of accommodating their beliefs and priorities; and of embracing peoples' cultural perspectives so they feel comfortable and included while also receiving high-quality 'technical care'. Culture might be argued as particularly important in dementia as it has such a deep-seated social as well as a 'technical' health dimension, touching fundamental aspects of being human and having dignity, belief systems, identity and 'fitting in' to social groups while also, in different ways, changing. The authors of Chapter 11 explain how, as researchers who are also community workers, they navigate the hybrid space between Indigenous belief and the biomedical health paradigm. This is made even more complex by Indigenous peoples' experiences of marginalisation, colonisation and intergenerational trauma with healthcare institutions 'regarded as a powerful symbol of a traumatic colonial history'. Forging an appropriate approach involves taking the perspective of 'two-eyed seeing' (that is, empathising with both a biomedical and Indigenous cultural perspective) and engaging with peoples' 'understandings of dementia, theories of causation, interpretation of symptoms, caregiving practices and treatment choices'.

Chapter 11 discusses the development of Indigenous-specific care tools and the process of adapting mainstream biomedical practices by involving people with dementia and their communities in design. Moving out from this specific Indigenous cultural focus, other chapters also pick up on the significance of engaging with culture in appropriate service design; for example, Chapter 2 shares reflections of Chen and colleagues (2014) on ideas of acceptable care for older rural Chinese people. Chen and colleagues (2014) consider that village-supported collective housing would be culturally acceptable whereas institutionalised residential care carries stigma. Extending this idea somewhat, Chapter 8 uses the example of engaging older men with dementia with computer gaming to highlight the importance of tailoring technological initiatives to the masculine cultural nuances of the group, while also providing enjoyment and a stimulating, educational experience.

Chapters 12 and 13 piercingly highlight the difficulties in maintaining 'the human' when discussing dementia services. Helen Rochford-Brennan and Nancy McAdam, two women living with dementia in rural areas, in Ireland and Scotland respectively, provide moving narratives of their lives and experiences. Helen Rochford-Brennan relates the deep loneliness not only of driving home for two hours following her diagnosis, but also of navigating how to deal with fear and sadness among her family members, and the embarrassment of talking about her diagnosis to people in her local community who had hitherto known her as an effective business and community leader. Similarly, Nancy McAdam depicts living for two years feeling 'foggy', worrying and thinking about death, after her diagnosis gave her two years to live. At this point, reflecting that several of the chapters highlight lack of early diagnosis as a problem (from a health systems perspective), it becomes easier to empathise with individuals and families who do not rush to gain a definitive diagnosis. We can understand how they might end up navigating and tolerating a 'field of tension' (as Stephanie Auer and colleagues depict the stages leading up to an initial consultation with a health professional, in Chapter 6) because a dementia diagnosis is a confronting, emotionally painful experience, often portrayed by health professionals as hopeless. Chapter 10 points to the particular devastation felt by rural dwellers having to give up driving due to a diagnosis of dementia. The authors cite Freund (2003), who described driving cessation as a 'painful, awkward, difficult, embarrassing, sad, frustrating, tearful, ugly experience'. In rural life, driving is often a strong part of identity, but there are also severe implications relating to loss of access to shopping, religious services and social activities when people with dementia have to stop driving. Nancy McAdam in Chapter 13 describes how she retains her car, which she 'loves'. She no longer drives it on public roads, but she drives it on her own land and it enables her to access public and community transport, reached at the end of the track to her house.

Maintaining the centrality of the human experience in a system centred on cost-efficiency and population-level service provision is challenging, suggesting that Kate Swaffer's (CEO of Dementia Alliance International) motto of 'nothing about us, without us' (raised in Chapter 2) should be kept central. Some of the innovations raised in this book do seem to highlight the human and social, such as the Austrian Dementia Service Centres co-run by social workers and psychologists, with an ethos of adapting to place and evolving in response to needs (see Chapter 6). The depiction in Chapter 9 of farms, animals and environments that engage people in exercise, planting, gardening and life routines, and the descriptions in Chapter 4 of engaging rural people in 'green' farming and 'blue' coastal activities emphasise aspects of individual wellbeing and the importance of continuing to enjoy beauty, nature and weather, rather than a focus on providing services for populations. Chapter 7 perhaps best sums this up, noting the over-emphasis on technical efficiency in health service provision and suggesting that people with dementia, and society, would be better served if dementia care was taken 'out of health and into social production'.

Chapter 2 was limited in its discussion of dementia practice innovations in LMIC settings by a lack of research material. This could be due to a lack of research published in English-language journals and there could also be a trove of grey literature covering rural dementia initiatives in a range of countries that has not made it into searchable databases. Fortunately, the work of the 10/66 Research Group is bringing international practice evidence to light, and is also stimulating practice initiatives such as translating key tools into a range of languages for use by health practitioners and communities. Some excellent summaries of emerging practices are provided by Alzheimer's Disease International, including those in sub-Saharan Africa, the Americas and the Asia-Pacific region.

Some central themes in recent research

Inherent in much of what is reported here is the notion of the relevance of place-based service planning and of involving local people with dementia and their communities in designing, and sometimes producing, services. While health regimes have traditionally tended towards a one-size-fits-all notion, as reflected in the opening quote of this chapter, more recently there is acceptance that the focus is on equitable outcomes and that services should be composed differently depending on place context (OECD, 2010). In this book, we see the ideas of place-appropriate services played out in different ways. Chapter 5, for example, provides a compelling narrative of 20 years of research in the Rural Dementia Action Research (RaDAR) initiative on providing dementia services in rural Saskatchewan, Canada – an area five times the size of England. From the start, the RaDAR team sought to generate research findings that translated into better services by engaging in community-based participatory research, involving all 30 regional health boards in the province of Saskatchewan. The authors note that there is considerable impact to be seen when working with communities and recommend this approach. A specific service model emerged through the researcher–community partnership in the Sun Country Health Region, where an exploration of strengths and weakness in current systems led to the co-development and implementation of rural primary healthcare memory clinics that operationalise the principles of best practice in dementia care in ways that fit the local context.

Continuing the place-based theme, several chapters describe capacity building to train people in the local community specifically to work with people with dementia and their carers. Sometimes, as well as being ways to provide holistic, relational, continuing local care, such initiatives are targeted at career development for practitioners. Chapters 4, 5 and 6 all contain examples of building local worker teams that meet together to learn and support each other formally and informally. In very remote places, these teams can be small (two to ten people). As Chapter 6 highlights, there may be 'fiscal challenges' where 'dementia trainers' (in their model) must meet the fluctuating needs of rural communities, working under a 'freelance contract' (meaning their work hours are not fixed). Considering funding for more innovative, alternative models of service provision raises a general issue for when community-based models involve local citizens and community members in producing or co-producing care. While, as Auer and colleagues note in Chapter 6, there is a need in dementia care for 'integrated, community-based services close to home' – as supported by the international literature (for example, Morgan et al, 2015) – there appears to be a gap in resourcing or funding models (apparently) beyond traditional health systems funding for standard health or social services workers, unless we turn to the social enterprise models mentioned in Chapters 9 and 10, where presumably services are provided through contracts with individuals, local councils or health services.

Building awareness about dementia in rural and remote communities seems particularly significant, as highlighted in Chapters 6 and 9. It is difficult for well-known local characters to change to more vulnerable identities in the face of neighbours who have known and respected them in previous 'able-bodied' personas. Community-based discussion about issues of shame and stigma, awareness and support, are central and clearly part of the rising discussion in several countries around dementia-friendly communities. Some of the aspects underpinning community discussions are already at hand in rural places. Such places traditionally feature communities where people know each other and look out for each other. Chapter 10 provides the example of Stornoway, in rural Scotland, where due to the small number of people using the airport and knowledge of the local community, airport staff are helpful and supportive of travellers with dementia and their families.

A second theme emerging across several chapters is the potential of technology as part of rural and remote dementia service provision. Chapter 5 depicts a mature, evaluated, technology-based service for providing Rural and Remote Memory Clinics in Saskatchewan,

Canada. Significantly, however, the authors' research shows that technology is only part of the model of care for rural people. Working to co-design services, the researchers have helped to develop a flexible service model based around needs of rural people. For example, in cases where people have to travel long distances to attend a city clinic, investigations and tests are carried out quickly so that health practitioners obtain the results while the person is in attendance, thus informing subsequent discussions. Furthermore, family or supporters who are unable to attend are contacted via telehealth facilities or phone. This is to ensure a supported environment for people with dementia, flexible to their circumstances – with the model fitting the person, not the person fitting the system. The researchers found that measures of satisfaction with telehealth and in-person follow-up were similar, but that telehealth was significantly more convenient and reduced travel, per person, by 426 km per round trip on average. The tested interventions, including a telehealth support group for spouses of people with frontotemporal dementia dispersed around the province, have now migrated from a research context to be run by local service providers, such as the Alzheimer Society. Advancing with changing technological capability and end-user experience, RaDAR researchers are now exploring the feasibility of service provision via the asynchronous app, RuralCARE.

Other examples of technology discussed in this book are the My Aged Care website, mentioned in Chapter 3, which is provided by the Australian government and designed to address accessibility to a complex service landscape. To customise this landscape for rural people with dementia, carers and practitioners, the Australian research team is developing the Verily Connect app specifically to enhance rural service accessibility.

Exploring the use of technology for social connection, fun and stimulation, Chapter 8 discuss the researchers' selection of computer games as 'gizmos' for rural men with dementia. Mainstream games technologies were selected rather than those specifically designed for people with dementia, as the latter can be stigmatising. Games can be played at a variety of levels and some also involve movement. The authors depict how engaging with gaming taps into men's inclinations to compete with each other. Interestingly, Nancy McAdam (a woman with lived experience of dementia in rural Scotland) discussed in Chapter 13 how she visited the local school for advice from school students about using her iPad and smartphone, highlighting a novel space of interaction between generations and a beneficial free service of up-to-date technological help.

While technology could present at least part of the solution for rural areas, the examples of technology deployment for service improvement, provided in this volume, highlight that uptake is laggardly unless there is sustained and adequate funding over long periods of time to translate technology use into service practice. Low rural internet connectivity, low digital literacy and health practitioner/health system reluctance continue to be marked in rural settings of many countries.

Although Chapter 10 highlights that driverless cars could be a boon for rural people with dementia, on the whole the contributions do not reveal futuristic applications of technology that could improve service delivery for rural and remote places. This perhaps suggests that technology can only ever be part of the solution for a challenge that is deeply personal and social, as well as involving technical health inputs. People will continue to be required in remote and rural dementia care, but as Chapters 8 and 13 indicate, technologies can also provide a bridge to community social connection. Chapter 2 discusses the generic technology-based tools developed by WHO that appear to have enormous potential as applicable across a range of resource-depleted to high-income settings; however, for these tools to be implemented, governments must first approach WHO and then support translation of the tools to local languages as well as actions to promote and implement them. As raised by Kate Swaffer of Dementia Alliance International, internet connectivity is a great potential boost to people with dementia and their carers, but people need basic access through connectivity, affordability and digital literacy before they can access these contemporary, online accessibility options.

A future research agenda: key research gaps raised

In this section, we list some of the research gaps and areas raised across the chapters that are particularly relevant to people with dementia in remote and rural areas.

Humanistic supports for the person with dementia. There appears to be a gap in research dealing with lived experiences of dementia in different parts of the world. To date, academic research may have focused on dementia as a medical and health 'problem', neglecting the idea that people with dementia have to navigate the lead-up to diagnosis, dealing with the diagnosis itself and with the practical, emotional and social issues that living with dementia brings. This can be a varyingly challenging process in diverse settings internationally, from the Black Isle in Scotland to sub-Saharan Africa, and it is vital to know 'how it feels' and how dementia is personally experienced in different contexts so as to inform the public as well as policy makers and practitioners. Specific gaps in research include:

- support for the person with dementia, at diagnosis and thereafter, including how to tell their family and people in their rural community;
- rural inclusion and continuing access to employment, social and cultural activities and community generally, as appropriate;
- support during and after giving up driving.

Cultural safety and sensitivity. As Indigenous peoples currently experience higher rates of incidence of dementia than non-Indigenous people, and generally experience less access to appropriate services, there is a need for research that engages and aligns with different cultural beliefs and practices. A particular issue raised in this book is how to align Western biomedical approaches with Indigenous cultural and belief-system approaches. Research needs include:

- population-based studies of incidence and prevalence in Indigenous populations;
- design and implementation of culturally relevant policy, supports and interventions;
- partnering with communities to develop local, culturally relevant teaching and awareness tools;
- exploring how to unite local cultural and community beliefs and practices with biomedical and health condition approaches, to achieve 'good combination approaches' to dementia in different country settings.

Advocacy. While WHO, Alzheimer's Disease International and the 10/66 Research Group have made great strides in systematising approaches to dementia planning and care, there are still gaps in approaches to dementia that are perhaps only brought to attention through advocacy, including advocacy by groups of people with their own lived experiences of dementia. Advocacy groups such as Dementia Alliance International have raised issues including the need for greater involvement of people with dementia in research and planning, attention to human rights and bringing dementia into national health and social priorities. Such groups have radically influenced the agenda and are likely to have further impacts, for example in dementia policy for low- and middle-income countries. One area useful to address, therefore, is research on the role of civil society in different countries as a force in remote and rural dementia service improvement. Studying and monitoring the rise of advocacy for dementia and the lived experience of dementia in developing country settings, including the role of technology in promoting or hindering civil society, is a crucial issue.

Roles of community. This book draws attention to dementia care as sitting at the nexus of health and social caring. It also shows that, particularly in rural areas, traditional types of specialist service systems are not available now, nor likely in the future. This all suggests that the community has a significant role to play in promoting awareness about dementia and collectively caring for, and about, people with dementia and their families. Specific research issues include:

- dementia-friendly communities in different remote and rural contexts;
- ways to resource or fund communities as collectives, for providing care and support;
- social enterprise, social entrepreneurship and volunteering as ways to provide services or support public health and social services in co-production;
- the benefits of, and funding models for, community rural social inclusion initiatives in different country contexts and settings.

Alternative workforce and upskilling. Attracting skilled workers to long-term work in rural areas is a well-known challenge in health and social services. Specialist personnel are also expensive and there is likely not sufficiently high volume to fund team models compliant with safety and quality requirements. Alternative models of providing services for rural areas are therefore required. Such models must be piloted, tested and scaled up. Some particular areas of potential research raised in the book are:

- appropriate roles in relation to providing services for people with dementia in rural and remote places, and training to counter the lack of a skilled rural professional workforce;
- adaptation and implementation of WHO tools such as iSupport (carer support and training) and mhGAP (education and training about key mental health conditions) in different rural and remote contexts;
- the impact of community and service provider awareness, education and training;

- new place-based, appropriate models of care, including hub and outreach models involving local people and those working in specialist centres.

Technology. While technology has long been proposed as significant in solving rural service accessibility challenges, it is perhaps only now starting to be taken up at scale in high-income country contexts. While existing innovations are likely to be increasingly diffused, extended and adapted for diverse rural and remote contexts, one particular research gap identified is around developing and testing appropriate technology for rural and remote areas with low internet connectivity and poorer access to sophisticated technical resources.

Policy and systems. In different countries around the world, dementia care is being adopted to various degrees as a national health priority. Its relative prominence often depends on the other health challenges in the relevant country. A key issue raised in this book is that policy makers, practitioners, communities and the public now perhaps need to move from identifying dementia as solely a biomedical and health challenge, to treating it as an issue that requires hybrid health and social approaches. To this end, research on dementia as a social challenge is missing, with particular policy and system issues raised in this book including the importance of measuring quality of life and social indicator benchmarking for people with dementia in rural areas, and, borrowing Chapter 11, adopting a 'two-eyed seeing' approach – that is, situating much more of dementia care within a social care model, rather than solely a technical health and medical model, and measuring the impact of such an approach.

Finally, overall we note that this book highlights a number of innovations occurring in different parts of the world. This draws attention to the question of whether, and how, good ideas can be transferred across settings, and subsequently implemented, sustained and scaled up. Rural places are each distinctive and, as emerges in this book, the rural initiatives developed need to align not just with the resources in the local context, but also with broader structural features of a country's health and social care system, such as funding arrangements and structures of provision. Finally, and crucially, initiatives need to align with belief systems and what is socially and culturally preferable or acceptable. Experimenting with how solutions to rural dementia care could be transferred across rural place and country contexts could be an interesting 'space' to explore designing a framework for how (or if) rural service solutions *can be* transferred and scaled up.

Limitations

The contributions to this book have, to an extent, been driven by our personal networks and the contributors' enthusiasm to write their chapters. We acknowledge gaps in themes we would have liked to include, such as experiences of implementing WHO initiatives in low- and middle-income countries and of providing services in communities that are highly 'hollowed out' (that is, populated mainly by the very old and very young) (Carr and Kefalas, 2010), as well as the experiences of communities participating in providing rural dementia care across the world, of service providers working in very remote and inaccessible communities, and of unpaid care providers. All of these ideas can be included in any follow-up book on remote and rural dementia services.

Conclusion

It is tempting, with the inspiring array of innovations portrayed in this book, to moot that these innovations now be translated and trialled across different countries and contexts. However, given our point about different innovations emerging in different systems and contexts, we wonder about the success of cross-national translation. Could the Austrian and Norwegian examples really translate to rural Australia? How would this occur? What research would be needed or is the challenge really about advocacy? Or is it a combination of sound research evidence, coupled with strong advocacy and including the real lived experiences of people with dementia, that is required?

From assembling this book, we note a lack of systematic research on the community health, social and rural services aspects of remote and rural dementia care. While considerable efforts are justified in gathering population-level information, we suggest that there is considerable room for more diverse and insightful evidence about living with dementia, providing services and making policy, in relation to remote and rural places around the world. In that respect, our work is novel and we hope it inspires a raft of new research and exploration, using mixed methods and further revealing international remote and rural experiences and solutions.

As noted by Helen Rochford-Brennan in Chapter 12, from the perspective of a rural woman living with dementia, 'I believe that a bespoke pathway of care that includes information, peer support, input from multidisciplinary healthcare professionals and the provision of a variety of services is critical'. Helen Rochford-Brennan lives in rural Ireland, but she believes this should be true wherever you live and we agree. We hope this book inspires more people to make this a reality with, and for, people with dementia in remote and rural areas of the world.

References

Carr, P.J. and Kefalas, M.J. (2010) *Hollowing out the middle: The rural brain drain and what it means for America*, Boston, MA: Beacon Press.

Chen, S., Boyle, L.L., Conwell, Y., Xiao, S. and Fung Kum Chiu, H. (2014) 'The challenges of dementia care in rural China', *International Psychogeriatrics*, 26(7): 1059–64.

Freund, K. (2003) 'Mobility and older people', *Generations*, 27(2): 68–9.

Go Upstream (2018) ' "Welcome" Aboard!', Go Upstream [Blog]. Available from: www.upstream.scot/blog/2018/10/12/welcome-aboard

Morgan, D., Kosteniuk, J., Stewart, N., O'Connell, M.E., Kirk, A., Crossley, M., Dal Bello-Haas, V., Forbes, D. and Innes, A. (2015) 'Availability and primary health care orientation of dementia-related services in rural Saskatchewan, Canada', *Home Health Care Services Quarterly*, 34(3–4): 137–58.

OECD (Organisation for Economic Co-operation and Development) (2010) *OECD Rural Policy Reviews: Strategies to improve rural service delivery*, Paris: OECD.

Prince, M., Wimo, A., Guerchet, M., Ali, G.C., Wu, Y.T. and Prina, M. (eds) (2015) *World Alzheimer Report 2015. The global impact of dementia: An analysis of prevalence, incidence, cost and trends*, London: Alzheimer's Disease International.

WHO (World Health Organization) (2017a) *Dementia: Toolkit for community workers in low- and middle-income countries. Guide for community-based management and care of people with dementia*, Manila: World Health Organization Regional Office for the Western Pacific.

WHO (World Health Organization) (eds) (2018) *Towards a dementia plan: A WHO guide*, Geneva: WHO.

WHO (World Health Organization) (2019) 'Global Dementia Observatory', [online]. Available at: www.who.int/mental_health/neurology/dementia/Global_Observatory/en

WHO (World Health Organization) (2020) iSupport for dementia. https://www.isupportfordementia.org/en

Index